Clinical and Forensic Applications
of Capillary Electrophoresis

PATHOLOGY AND LABORATORY MEDICINE

Series Editors: Stewart Sell and Alan Wu

PATHOLOGY AND LABORATORY MEDICINE

Clinical and Forensic Applications of Capillary Electrophoresis

Edited by

John R. Petersen

and

Amin A. Mohammad

University of Texas Medical Branch, Galveston, TX

Humana Press Totowa, New Jersey

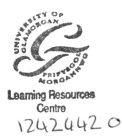

© 2001 Humana Press Inc.
999 Riverview Drive, Suite 208
Totowa, New Jersey 07512

For additional copies, pricing for bulk purchases, and/or information about other Humana titles, contact Humana at the above address or at any of the following numbers: Tel.: 973-256-1699; Fax: 973-256-8341; E-mail: humana@humanapr.com or visit our Website: http://humanapress.com

This publication is printed on acid-free paper. ∞
ANSI Z39.48-1984 (American Standards Institute) Permanence of Paper for Printed Library Materials.

Cover design by Patricia F. Cleary.

Production Editor: Mark J. Breaugh.

Photocopy Authorization Policy:

Printed in the United States of America. 10 9 8 7 6 5 4 3 2 1

Library of Congress Cataloging-in-Publication Data

Clinical and forensic applications of capillary electrophoresis / edited by John R. Petersen and Amin A. Mohammad.
    p. ; cm.
  Includes bibliographical references and index.
  ISBN 0-89603-645-6 (alk. paper)
 1. Capillary electrophoresis. 2. Clinical chemistry. 3. Chemistry, Forensic. I. Petersen, John R. II. Mohammad, Amin A.
  [DNLM: 1. Clinical Laboratory Techniques. 2. Electrophoresis, Capillary--methods. 3. Amino Acids--blood. 4. Blood Proteins--analysis. 5. Forensic Medicine--methods. 6. Immunoassay--methods. QU 25 C6408 2001]
RB43.8.C36 C54 2001
616.07'56--dc21
                                                                          2001016677

Preface

Since the advent of the clinical laboratory in the 20th century, the need to report more accurate results, faster, and at a lower cost has driven technology. One area that has lagged behind the rest of the laboratory is electrophoretic separations of analytes that are clinically relevant. Because of this, electrophoresis has been relegated to the very specialized sections of the laboratory, limiting its use in patient care.

Electrophoresis, as we use it today, was first described by Tiselius in his PhD thesis in 1937. In pioneering experiments that have led to the methods used today, he used a U-shaped quartz tube to show the zonal separation of serum in free solution using Schlieren optics to monitor the migration of the protein bands. Driven by the desire to make electrophoresis easier, a number of matrixes—such as paper, cellulose acetate, agarose, starch gel, and polyacrylamide—were investigated and, in one form or another, are still used today. From the basic method described by Tiselius a number of innovative electrophoretic methods have now been developed, including immunoelectrophoresis, isoelectric focusing (IEF), isotachophoresis (ITP), and size separation by gradient electrophoresis.

Tiselius's basic concept of using a tube for electrophoretic separation received little notice until the late 1960s when Hjerten described the first capillary electrophoresis (CE) apparatus. In spite of the pioneering work by Hjerten, CE remained relatively unknown until 1981 when Jorgenson and Lukacs described the separation and fluorescent detection of amino acids, peptides, and urine proteins by capillary zone electrophoresis. Since then, all of the classical separation techniques—IEF, ITP, zone electrophoresis, and micellar electrokinetic chromatography (MEKC)—have allowed CE to rival the versatility of high pressure liquid chromatography (HPLC). MEKC, which in its simplest form is the addition of detergent to the buffer, has enabled CE to be used in an area once thought impossible for electrophoresis techniques, the separation of small, electrically neutral molecules.

CE has come a long way since it was first described. Current methods are capable of being automated, and, because it is a microtechnique, the method conserves precious samples and minimizes the use of hazardous organic chemicals. Although CE has not made inroads into the clinical laboratory that many anticipated, we expect that, in the future, it will find its "proper" place. Because this "proper" place may surprise everyone involved in the clinical applications of CE, this book is not meant to give an in-depth methodological description of the use of CE in the clinical laboratory, but to give an overview of its current use.

We arranged *Clinical and Forensic Applications of Capillary Electrophoresis* into six main sections. Section I covers the history and some of the potential applications of CE. This section also covers the principles necessary for the clinical laboratory scientist to understand the basics of CE. Section II covers the separation of proteins, probably the first use of CE in the clinical laboratory. The section describes the potential problems and solutions when using CE to separate proteins, along with outlining how CE has been used to separate serum and CSF proteins, detect serum and urine paraproteins, and separate lipoproteins and hemoglobin variants. Section III covers metabolic diseases, which are usually detected by abnormalities in small molecules, such as amino acids, organic acids, or steroids. Section IV covers the use of CE in immunoassay, where CE is used as a separation method. Although this may seem trivial at first glance, it opens up the possibility of simple, yet highly sensitive, analysis at the point of care. Section V describes what may be the future of CE in the clinical laboratory, the use of CE in molecular diagnostics, both for the detection of diseases and quantiation of viral loads and its use in the forensic DNA identification laboratory. Finally, Section VI describes how CE can be used in conjunction with mass spectrometry, its potential use in detection of heavy metal poisoning, therapeutic drug monitoring, and clinical and forensic toxicology.

John R. Petersen
Amin A. Mohammad

Contents

Contributors

BODE ADESOJI • *Department of Pathology, University of Texas Medical Branch, Galveston, TX*

NEBOJSA AVDALOVIC • *Dionex Corporation, Sunnyvale, CA*

JOHN M. BUTLER • *GeneTrace Systems Inc., Alameda, CA*

JITKA CASLAVSKA • *Department of Clinical Pharmacology, University of Bern, Bern, Switzerland*

SAMIR CHERKAOUI • *Laboratory of Pharmaceutical Analytical Chemistry, University of Geneva, Switzerland*

RANDALL D. CRAVER • *Department of Pediatrics, Louisiana State University School of Medicine, New Orleans, LA*

MAURO GOLIN • *Forensic Laboratory, Royal Canadian Mounted Police, Regina, Saskatchewan, Canada*

NORBERTO A. GUZMAN • *The R.W. Johnson Pharmaceutical Research Institute, Raritan, NJ*

JAMES M. HEMPE • *Department of Pediatrics, Louisiana State University School of Medicine, New Orleans, LA*

JOHN C. HUDSON • *Forensic Laboratory, Royal Canadian Mounted Police, Regina, Saskatchewan, Canada*

CARL R. JOLLIFF • *Physician's Laboratory Services Inc., Lincoln, NE*

JILL M. KOLESAR • *Department of Pharmacy (CHS), University of Wisconsin-Madison, Madison, WI*

RAINER LEHMANN • *Department of Internal Medicine IV, Division of Endocrinology, Metabolism and Pathobiochemistry, Medical Center Hospital, University of Tübingen, Tübingen, Germany*

MANJIRI LELE • *Department of Pathology, University of Texas Medical Branch, Galveston, TX*

SUBODH M. LELE • *Department of Pathology, University of Texas Medical Branch, Galveston, TX*

MARY KATHRYN LINDE • *College of Professional Studies, Shawnee State University, Portsmouth, OH*

MURRAY J. MALCOLM • *Forensic Laboratory, Royal Canadian Mounted Police, Regina, Saskatchewan, Canada*

BRUCE R. MCCORD • *Deparment of Chemistry, Clippinger Laboratories, Ohio University, Athens, OH*

AMIN A. MOHAMMAD • *Department of Pathology, University of Texas Medical Branch, Galveston, TX*

STEPHEN NAYLOR • *Department of Biochemistry and Molecular Biology, Department of Pharmacology, Mayo Foundation, Rochester, MN*

KERN L. NUTTALL • *Department of Pathology, University of Utah School of Medicine, Salt Lake City, UT*

ANTHONY O. OKORODUDU • *Department of Pathology, University of Texas Medical Branch, Galveston, TX*

JOHN R. PETERSEN • *Department of Pathology, University of Texas Medical Branch, Galveston, TX*

CHRIS POHL • *Dionex Corporation, Sunnyvale, CA*

LOKINENDI V. RAO • *University of Texas Medical Branch/Texas Department of Criminal Justice Laboratory Services, Huntsville, TX*

ZACK K. SHIHABI • *Department of Pathology, Bowman Gray School of Medicine, Wake Forest University Baptist Medical Center, Winston-Salem, NC*

KANNAN SRINIVASAN • *Dionex Corporation, Sunnyvale, CA*

WOLFGANG THORMANN • *Department of Clinical Pharmacology, University of Bern, Bern, Switzerland*

ANDY J. TOMLINSON • *Department of Biochemistry and Molecular Biology, Department of Pharmacology, Mayo Foundation, Rochester, MN*

ALFONSO VARGAS • *Department of Pediatrics, Louisiana State University School of Medicine, New Orleans, LA*

HARRY WHATLEY • *Beckman Coulter, Fullerton, CA*

CECILLA YOUH • *Department of Pathology, University of Texas Medical Branch, Galveston, TX*

I
Introduction

Capillary Electrophoresis
General Overview and Applications in the Clinical Laboratory

Manjiri Lele, Subodh M. Lele, John R. Petersen, and Amin Mohammad

1. INTRODUCTION

Electrophoresis was first described by Arne Tiselius *(1)* in 1930, for which he received a Nobel Prize in 1948. In this pioneering experiment, he used a U-shaped quartz tube to show the separation of different proteins in free solution as contiguous bands. His work was published in 1937 *(1)* but received little notice until the late 1960s, when Hjerten *(2)* described the first capillary electrophoresis (CE) apparatus. Hjerten's apparatus consisted of three units: 1) a high voltage power supply; 2) a detector; and 3) a unit holding a 1–3 mm ID quartz capillary tube, which was immersed in a cooling bath *(2)*. He used this apparatus to prove numerous theoretical concepts in CE and was able to separate inorganic ions, proteins, nucleic acid, and microorganisms by capillary zone electrophoresis (CZE) or capillary isoelectric focusing (CIEF). In spite of the pioneering work by Hjerten, CE was still relatively unknown until Jorgenson and Lukacs *(3–5)* published a series of papers in 1980. The availability of polyiimide-coated fused silica capillaries with a 75–100-μm internal diameter, in addition to sensitive absorbance detectors developed for micro-bore high-performance liquid chromatography (HPLC), were instrumental in the development of commercial CE applications. The smaller internal diameter eliminated band broadening caused by convection, whereas the plug flow characteristics of the electroosmotic flow (EOF) allowed efficiencies reaching hundreds of thousand of theoretical plates. Since the landmark publication in 1980 by Jorgenson and Lukacs research dealing with the applications of CE has grown exponentially. Consistent with the theme of this book, this chapter will try to provide a general overview of current and future applications of CE in clinical chemistry. It is not meant to be a comprehensive review of

From: *Clinical and Forensic Applications of Capillary Electrophoresis*
Edited by: J. R. Petersen and A. A. Mohammad © Humana Press Inc., Totowa, NJ

general literature, but instead an attempt to give a reader a flavor of its potential power in solving some of the challenging problems that arise in a clinical laboratory.

2. INTERGRATION OF CE INTO THE CLINICAL LABORATORY

Clinical laboratories had evolved considerably since the early 1980s and will continue to do so during the next millennium. Reduced turnaround time, convenience, patient satisfaction (quick diagnosis), and physician satisfaction (improved real-time clinical decision-making) are some of the benefits gained from having more clinical testing to be done in the hospital laboratory. At the same time economies of scale, reduced cost, regionalization, and continuity of care are responsible for outsourcing laboratory testing to reference laboratories. These two opposing forces have placed tremendous pressure on clinical chemists to develop assays that are inexpensive, fast, amenable to laboratory automation, while still being accurate and precise. Thus the million dollar question is: "Can capillary electrophoresis fulfill some or any of these conditions?" This is a key question that every laboratory director, laboratory manager, or administrative director must answer before introducing a new technology for patient testing. Let us now examine applications of CE from this perspective.

2.1. Cost

Because CE is a separation technique, it will compete with more traditional chromatographic techniques such as gas chromatography (GC) and HPLC. However, unlike the classical chromatographic techniques, CE can also compete with classical electrophoresis, such as agarose gel and isoelectric focusing. Table 1 gives a typical cost comparison for the procedures that CE could replace in a clinical laboratory. As shown in this table, in certain instances CE can be less expensive. The main cost savings comes from the use of fused silica capillaries, which are less expensive than HPLC or GC columns. For instance, the cost of an HPLC column used for clinical testing can range from $250 to 300, whereas a 10-m piece of CE fused silica capillary will cost about $80. Assuming that a CE method will use a 57-cm piece of fused silica capillary and that the capillary will last ~200 injections, a very conservative estimate, one can expect at least 1800 injections from 10 m of fused silica capillary instead of 800 injections for an HPLC column. Even neutral-coated capillaries, which are appreciably more expensive than uncoated, fused silica capillaries, are less expensive than reverse-phase (RP) or ion exchange HPLC columns. It should be noted that in this analysis we did not account for the labor component because in our experience, the hands-on labor for CE is comparable to traditional chromatographic and electrophoretic techniques.

Table 1
Comparison of Cost of Capillary Electrophoresis Methods
vs. Current Clinical Methodology

	Technique	Instrument cost	Technical service	Reagent cost (per 100 tests)
Tricyclic antidepressant	HPLC	$46,000.00	$5000.00	$1150.00
	CE	$45,000.00	$5000.00	$700.00
Serum protein electrophoresis	Gel electrophoresis	$20,000.00	$2200.00	$200.00
	CE	$45,000.00	$5000.00	$20.00
Immuno fixation electrophoresis	Gel electrophoresis	$10,000.00	$1200.00	$360.00
Immuno subtraction	CE	$45,000.00	$5000.00	$400.00
Hemoglobin variant	HPLC	$46,000.00	$5000.00	$140.00
	CE	$45,000.00	$5000.00	$20.00

2.2. Speed

It is well-established that capillary electrophoretic separations are much faster than routine gel electrophoresis. This is because of the high electric field (800 V/cm) that can be reached in CE, whereas in slab gel electrophoresis the electric fields are limited to 15–40 V/cm. The field strength that can be applied to slab gels is low owing to Joule heating (for a detailed discussion of Joule heating, *see* Subheading 1.2.3. in Chapter 2), which is directly related to surface-to-volume ratio. Applying higher field strengths in slab-gel electrophoresis results in a significant increase in temperature, causing irreproducible separations. For example, a $14 \times 11.5 \times 0.15$-cm slab gel will have a surface to volume ratio that is 40 times greater than that of a typical 57 cm $\times 75$ μm ID fused silica capillary. This high surface-to-volume ratio in CE allows efficient dissipation of joule heat allowing the use of very high electrical fields. This is best illustrated by comparing the ability of CE to perform a serum protein electrophoretic separation in less than 1 min whereas a similar separation by agarose gel electrophoresis requires 20–25 min. The one advantage that gel electrophoresis holds over CE is the ability to analyze as many as 90 samples simultaneously, overcoming the limitation of slow separation speed. This is probably the main reason why CE has not been widely used for routine analysis of serum proteins in clinical laboratories.

2.3. Potential for Automation

Commercially available capillary electrophoresis systems are remarkably simple from an instrumentation point of view. The basic instrument consists of four parts: 1) a fused silica capillary holder, 2) a high voltage power supply, 3) a detector, and 4) a safety interlock. Most instruments also provide a mechanism to control the temperature in the capillary. This may be controlled either by air cooling, using a peltier device, or by enclosing the capillary in a cartridge, which is filled with a coolant that is maintained at a constant temperature. All components of the CE are monitored or controlled by computer software. This allows the end user to develop methods and then analyze the separated components, post-electrophoresis. In this respect current CE instruments compare favorably with automated HPLC systems used in the clinical laboratory. However, unlike the highly automated instruments found in a clinical laboratory, the operation of CE instruments requires an above average amount of technical expertise. In other words, these instruments are not black boxes that just require an operator to push a switch and then wait for a result to be generated. Most importantly, in order for CE to be used routinely in the highly automated clinical laboratory, primary sample tube sampling, the ability to read a bar code, and a bidirectional interface to Laboratory Information System are required. With the exception of Beckman Paragon CZE 2000®, no other CE system has this capability.

2.4. Accuracy, Sensitivity, and Precision

In CE, accuracy has never been an issue because the analyte is usually separated from interfering substances. However, the limit of detection (LOD) has been and still is the main problem with CE. Various manufacturers of commercial CE units have tried to address this problem by using modified capillaries (i.e., bubble-cell or z-shaped cells) or by using laser-induced fluorescence (LIF). Typical detection limits range from 1×10^{-6} M for UV detection to 1×10^{-9} M for LIF. Alternatively, sensitivity can also be enhanced by sample stacking. Chien et al. *(6)* has comprehensively reviewed sample stacking in capillary zone electrophoresis and its applications for routine analysis. Typically, sample stacking involves a movement of sample ions across a boundary, which divides regions into high (low-conductivity sample solution or water plug) and low (high-conductivity separation solution) electric fields inside the capillary. The sample is usually dissolved in a buffer having an ionic strength that is 1/10 that of the run buffer. As a result, the electric-field gradient across the sample zone is relatively high, causing the analyte ions to migrate rapidly until they reach the interface between the sample buffer and the run buffer. On reaching the interface, the ion mobility drops, causing stacking of sample at the boundary of two solutions giving a 5- to 10-fold increase in signal-to-noise ratio. Because sample stacking relies on the enhanced electrophoretic velocities of ionic species in the low-conductivity or high-electric field region, neutral analytes are not concentrated unless they are compartmentalized in an ionic micelle. Quirino et al. *(7)*

described an exceptional narrowing of neutral analytes zones in electrokinetic chromatography that allowed a 5000-fold concentration of neutral analytes, such as steroids, racemic herbicides, and other biologically important compounds. This special preconcentration phenomenon, dubbed as sweeping, works for all charged and neutral compounds. Detection limits ranging from 1.7 to 9.6 ng/mL have been reported by these authors for various clinically important steroids. Although very promising, the technique needs to be applied to real patient samples. It may also require a prior sample clean up in order prevent the interference of unwanted proteins and other analytes present in the sample that also under go preconcentration.

The ability to measure precisely (analytical imprecision) an analyte is very important in a clinical laboratory. Coefficients of variation (CV) <5% are routinely observed for various analytes, such as electrolytes, enzymes, proteins, and so forth, on automated analyzers. The various factors that can affect both with in- and between-run imprecision in CE are listed here (a more in-depth discussion on these factors can be found in Chapter 2):

1. Capillary surface: The inner surface of the capillary, which participates in the separation process, can be a major factor in the cause of imprecision in CE. Not only does the sample, and therefore the various analytes, come in contact with the surface, but the analytes can also bind to the surface, changing the properties of the capillary. For the most part, it is best to try and eliminate any interaction of the analyte with the surface of the capillary. This can be done by deliberately changing the surface by treating with polymers, various detergents, or simply by changing the buffer or buffer concentration.

2. Current: When a CE instrument is "turned on" a current is generated. It is extremely important to control this current, because a variation in the current can cause a change in the temperature. A change in the temperature can result in a change in pH, which can then lead to a change in the current, the original variable that was being controlled. With the power sources available today, controlling the current is not an issue.

3. Capillary conditioning: In order to ensure good reproducibility in bare and coated fused silica capillaries, daily conditioning with a series of buffers is required before a capillary is used. In our experience, a daily rinse of 30 min for serum protein electrophoresis, 30 min for hemoglobin variants using capillary isoelectric focusing, 15 min for steroids using coated capillary, and 45 min on a bare fused silica capillary are very typical. Furthermore, the rinsing time is very dependent on the capillary surface and can change from one lot of capillaries to another. Most of the buffers used for capillary conditioning are quite stable if protected from the atmosphere and stored at 4°C. Hence, buffer stability is not much of an issue. For IEF, preconditioning the capillary with a 0.04% methylcellulose and ampholine solution is extremely important to ensure reproducible migration times. In our hands, the CV for migration time increased from <5 to >20% when the pre-rinsing time is shortened from

30 min to 10 min for the analysis of hemoglobin variants using capillary iso-electric focusing on a bare fused silica capillary.

4. Buffer: Although the capillary wall can significantly affect the separation, the separation also takes place in the presence of a buffer. This buffer has multiple purposes, one of which is to control the pH. It is extremely important to control pH because analyte charge, EOF, and heat production all change with even small changes in pH. The actual buffer used can also have an affect on the separation process because of interaction between the buffer and the analyte. In addition some buffers, i.e., borate or zwitterionic buffers, carry less current than mono-functional buffers like phosphate. Buffer concentration is also important because higher buffer concentrations will lessen the interaction of the analyte with the capillary wall.

5. Temperature: Control of the temperature within the capillary is extremely important. However, temperature control is complicated by the generation of heat (Joule heating) when current passes through a buffered solution. As mentioned previously, multiple factors (temperature, pH, and current) are interrelated. In other words, what affects one will potentially affect the other. With current instruments, the temperature is controlled either by air cooling, a peltier device, or by enclosing the capillary in a cartridge, which is filled with a coolant maintained at a constant temperature. For most applications, the use of a coolant will control temperature better than air-cooling.

6. Sample Injection: In the past, sample injection was a major source of error for traditional CE systems. However, with the use of high-precision pressure valves, this problem has been significantly reduced.

2.5. Modes of CE

CE is highly versatile, with numerous modes of operation, which are accessed, in many instances, by altering the buffer composition. The commonly used modes of CE include CZE, capillary gel electrophoresis (CGE), CIEF, and capillary isotachophoresis (CITP) *(8)*.

2.5.1. Capillary Zone Electrophoresis (CZE)

CZE, the simplest form of CE, requires filling the capillary with only running buffer. In this form of CE, the ionic solutes migrate with different velocities (as determined by their charge-to-mass ratio) forming discrete zones in the running buffer. By using the electroosmotic flow (EOF), separation of many of the cationic and anionic solutes is possible. Neutral solutes, which move with the EOF, are not separated *(8)*. Applications of CZE include analysis of amino acids (*see* Chapter 9), peptides (*see* Chapter 16), protein analysis (*see* Chapters 4, 5, 6, 7, and 8)—including screening of proteins variants and evaluating protein purity—and forensic applications (*see* Chapter 20).

2.5.2. Micellar Electrokinetic Chromatography (MEKC or MECC)

MEKC is a combination of electrophoresis and chromatography in which both neutral and charged solutes can be separated *(9)*. This form of CE takes advantage of a property that when the concentration of some surfactants reach the critical micelle concentration, aggregates (micelles) are formed that help separate neutral species. These spherical micelles contain the hydrophobic tails of the surfactant molecules directed towards the center and charged heads directed toward the outside buffer. The micelles are thus charged and migrate, depending on their charge, after application of a potential field across the capillary. Solutes are partitioned between the micelles and liquid phase leading to differential retention and separation of the solutes *(10)*. The physical nature of the micelle can be changed using different types of surfactant thus altering the selectivity of the micelle. Some applications of MEKC include separation of amino acids (*see* Chapter 9), heavy metals (*see* Chapter 18), nucleotides, vitamins, drugs (*see* Chapters 17 and 18).

2.5.3. Capillary Gel Electrophoresis (CGE)

"Gels" used in CGE are a polymer network of compounds such as bis-polyacrylamide, agarose, or methylcellulose, and separate high molecular weight compounds by the sieving effect of the polymer network. CGE can separate DNA and denatured proteins *(11)*. CGE has been applied in the analysis of polymerase chain reaction (PCR) products (*see* Chapters 13 and 14), purity of oligonucleotides, sequencing of DNA, and so forth.

2.5.4. Capillary Isoelectric Focusing (CIEF)

CIEF is a technique that separates peptides and proteins on the basis of isoelectric point (pI) and can separate proteins with a pI difference of as little as 0.005 pI units *(12)*. This technique is applied to the separation of hemoglobins and hemoglobin variants (*see* Chapter 8), protein isoforms, and immunoglobulins that are difficult to separate by other methods.

2.5.5. Capillary Isotachophoresis (CITP)

CITP is a moving boundary electrophoretic technique that uses a combination of two buffer systems to create a state where the separated zones move at the same velocity. These zones are sandwiched between leading and terminating electrolytes, making it possible to separate either anions or cations, but not both, in a single experiment. CITP can be used to concentrate the solutes before CZE, MEKC, or CGE *(13)*. When used in this manner it is known as transient CITP.

3. APPLICATIONS OF CAPILLARY ELECTROPHORESIS IN CLINICAL SETTINGS

3.1. Serum and Urinary Proteins

Serum proteins that are routinely analyzed by thin-layer agarose gels can be separated and analyzed with greater precision by CZE (*see* Chapters 4 and 5). A combination of CZE and immunosubstraction has been shown to be well suited for routine serum protein analysis in the clinical laboratory. This system can detect different paraproteins at levels of 500 mg/L for IgG, 750 mg/L for IgA, and 750 mg/L for IgM. Using computer software available with current CE instrumentation, it is possible to magnify different regions of the electropherogram, improving the ability to distinguish abnormal peaks in the β-globulin region. One drawback of this system, however, is inability to detect β-lipoproteins and mini monoclonal bands that show up as faint bands on agarose gels *(14)*. Ethanol precipitation for concentrating urine samples has been found to be an effective method to analyze urine proteins, including Bence-Jones proteins by CZE *(15)*. It is also possible to detect Bence-Jones proteinuria (range 0.04–9.7 g/L), intact immunoglobulins, and Tamm Horsfall proteins in unconcentrated urine samples by CE *(16)*.

3.2. Lipoproteins

CITP has been used to perform serum lipoprotein analysis *(17)* and is discussed in more detail in Chapter 7. CITP can be used to directly identify apolipoprotein A-I (apoA-I) from serum, although identification of apolipoprotein A-II (apoA-II) requires some sample preparation because it migrates with the albumin. By plotting a graph of peak areas vs standard concentration it is possible to quantitate the two apolipoproteins. Thus, it is possible to predict the risk of development of premature atherosclerosis by determining the ratio of apoA-I and apoA-II *(18)*. Although useful in research studies, the method lacks the simplicity offered by photometric or immunoassays available in the clinical laboratory.

3.3. Analysis of Organ Function Tests

MEKC has been used to determine antipyrine levels in saliva or plasma after oral administration to assess liver microsomal enzyme activity *(19,20)*. CZE and MEKC methods have been developed to identify different phenotypes for hydroxylation and acetylation enzymes involved in metabolism of drugs by determining levels of different drug metabolites in urine *(21,22)*.

3.4. Serum and Urine Steroid Levels

Determination of levels of different hormones in serum is important for diagnosing various endocrinological disorders. MEKC can effectively separate and quantify a variety of corticosteroids such as corticosterone, cortisone, cortisol, aldosterone, 21-deoxycortisol, 1-dehydroaldosterone, and 17-isoaldosterone *(23)*. CE can also identify and separate estrogens such as urinary estrone and estriol, but not 17 β-estradiol, because its concentration is too low to be detected by this method *(24)*. A competitive solution-phase immunoassay has been developed for separation and quantitation of serum cortisol by CE combined with laser-induced fluorescence *(25,26)*. An assay for urinary free cortisol, unaffected by other urinary metabolites, has also been shown to detect cortisol concentrations as low as 10 µg/L *(27)*. Chapter 11 contains a detailed discussion of the use of CE in the detection of steroids whose levels, when measured, are clinically useful.

3.5. Vitamins and Minerals

By using CZE, vitamin A and vitamin A binding protein can be detected from one or two drops of blood or from air-dried blood samples that have been collected on filter paper. This can be a useful tool for screening vitamin A levels in infants and young children *(28,29)*. CE can detect vitamin C levels in urine, serum, and even fruit beverages *(30)*. It is also possible to identify and quantitate trace amounts of iron in human serum by CE. This method, which is sensitive enough to detect iron in as little as a single drop (10 µL) of serum, could be suitable for diagnosing iron-deficiency anemia *(31)*.

3.6. Serum Bilirubin

MECC in conjunction with LIF can separate and detect four bilirubin species, the unconjugated form, monoester and diester conjugates of bilirubin, and bilirubin covalently linked to albumin, directly from human serum. This method can also detect bilirubin at concentrations much lower than that detected by routine visible light absorption methods *(32)*. Although it is possible to use CE to separate and detect various forms of bilirubin, it is unlikely that a CE assay will be used in the clinical laboratory. This is because at present, CE methods cost appreciably more than current automated methods.

3.7. Cytokines

Detection of cytokines involved in inflammation in pathological tissue samples can be a good indicator of persistence of disease in addition to help gauge its severity. Microdissection followed by CZE of frozen sections of renal biopsy material obtained from patients with acquired immune deficiency syndrome (AIDS) has been developed to identify tissue bound inflammatory cytokines, such as interleukin-1 (IL-1), interleukin-2 (IL-2), tumor necrosis factor-α (INF-α), and so on. This was done to study the pathobiology of renal disease in AIDS and showed higher levels of IL-1, TNF-α and IL-6 in the glomerular and interstitial tissue of patients with HIV-associated glomerulonephritis as compared to non-HIV associated glomerulonephritis *(33)*. Although useful in research, cytokine assays have not found a routine use in the clinical laboratory.

3.8. Hemoglobin and Its Variants

Capillary isoelectric focusing (CIEF) has been helpful in making the differential diagnosis of S/beta thalassemia, G-Philadelphia trait, S/C-Harlem disease, and HbH disease (*see* Chapter 8). In addition, CIEF can identify hemoglobin-oxidation products, which can bias HbA1c results, produced by improper storage. Another important use of this method was in the detection of minor hemoglobin variants like HbA2', an indicator of an alpha globin mutation. CIEF has also been shown to be useful in the neonatal screening for hemoglobin variants using blood samples collected on filter paper *(34)*.

3.9. Porphyrins

CZE or MECC with fluorescence detection can separate and quantitate porphyrin and its precursors in urine *(35)*. Although cost-effective and potentially useful in the diagnosis of porphyria, CE has not yet found its way into laboratories involved in the study of porphyrin metabolism.

3.10. Inorganic Ions

CE can separate inorganic cations such as potassium, calcium, sodium, and magnesium in a single run from serum. It can also detect calcium, ammonia, sodium, magnesium, lithium, barium, and creatinine in urine. Biologically active ionized calcium and total calcium can also be identified and quantitated by CZE in human serum using indirect photometric detection in a single run *(38)*. The ability to detect many components in one run can give CE an advantage over autoanalyzers *(36,37)*. However, owing to the highly automated nature and speed of analyzers present in the clinical laboratory, it is highly unlikely that CE will be used as the method of choice for these analytes.

Nitrite and nitrate, oxidation products of nitric oxide, which is an important agent in shock and organ failure in critically ill patients, can be determined by CZE in plasma and urine samples without any pre-treatment of the samples *(39,40)*. The clinical usefulness of such an assay is still to be determined.

3.11. Inborn Errors of Metabolism

CE allows easy, rapid identification and quantitation of organic acids (*see* Chapter 10) such as methylmalonic, pyroglutamic, and glutaric acids in urine or serum. These organic acids can be increased owing to deficiency of enzymes in amino-acid metabolism *(41)*. Methylmalonic acid can also be increased when there is a deficiency of folate or Vitamin B_{12}.

CZE can also effectively separate purine bases and nucleosides, such as adenine, guanine, hypoxanthine, and uric acid from neonatal plasma *(42)*. Deficiency of adenylosuccinate lyase in the purine metabolism pathway leads to accumulation of succinyladenosine and succinylaminoimidazole carboxamide riboside in body fluids that can be identified by CE *(43)*.

3.12. Serum and Urine Analysis of Drugs

MEKC has been applied to therapeutic drug monitoring. Using MEKC theophylline and its analogues have been separated in plasma. In addition, it has been used to detect and quantitate serum levels of digoxin *(44,45)*. MEKC can also efficiently separate and quantitate antiepileptic drugs that are used in combination, especially ethosuxamide, phenobarbitol, phenytoin, and carbamazepine *(46)*. (See Chapter 17 for a detailed discussion of the use of CE in therapeutic drug monitoring.) CE has also been used in the clinical and forensic arena (*see* Chapter 19). In these cases, the use of urine to identify intoxication and/or drug abuse of opiates, barbiturates, benzodiazepines, stimulants, and doping screening is possible within a few minutes *(47–51)*. It is also possible to use CE to screen post mortem fluids for illicit drugs or elevated levels of legal drugs (*see* Chapter 20). CE has also been applied to determine the tissue concentration of 5-Fluorouracil (5-Fl) in tumor and subcutaneous adipose tissue microdialysates from patients with primary breast cancer *(52)*.

3.13. Urine Myoglobin

CE has been used separate myoglobin from hemoglobin, another pigmented protein in urine. It can detect and quantitate myoglobin in urine obtained from patients with muscular dystrophy, severe trauma, infections, and intoxication. This helps in monitoring muscle dystrophies, trauma, and acute myocardial infarction *(53)*.

3.14. Cerebrospinal Fluid (CSF)

CZE can play an important role in the biochemical diagnosis of central nervous system (CNS) diseases identifying and quantitating lactate, pyruvate oxalate, fumarate, acetate, glutamate, and ascorbate in CSF. Increased ratios of lactate and pyruvate have been observed in cerebral infarction and bacterial meningitis. CZE can also identify ascorbic acid in CSF, which is decreased in inflammatory conditions of CNS *(54)*. In addition, CZE has been shown to useful in detecting oligoclonal banding in unconcentrated CSF (*see* Chapter 6).

3.15. Analysis of PCR Products

Future trends are toward using combined PCR and CE for clinical analysis of PCR products. PCR can be used to amplify genomic material; however, it can not quantitate it. In conjunction with CE, reasonably rapid quantitation is possible. A good example of this is how CE has been used along with PCR to quantitate the viral load in HIV patients (*see* Chapter 13). CGE can also effectively separate DNA restriction fragments and specific amplified DNA sequences from HIV-1 virus in blood *(55)*. Reverse transcription products generated from the RNA of poliovirus can be separated and quantitated by CGE *(56)*. DNA sequencing by CGE is one of the fastest techniques in DNA analysis *(57)*.

4. CONCLUSION

CE is a sensitive and versatile technique and represents an inexpensive and practical method for the determination of many clinically important analytes. Body fluids represent a complex matrix with high levels of proteins and salt that can modify the capillary surface, resulting in variable migration times. In addition to the problems associated with migration times, CE has the additional problem of sensitivity. For the most part this can be overcome by pre-concentration (either on or before the capillary) or by the use of special flow cells. Using these methods, sensitivities close to that of the HPLC can be obtained. In addition, several relatively simple methods for sample stacking on the capillary for CZE and MEKC have been described in the last few years. However, owing to the need to measure drugs at lower and lower serum levels there is still a need for further studies addressing new stacking methods, flow cells, and detectors (i.e., LIF).

The use of CE in combination with immunoassay opens up some interesting avenues of investigation, specifically in the ability to screen and detect multiple analytes simultaneously. The development of CE-based multianalyte immunoassays is limited only by the ability to separate the analytes from each other and from the Ab-Ag complex. In combination with microchips and LIF, the multianalyte CE-based immunoassay could be extremely rapid and sensitive.

CE use in molecular biology and forensic DNA laboratories is also increasing because of its speed and automation. In fact, multichannel fluorescence CE systems have become the instrument of choice for STR analysis in many DNA-typing laboratories primarily because of the appealing aspect of unattended operation, freeing forensic scientists for other duties.

For therapeutic drug monitoring, CE has been found to be most useful in the analysis of new drugs rather than for those with established immunoassays. This is because the cost to operate a CE is much less than that of HPLC. In addition to analyzing a drug and its metabolites, CE can be used for analysis of the bound, free drugs, isomers, and measure the physicochemical properties. Overall, it is our opinion that analysis of newly developed drugs by CE will be an area of growth, owing to the need to monitor serum levels of these new drugs.

Serum protein electrophoresis by CE offers many advantages in labor-saving cost per test and reproducibility compared to the agarose gel procedures. It also offers an alternative way of evaluating serum samples for paraproteinemias. The main advantage of CZE is its ability to screen large numbers of specimens with very little hands-on time at a relatively low cost per test. This is because only buffer and rinse solutions are needed to separate proteins.

CE has made significant progress in the field of bio-separations. With the recent advances in coating chemistries and capillaries, the technique has become more robust, particularly for protein analysis. The benefit of improved separation efficiencies, recovery, and reproducibility of protein separations using coated capillaries translates into wider acceptability of CE. As the demand for recombinant drugs increases, the need for analytical techniques that give complementary results increases and the utility of CE in this area is anticipated.

CE has the advantage of extreme analytical flexibility, using small quantities of low-cost separation buffer, ability to use a variety of detection modes, small sample size (nanoliter), high speed, efficiency, and reproducibility. It is also possible to install fully automated procedures. Furthermore, CE allows a rapid change from one buffer system to another; in other words, changing from one analytical procedure to another. In the future, with a multi-capillary instrument and on-line sample pretreatment, it could be more competitive than other separation methods, such as electrophoresis, HPLC, and GC, in the analysis of clinical relevant analytes. However, for broader acceptance of CE, three things are needed: 1) The development of chemical reagent kits, instruments and software suitable for daily clinical laboratory use; 2) An increase of sensitivity and sample throughput; and 3) Comparison and evaluation of various applications with current laboratory methods under daily laboratory conditions. Many of these areas are being investigated. For example, commercial 96-capillary array instruments will soon be available, which should dramatically improve sample throughput capabilities. Thus, as the number and variety of applications increase, a greater role for CE in the future of the clinical laboratory can be anticipated.

REFERENCES

1. Tiselius, A. (1930) The moving boundary method of studying the electrophoresis of proteins. Ph.D. thesis, Nova Acta Regiae Societatis Scientiarum Upsaliensis, Ser IV, Vol. 17, No. 4, Almqvist & Wiksell, Uppsala, Sweden, pp. 1–107.
2. Hjerten, S. (1967) Free zone electrophoresis. Chromatogr. Rev. 9, 122–219.
3. Jorgenson, J. W. and Lukacs, K. D. (1981) Zone electrophoresis in open tubular glass capillaries. Anal. Chem. 53, 1298–1302.

4. Jorgenson, J. W. and Lukacs, K. D. (1981) High-resolution separation based on electrophoresis and electroosmosis. J. Chromatogr. 218, 209.

5. Jorgenson, J. W. and Lukacs, K. D. (1983) Capillary zone electrophoresis. Science 222, 266–272.

6. Burgi, D. S. and Chien, R. L. (1996) Applications and limits of sample stacking in capillary electrophoresis. Methods Molec. Biol. 52, 211–226.

7. Quirino, J. P. and Terabe S. (1998) Exceeding 5000-fold concentration of dilute analytes in micellar electrokinetic chromatography. Science 282, 465–468.

8. Ewing, A. G., Wallingford, R. A., and Olefirowicz, T. M. (1989) Capillary electrophoresis. Anal. Chem. 61, 292A–303A.

9. Wallingford, R. A. and Ewing, A. G. (1988) Retention of ionic and nonionic catechols in capillary zone electrophoresis with micellar solutions. J. Chromatogr. 441, 299–309.

10. Cohen, A. S., Terabe, S., Smith, J. A., and Karger, B. L. (1987) High performance capillary electrophoretic separation of bases, nucleosides and oligonucleotides: retention manipulation via micellar solutions and metal additives. Anal. Chem. 59, 1021–1027.

11. Cohen, A. S. and Karger, B. L. (1987) High performance sodium dodecyl polyacrylamide gel capillary electrophoresis of peptides and proteins. J. Chromatogr. 397, 409–417.

12. Jorgenson, J. W. (1986) Electrophoresis. Anal. Chem. 58, 743A–760A.

13. Everaerts, F. M., Beckers, J. L., and Vehrggen, T. (1976) Isotachophoresis: Theory, Instrumentation and Applications: Elsevier; Amsterdam, The Netherlands.

14. Jollif, C. R. and Blessum, C. R. (1997) Comparison of serum protein electrophoresis by agarose gel and capillary zone electrophoresis in a clinical setting. Electrophoresis 18, 1781–1784.

15. Friedberg, M. A. and Shahabi, Z. K. (1997) Urine protein analysis by capillary electrophoresis. Electrophoresis 18, 1836–1841.

16. Jenkins, M. A. (1997) Clinical application of capillary electrophoresis to unconcentrated human urine proteins. Electrophoresis 18, 1842–1846.

17. Schimtz, G., Borgmann, U., and Assmann, G. (1985) Analytical capillary isotachophoresis: a routine technique for the analysis of lipoproteins and lipoprotein subfractions in whole serum. J. Chromatogr. 320, 253–262.

18. Lehmann, R., Liebich, H., Grubler, G., and Voelter, W. (1995) Capillary electrophoresis of human serum proteins and apolipoproteins. Electrophoresis 16, 998–1001.

19. Wolfishberg, H., Schmutz, A., Stotzer, R., and Thormann, W. (1993) Assessment of automated capillary electrophoresis for therapeutic and diagnostic drug monitoring: determination of bupvacaine in drain fluid and antipyrine in plasma. J. Chromatogr. A 652, 407–416.

20. Perrett, D. and Ross, G. A. (1995) Rapid determination of drugs in biofluids by capillary electrophoresis-measurement of antipyrine in saliva for pharmacokinetic studies. J. Chromatogr. A 700, 179–186.

21. Caslavska, J., Hufschmid, E., Theurillat, R., Desiderio, C., Wokfishberg, H., and Thormann, W. (1994) Screening for hydroxylation and acetylation poly-

morphisms in man via simultaneous analysis of urinary metabolites of mephenytoin, dextomethorphan and caffeine by capillary electrophoretic procedures. J. Chromatogr. B 656, 219–231.

22. Guo, R. and Thormann, W. (1993) Acetylator phenotyping via analysis of four caffeine metabolites in human urine by micellar electrokinetic capillary chromatography with multiwavelength detection. Electrophoresis 14, 547–553.

23. Jumppanen, J. H., Wiedmer, S. K., Siren, H., Riekkola, M-L, and Haario, H. (1994) Optimized separation of seven corticosteroids by micellar electrokinetic chromatography. Electrophoresis 15, 1267–1272.

24. Ji, A. J., Nunez, M. F., Machacek, D., Ferguson, J. E., Iossi, M. F., Kao, P. C., and Landers, J. P. (1995) Separation of urinary estrogens by micellar electrokinetic chromatography. J. Chromatogr. B 669, 15–26.

25. Schmalzing, D., Nashabeh, W., Yao, X-W, Mhatre, R., Regnier, F. E., Afeyan, N. B., and Fuchs M. (1995) Capillary electrophoresis based immunoassays for cortisol in serum. Anal. Chem. 67, 606–612.

26. Schmalzing, D., Nashabeh, W., and Fuchs, M. (1995) Solution-phase immunoassay for determination of cortisol in serum by capillary electrophoresis. Clin. Chem. 41, 1403–1406.

27. Rao, L. V., Peterson, J. R., Bissell, M. G., Okorodudu, A. O., and Mohammad, A. A. (1999) Development of a urinary free cortisol assay using solid-phase extraction capillary electrophoresis. J. Chromatogr. B 730, 123–128.

28. Ma, Y., Wu, Z., Furr, H. C., Lammi-Keefe, C., and Craft, N. E. (1993) Fast mini-microassay of serum retinol (vitamin A) by capillary zone electrophoresis with laser-excited fluorescence detection. J. Chromatogr. 616, 31–37.

29. Shi, H., Ma, Y., Humphrey, J. H., and Craft, N. E. (1995) Determination of vitamin A in dried human blood spots by high-performance capillary electrophoresis with laser-excited fluorescence detection. J. Chromatogr. B 665, 89–96.

30. Koh, E. V., Bissell, M. G., and Ito, R. K. (1993) Measurement of vitamin C by capillary electrophoresis in biological fluids and fruit beverages using a stereoisomer as an internal standard. J. Chromatogr. 633, 245–250.

31. Che, P., Xu, J., Shi, H., and Ma, Y. (1995) Quantitative determination of serum iron in human blood by high-performance capillary electrophoresis. J. Chromatogr. B 669, 45–51.

32. Wu, N., Sweedler, J. V., and Lin, M. (1994) Enhanced separation and detection of serum bilirubin species by capillary electrophoresis using a mixed anionic surfactant-protein buffer system with laser-induced fluorescence detection J. Chromatogr. B 654, 185–191.

33. Phillips, T. M. and Kimmel, P. L. (1994) High performance capillary electrophoretic analysis of inflammatory cytokines in human biopsies. J. Chromatogr. B 656, 259–266.

34. Hempe, J. M., Granger, J. N., and Craver, R. D. (1997) Capillary isoelectric focusing of hemoglobin variants in the pediatric clinical laboratory. Electrophoresis 18, 1785–1795.

35. Weinberger, R., Sapp, E., and Moring, S. (1990) Capillary electrophoresis of urinary porphyrins with absorbance and fluorescence detection. J. Chromatogr. 516, 271–285.

36. Buchberger, W., Winna, K., and Turner, M. (1994) Applications of capillary zone electrophoresis in clinical chemistry: determination of low-molecular mass ions in body fluids. J. Chromatogr. A 671, 375–382.
37. Xu, X., Kok, W. T., Kraak, J. C., and Poppe, H. (1994) Simultaneous determination of urinary creatinine, calcium and other inorganic cations by capillary zone electrophoresis with indirect UV detection. J. Chromatogr. B 661, 35–45.
38. Zhang, R., Shi, H., and Ma, Y. (1994) Quantitative determination of ionized and total calcium in human serum by capillary zone electrophoresis with indirect photometric detection. J. Microcolumn 6, 217–221.
39. Ueda, T., Maekawa, T., Sadamitsu, D., Oshita, S., Ogino, K., and Nakamura, K. (1995) The determination of nitrite and nitrate in human blood plasma by capillary zone electrophoresis. Electrophoresis 16, 1002–1004.
40. Janini, G. M., Chan, K. C., Muschick, G. M., and Issaaq, H. J. (1994) Analysis of nitrate and nitrite in water and urine by capillary zone electrophoresis. J. Chromatogr. B 657, 419–423.
41. Garcia, A., Barbas, C., Aguila, R., and Castro, M. (1998) Capillary electrophoresis profiling of organic acidurias. Clin. Chem. 44, 1905–1911.
42. Grune, T., Ross, G. A., Schimdt, H., Siems, W., and Perrett, D. (1993) Optimized separation of purine bases and nucleosides in human cord plasma by capillary zone electrophoresis. J. Chromatogr. 636, 105–111.
43. Gross, M., Gathof, B. F., Kolle, P., and Gresser, U. (1995) Capillary electrophoresis for screening of adenylosuccinate lyase deficiency. Electrophoresis 16, 1927–1929.
44. Liu, X., Xu, Y., and Ip, M. P. C. (1995) Capillary electrophoretic enzyme immunoassay for digoxin in human serum. Anal. Chem. 67, 3211–3218.
45. Steinmann, L., Caslavaska, J., and Thormann, W. (1995) Feasibility study of a drug immunoassay based on micellar electrokinetic capillary chromatography with laser induced fluorescence detection: Determination of theophylline in serum. Electrophoresis 16, 1912–1926.
46. Kataoka, Y., Makino, K., and Oishi, R. (1998) Capillary electrophoresis for therapeutic drug monitoring of antiepileptics. Electrophoresis 19, 2856–2860.
47. Wernly, P. and Thormann, W. (1991) Analysis of illicit drugs in human urine by micellar electrokinetic capillary chromatography with one-column fast scanning polychrome absorption detection. Anal. Chem. 63, 2878–2882.
48. Thormann, W., Meier, P., Marcolli, C., and Binder, F. (1991) Analysis of barbiturates in human serum and urine by high-performance capillary electrophoresis-micellar electrokinetic capillary chromatography with on-column multiwavelength detection. J. Chromatogr. 545, 445–460.
49. Schafroth, M., Thormann, W., and Allenmann, D. (1994) Micellar electrokinetic capillary chromatography of benzodiazepines in human urine. Electrophoresis 15, 72–78.
50. Chee, G.L. and Wan, T. S. M. (1993) Reproducible and high-speed separation of basic drugs by capillary zone electrophoresis. J. Chromatogr. 612, 172–177.
51. Chicharro, M., Zapardiel, A., Bermejo, E., Perez, J. A., and Hernandez, L. (1993) Direct determination of ephedrine and norephedrine in human urine by capillary zone electrophoresis. J. Chromatogr. 622, 103–108.

52. Mader, R. M., Brunner, M., Rizovski, B., Mensik, C., Steger, G. G., Eichler, H-G., and Muller, M. (1998) Analysis of microdialysates from cancer patients by capillary electrophoresis. Electrophoresis 19, 2981–2985.
53. Shihabi, Z. K. (1995) Myoglobulinuria detection by capillary electrophoresis. J. Chromatogr. B 669, 53–58.
54. Hiroaka, A., Akai, J., Tominaga, I., Hattori, M., Sasaki, H., and Arato, T. (1994) Capillary zone electrophoretic determination of organic acids in CSF from patients with central nervous system diseases. J. Chromatogr. A 680, 243–246.
55. Schwartz, H. E., Ulfelder, K. J., Sunzeri, F. J., Busch, M.P., and Brownlee, R.G. (1991) Analysis of DNA restriction fragments and polymerase chain reaction products towards detection of the AIDS (HIV-1) virus in blood. J. Chromatogr. 559, 267–283.
56. Rossomando, E. F., White, L., and Ulfelder, K. J. (1994) Capillary electrophoresis separation and quantitation of reverse transcriptase PCR products from poliovirus. J. Chromatogr. B 656, 159–168.
57. Smith, L. M. (1991) High-speed DNA sequencing by capillary gel electrophoresis. Nature 349, 812,813.

2

Basic Principles and Modes of Capillary Electrophoresis

Harry Whatley

1. BASIC PRINCIPLES OF CAPILLARY ELECTROPHORESIS

1.1. Fundamentals of Electrophoresis

Capillary electrophoresis (CE) is a special case of using an electrical field to separate the components of a mixture. Electrophoresis in a capillary is differentiated from other forms of electrophoresis in that it is carried out within the confines of a narrow tube. To understand the behavior of molecules under the influence of an electrical field inside a capillary it is essential to understand the phenomena that result from the geometry of a capillary.

1.1.1. Basic Principles

It has long been known that molecules can be either positively or negatively electrically charged. When the numbers of positive and negative charges are the same, the charges cancel, creating a neutral (uncharged) molecule. If given the freedom to move, charged particles will seek regions, such as an electrode, having an opposing charge; in other words, opposites attract. Figure 1 illustrates a simple example of electrophoresis. In this example a mixture of ionic substances is dissolved in a suitable solvent, such as water. In the absence of an electrical field, the motion of these ions is essentially random. When the electrical field is applied, charged species begin to move. A crude separation occurs, resulting in a less random distribution of charged particles. Cations (positively charged ions) move toward the cathode (negatively charged electrode), and anions (negatively charged ions) move toward the anode (positively charged electrode).

Figure 1 also illustrates another aspect of electrophoresis in solution, the significance of the mass charge ratio (m/z). In this figure there are actually four types of charged particles: large and small positively charged and large

From: *Clinical and Forensic Applications of Capillary Electrophoresis*
Edited by: J. R. Petersen and A. A. Mohammad © Humana Press Inc., Totowa, NJ

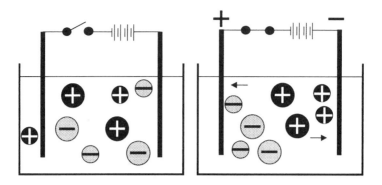

Fig. 1. Simple electrophoresis.

and small negatively charged. If each particle has only a single charge, then the absolute value of the force on each particle will be the same. The acceleration created by this force can be determined by the relationship Force = mass × acceleration (F = ma). The viscosity of the separation medium opposes the acceleration with the result that a steady velocity is achieved under constant conditions. This means that the system can not only separate particles having opposite charges, but can also separate particles of the same charge if there are other differences between them. The science of electrophoresis is largely concerned with creating systems that exploit the differences between the molecules. Alternatively, the analyst may wish to develop a system that creates differences between molecules. Varying the pH of the separation method is an example. At pH = 10.0, glycine and acetic acid will have the same charge (–1). At pH = 7.0, glycine will have a very small net charge whereas acetic acid will still have a charge of –1. Separation of these two molecules would therefore be different at pH = 7.0 and at pH = 10.0.

Numerous other factors besides pH affect electrophoretic separations. These include the hydrodynamic radius of the molecules, the viscosity of the separation medium, and temperature. In real systems there are other forces, in addition to the electrical field, acting on the charged molecules, e.g., the entire fluid mass may be moving relative to the vessel in which it is contained. Some of these factors can affect the electrophoresis in a very complex manner; for example, the passage of current through a liquid can raise the temperature of that liquid. This change in temperature can influence the electrical resistance of the system (and hence the current), the viscosity, and the velocity of the molecules moving in the field. These factors will be discussed later in the specific context of CE. Janini and Issaq presented a detailed discussion of the theoretical underpinnings of these factors *(1)*.

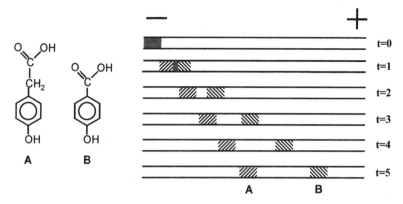

Fig. 2. Capillary electrophoresis.

1.1.2. Electrophoresis in a Capillary

The electrophoretic process in a capillary has all of the features previously described. In addition, the small diameter of the capillary and its large aspect ratio (length/width) contribute additional factors. What actually defines a capillary? For this chapter the discussion will be limited to capillaries formed from fused silica and having an inner diameter (i.d.) of 100 μm or less. The usual range of inner diameters is from 20–100 μm. Typically the capillaries that are used in CE are circular in cross-section. However, capillaries with square cross-sections have been produced. These may offer some advantages in terms of thermal regulation and detection sensitivity *(2)*, but to date they have not been widely used.

1.1.2.1. ADVANTAGES OF THE CAPILLARY

Capillaries were introduced into electrophoresis as an anti-convective and heat controlling innovation. In wide tubes thermal gradients cause band mixing and loss of resolution. The use of glass capillaries of 200–500-μm i.d. was reported by Virtanen *(3)* in 1969. Jorgensen's *(4)* introduction of 75 μm capillary tubes was the start of modern "high-performance" CE.

Figure 2 illustrates the separation of a mixture of two components (both negatively charged) in a capillary. A small plug of sample is introduced into one end. When an electrical field is applied, the components begin to move in the field as previously described. The narrow capillary reduces lateral diffusion and insures that temperature differences between the center of the capillary and the wall are quite small. Because the two components in this example move at different velocities, they can be separated. The geometry and other properties of the capillary electrophoretic separation also lead to a condition known as plug flow. Under ideal plug flow conditions, the only factor leading to sample dispersion is diffusion. This contributes to the high efficiency of CE separations.

1.1.2.2. ELECTROOSMOSIS

The small diameter of the capillary contributes to another aspect of the separation process. This is the phenomenon known as electroosmosis, electroendoosmotic flow, or simply EOF. EOF exists in any electrophoretic system. It will occur whenever the liquid near a charged surface is placed in an electrical field resulting in the bulk movement of fluid near that surface. Because the surface to volume ratio is very high inside a capillary, EOF becomes a significant factor in CE.

The velocity of the electroosmotic flow through a capillary is given by the Smoluchowski equation *(5)* (Eq. 1),

$$v_{eof} = -(\varepsilon \zeta / 4\pi \eta)E \tag{1}$$

where ε is the dielectric constant of the electrolyte, ζ is the zeta potential (Volts), η is the viscosity (Poise), and E is the potential applied (Volts/cm). In CE the zeta potential (ζ) is a measure of the charge on the wall of the capillary. This charge arises from both the nature of the material that composes the capillary and the composition of the electrolyte (buffer). The most commonly employed capillary material is fused silica. The surface of a fused silica capillary can be hydrolyzed to yield a negatively charged surface as described in Section 1.2.1. The negatively charged wall attracts cations that are hydrated from the electrolyte solution, creating an electrical double layer. In an electrical field they migrate toward the cathode, pulling water along and creating a pumping action. The zeta potential increases with the density of the charge on the surface. For fused silica and many other materials charge density will vary with pH *(6)*. Bare fused silica behaves much like a weak acid with a pKa of 6.25. The relationship between EOF and pH is shown in Fig. 3. EOF also decreases with the square root of the concentration of the electrolyte, i.e., increasing buffer concentration decreases the velocity of EOF. Although the aforementioned discussion has focused on bare fused silica capillaries, other types of surfaces can be chemically created from fused silica. The new surface may be positive, negative, or neutral. The direction of the electroosmotic flow will therefore depend on the sign of the charge on the wall of the capillary. Flow is always toward the electrode that has the same charge as the capillary wall. Thus an uncharged wall will have, in theory, no EOF. In reality this is difficult to accomplish.

In the narrow confines of the capillary the velocity of liquid is nearly uniform across the i.d. of the capillary resulting in what has been termed "plug flow" *(4)*. This is in contrast to the laminar flow exhibited by pumped

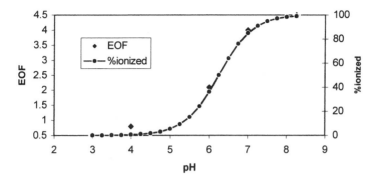

Fig. 3. EOF as a function of pH.

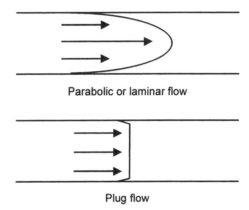

Parabolic or laminar flow

Plug flow

Fig. 4. Flow profiles.

systems, which creates a velocity profile across the diameter of the tube. On the other hand, plug flow greatly reduces the band broadening seen in systems (such as high-performance liquid chromatography [HPLC]) that are pumped by a pressure differential. A comparison of laminar flow and plug flow is shown in Fig. 4.

In the example shown in Fig. 2 the EOF is assumed to be zero. In practice it is very difficult to completely eliminate EOF, although it can be reduced to a value near zero. In many separations it is a significant factor, and it may affect the net movement of the analyte molecules more than does the electrophoretic force. The movement (vectors) due to the electrophoretic and electroosmotic forces may even be in opposite directions. Figure 5A shows a separation of two negatively charged species in a fused silica capillary at pH 8.3. Both analytes have a charge of −1 under these conditions. The EOF

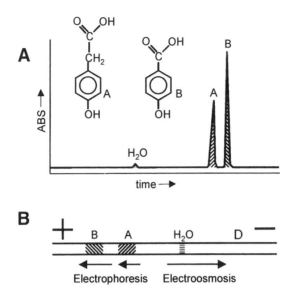

Fig. 5. Separation with EOF.

in this case is toward the cathode, while the analytes are moved electro-phoretically toward the anode. The EOF contribution is larger than the electrophoretic, so that the net movement is toward the cathode. The small peak labeled H_2O represents the water in which the sample was dissolved. This water plug does not have any electrophoretic mobility; the movement of this plug is due solely to electroosmotic flow, and it is the first peak to pass the detector. The next peak to emerge, A, has the higher mass/charge ratio of the two analytes. This is in contrast to the case of Fig. 1 (no EOF) where the first peak to emerge had the lower mass/charge ratio. Note also that the polarity of the electrodes has been reversed compared to Fig. 1. Figure 5B shows a snapshot of the inside of the capillary during the separation but prior to any peak reaching the detector (D). Because A and B are influenced by both the EOF and the electrophoretic force, their net movement is the sum of the electroosmotic and electrophoretic vectors.

1.1.2.3. CAPILLARIES

Many materials have been suggested and tested for the construction of capillaries for CE. These include fused silica, borosilicate glass, and polytetrafluoroethylene (Teflon*). Fused silica is now the preferred material for the construction of capillaries. The silica used is of very high purity,

---

*Teflon is a registered trademark of DuPont.

similar to that used to produce silicon chips for electronic components. Tubes of silica are heated to over 1000°C, then stretched to produce the final dimensions. Fused silica capillaries are extremely brittle. To facilitate handling they are coated with a layer of polyimide 10–25 μm thick, rendering the capillary very flexible. It can easily be wound on a spool 2.5 cm in diameter without breaking. The coating, however, has the disadvantage of being virtually opaque to UV light. It must be removed to create a "window" to allow on-capillary detection. This makes an area that is very fragile, warranting careful handling to prevent breakage.

The thickness of the wall of the capillary and the polyimide coating is generally much greater than the i.d. of the capillary *(7)*. A typical capillary will have an external diameter of 350 μm. If the internal diameter is 50 μm, this leaves a wall thickness of 150 μm. The thickness of the wall is critical, because the heat that is produced when an electrical current passes through the electrolyte must be removed through this wall. Reducing the wall thickness increases the fragility of the capillary at the same time as it increases the heat transfer capacity. External diameter is thus a trade-off between strength and heat transfer. Heat transfer will be discussed in more detail in Subheading 1.2.3.

1.2. Variables in CE

CE offers many directions from which to approach an analytical problem. This can be advantageous because as the number of options available increases, the likelihood that a solution to the analytical problem can be found also increases. This can also be a disadvantage, particularly to the newcomer, because the wide choice of options can appear daunting. This is compounded by the interactive nature of some of these factors. For example, a change in pH can affect the current; a change in current can affect temperature; a change in temperature can affect pH, the factor we were trying to vary in our experiment. Understanding these key factors will contribute to successful analysis.

1.2.1. The Capillary Surface

The inner surface of a capillary is an extremely important factor in CE. The inner wall is in contact with the separation chemistry and the samples. As noted earlier, the capillary wall is the site of the mechanism by which EOF is created. In order to understand how to control the effect of the surface on the separation, it important to understand the behavior of the capillary surface. The inner surface of a CE capillary is more analogous to the surface of the particles packed inside an HPLC column than it is to the HPLC column wall. Unlike the wall of an HPLC column, the capillary wall partici-

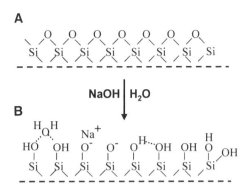

Fig. 6. Silica surface chemistry. Surface of fused silica before (**A**) and after (**B**) NaOH hydrolysis.

pates in the separation process. In CE the goal is usually to prevent interaction between the analytes and the inner wall of the capillary while simultaneously controlling EOF. In order to have control over the separation process it is necessary to have control over this surface.

1.2.1.1. SURFACE MODIFICATIONS

The nature of the surface of a bare fused silica capillary depends somewhat on the treatment it has experienced *(8)*. A freshly manufactured silica capillary has a surface similar to that shown in Fig. 6A. Most of the surface is in a siloxane form; there are few groups present that can create a charged surface. Treatment with base (NaOH or KOH) causes the hydrolysis of the siloxane group, creating the surface shown in Fig. 6B. Sometimes referred to as an etched surface, this layer is rich in silanol groups, which are the weak acids referred to in the discussion of EOF. To convert completely the surface of the capillary into this form may require long periods of exposure with 0.1–1.0 *M* base at elevated temperatures. Incomplete conversion may lead to poor reproducibility in peak migration times.

Not all separations can be optimized using bare silica. However, the silica surface is chemically reactive and can be derivatized in a variety of ways. Silane derivatization reactions are commonly employed to link other groups to silica. This can result in a linkage through a Si-O-Si-C bond or through a Si-C bond depending on the chemistry employed. The Si-C bond is said to be the more stable of the two at high pH values *(9)*. Using a molecule that has a silane at one end and a second functional group at the other allows a second layer to bond. This approach allows more complex coatings to be applied in layers. In this way many types of coatings have been created including polyacrylamide *(9,10)*, polyvinyl alcohol, polyethylene glycol *(11)*, and polyvinylpyrolidone *(12)*. Each of these coatings will have different properties of charge and adsorptivity. Most were designed to reduce protein binding to the capillary wall. Basic proteins, being positively charged, are particularly difficult to analyze in untreated capillaries because they bind tightly to the negatively charged wall *(13)*. Coatings are also employed to modify the charge of the wall such that EOF is drastically altered or reversed.

Presently, the analyst seldom prepares covalently coated capillaries, as many types are commercially available. With commercially available fixed coatings, it is possible to obtain charges ranging from acidic to neutral to basic and from hydrophilic to hydrophobic. The analyst may also wish to incorporate noncovalent coatings into a separation method using a bare silica capillary. These transient or dynamic coatings rely on ionic interactions to hold them on the capillary wall. Polyamines will stick to the negatively charged silica, effectively shielding the negatively charged wall from the solution and creating a positively charged surface *(14)*. In such a capillary, the EOF will be toward the anode. Coatings of this type may be stable for several runs. Cationic detergents such as tetradecyltrimethylammonium bromide (TTAB) can be used to form a positively charged surface as well *(15)*. Such coatings are actually bilayers. The first layer has the positively charged head of the detergent attached to the negatively charged silanol surface. The hydrophobic tails of the molecules extend radially inward, forming a hydrophobic surface. A second layer of detergent forms with the hydrophobic tails in contact with the tails of the first layer and the positively charged heads forming the inner surface of the capillary. Again, EOF will be toward the anode. These detergent bilayers are easy to form but lack stability. They are easily disrupted by organic solvents and usually require that the detergent be added to the run buffer (where it may interact with analytes).

Whenever a capillary is used, the buffer being used modifies the surface. Most workers have come to recognize that capillaries perform best when they are "dedicated" to a specific type of buffer species. For example, if a capillary that has been equilibrated with a phosphate buffer is used with a borate buffer of similar concentration and pH the migration times will drift from run to run until a new equilibrium condition has been established. Although neither borate nor phosphate would be expected to form a coating on the capillary wall, it is apparent that the capillary does "remember" the buffer it has held. This dedication of a capillary to one type of system is a relatively inexpensive way to improve results.

1.2.1.2. CAPILLARY REGENERATION

Regeneration is the process of creating the same surface on the inner wall of the capillary prior to the start of every analytical run with a given method. Although it is only necessary to recreate the same surface condition every time, it is in fact easier in the long run to fully regenerate the surface. There are two goals to regeneration: 1) to clean the capillary of any residual buffer and sample from the previous analysis; and 2) to create the same surface from run to run, thereby enhancing reproducibility. If the method has been properly designed these steps should not be necessary. If sample components are sticking to the capillary wall in sufficient quantity to affect subsequent runs, it is advisable to change the method to prevent the sample from sticking (perhaps by using a coating or by increasing the buffer concentration) rather than incorporating a cleaning procedure. In practice this can be difficult to accomplish, particularly with samples containing protein (such as serum) that is inherently troublesome.

This chapter will focus on the regeneration of bare silica capillaries. The special handling of coated surfaces will be discussed in Chapter 3. However, when using commercially coated capillaries, it is important to follow the manufacturer's instructions for cleaning and regeneration. This is because coated capillaries are easily converted into bare silica capillaries.

Freshly purchased fused silica capillaries, even those sold as "ready to use," may not be clean when first received. Therefore, some variation of the following procedure should be used whenever a new piece of bare silica capillary is used.

1. Flush the capillary with methanol. This will remove any organic residues (such as oil) and will aid in the subsequent wetting of the surface.
2. Flush with water.
3. Flush with 1 N hydrochloric acid. This removes any residual cations.
4. Flush with water.
5. Flush with 1 N NaOH. This step hydrolyzes the siloxanes to create the charged silanol groups that provide EOF.
6. Flush with water.
7. Flush with electrolyte.

Many variations on this procedure exist. For example, a second hydrochloric acid wash can be added after the NaOH if the removal of residual sodium is desired (as prior to a sodium analysis). The time and temperature of each step is important. A minimum of three capillary volumes should be used over at least 5 min (Section 1.3.1. will describe how to calculate fluid delivery). Static soaking should be avoided in favor of a continuous flow. As expected, the use of elevated temperature (35–40°C) will enhance the cleaning rate. The final flush with electrolyte, although critical to obtain assay reproducibility, is often neglected. The procedure described above creates a virgin surface that may change as analysis proceeds. There is usually an equilibration between the capillary wall and even simple buffers, such as sodium phosphate. Applying voltage to the capillary facilitates the exchange of ions at the surface after filling with the electrolyte.

The regeneration process between sample runs can be milder than the initial cleaning, particularly if the method is not detrimental to the surface and the samples are not sticky. In the best of cases it is only necessary to flush with fresh run buffer. At other times exposure to acid or base, or even an organic solvent, may be required to restore the surface to the original condition. The regeneration procedure, however, should be matched to the separation method. For separations using sodium borate buffer, pH 8.3, regeneration with NaOH is appropriate. For separations using phosphate buffer, pH 2.5, the use of NaOH or other base rinses should be avoided. At low pH, EOF is suppressed because the silanol groups are poorly ionized. Using NaOH to regenerate the capillary will increase the time needed to re-equilibrate the surface with the low pH electrolyte (phosphate), thus rinsing with a higher concentration of low pH buffer or even with 1 N acid (i.e., phosphoric) will generally give better results.

Rinsing coated capillaries adds a further complication, in that the coating itself may be labile in the presence of the cleaning solution. Exposure to NaOH will strip many covalently bonded phases from the capillary surface. It is critical to follow the manufacturer's recommendations for cleaning and regenerating coated capillaries. Dynamic coatings such as TTAB should be reconstructed by rinsing with a more concentrated solution of the coating material than is used in the run buffer. For example, if the running buffer contains 0.5 mM of detergent, a pre-rinse with 20 mM detergent followed by the actual running buffer would be appropriate.

1.2.2. Separation Buffers

The significance of the capillary wall in controlling the process of separation in CE cannot be overstated. The separation, however, takes place in the separation buffer. It is here that the conditions are such that the differences in mobility can exist. Buffers can either be made or purchased. Buffer quality is independent of the instrument system used. However, even the best instrument system will not perform properly with a poorly prepared buffer.

1.2.2.1. SIGNIFICANCE OF pH

The most common measurement in analytical chemistry is probably the measurement of pH. It is also the measurement that is most often made improperly. In CE it is extremely important to properly control pH since it affects analyte charge, electroosmotic flow, and, by affecting current, heat production. Thus small changes in pH tend to have greater impact in CE than do comparable pH variations in HPLC.

Figure 3 shows the titration curve of the silica surface, which behaves as a typical weak acid (e.g., acetic acid). The ionization of acetic acid (pK_a = 4.76) is shown in Eq. 2. At the pK_a, the analyte will be 50% charged. This does not mean that each molecule carries one-half of a charge, but rather that at any point in time one half of the molecules are charged and the other half are uncharged. A titration curve like that shown in Fig. 3 represents the probability than any given molecule will be charged at a given pH.

$$H_3C\text{-}COOH \rightleftarrows H_3C\text{-}COO^{(-)} + H^{(+)} \tag{2}$$

When the molecule is uncharged it is under the influence of the electroosmotic flow but not the electrical field. When charged the molecule responds to both forces. As the fraction of the time the molecule spends in each state varies with pH, the net migration velocity will change. As discussed earlier, the EOF also changes with pH. Failure to properly control pH is one of the major causes of poor reproducibility in CE.

1.2.2.2. BUFFER SPECIES

Buffers are compounds that are used to control the pH of a solution. They are generally weak acid or bases that can accept or donate protons. Buffers reduce the change in pH that is caused by the introduction of additional acid or base; CE buffers are selected on the basis of the pH range that is to be maintained, as well as other factors.

A wide range of buffers has been employed in CE systems. The most commonly employed are phosphate, borate, citrate, acetate, and Tris (trishydroxymethylamino methane). The zwitterionic buffers that have been recommended by several authors have the advantage of carrying less current than do mono-functional buffer molecules. However, the selection of a buffer for CE should be based on several factors, including: 1) pH value desired; 2) operating temperature; 3) charge of the buffer relative to the analytes and the capillary wall; and 4) effects on detection. These factors are further described as follows:

1. For any buffer the effective buffering range is defined as within one pH unit of the buffers pK_a. Thus a buffer with a pK_a of 5 would be usable from pH 4.0 to pH 6.0. For CE it is much better to have the pH as close to the pK_a of the buffer as possible, certainly within ± 0.5 pH units, to reduce the buffer's contribution to variability.

2. Buffer molecules exhibit a temperature coefficient. The pH of a buffered system will tend to change with temperature. In addition, buffers tend to differ in their sensitivity to temperature. For example, phosphate has a low temperature coefficient compared to Tris. The temperature coefficient of the buffer is also important because during electrophoresis the analyst has only limited control of the temperature inside the capillary. This is discussed in more detail in Subheading 1.2.3.

3. Interaction between the buffer and the analytes can change the effective charge on the analyte molecules, changing their migration velocity. Ion pairing can also occur between the buffer molecules and the analytes affecting the separation.

4. Buffers differ widely in their absorbance spectra. This is much less of a problem in CE than in HPLC because of the short path-length in CE detection. However, for high-sensitivity work the background absorbance may become an issue.

Once the buffer composition has been selected, it is essential that it be prepared properly. In order to make a buffer consistent it is critical to make the buffer the same way every time. For example, preparing a 50 mM sodium phosphate buffer by starting with 50 mM sodium phosphate and adjusting the pH with phosphoric acid will result in a buffer with a phosphate concentration higher than 50 mM. Such a buffer is best prepared by titration of phosphoric acid with NaOH.

A buffer that has found wide application in CE is sodium borate. However, the preparation of borate buffers can be confusing because boric acid combines with sodium hydroxide according to Eq. 3.

$$4\ H_3BO_3 + 2\ NaOH \rightleftarrows Na_2B_4O_7 + 7\ H_2O \tag{3}$$

Four moles of boric acid react with sodium hydroxide to form one mole of sodium tetraborate. A borate buffer will contain both boric acid and tetraborate. In discussing these systems it is customary to refer to the concentration of Boron. Thus, 4 M boric acid and 1 M sodium tetraborate have the same concentration of boron.

1.2.2.3. BUFFER CONCENTRATION

Increasing the concentration of a buffer will increase the buffering capacity of the system, making it less likely to change pH with the addition of acid or base. In addition, there are other factors in CE that can be affected by the concentration of the buffer *(16,17)*. These factors can be critical when trying to achieve optimum resolution and reproducibility.

If the composition of the sample plug is different from the composition of the buffer in the capillary, the phenomenon of stacking may occur *(18,19)*. Properly exploited stacking can result in sharper peaks and greater sensitivity. One way to achieve stacking is to keep the conductivity of the sample lower than the conductivity of the running buffer by reducing the concentration of the sample buffer relative to the run buffer. To understand this phenomenon, consider the buffer filled capillary as a wire. If the buffer concentration is uniform from one end of the capillary to the other end, the voltage drop will be linear. Inserting a plug of dilute sample is like inserting a resistor into the wire. The voltage drop now becomes steeper in the region of the plug than it is elsewhere. Since velocity is proportional to the voltage gradient, the velocity of the analytes will be faster in this region. Analytes will move rapidly until they reach the boundary between the dilute sample plug and the more concentrated running buffer. On reaching this point they

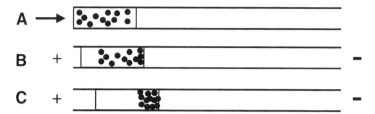

Fig. 7. Sample stacking. (**A**) In an injected sample plug the analyte molecules are distributed randomly. (**B**) When the voltage is applied the entire sample plug begins to move under EOF. The analytes in the sample move more rapidly than the bulk flow due to the difference in ionic strength between the sample plug and the run buffer. (**C**) Before the analytes begin to migrate out of the sample plug they have been concentrated. Note that the length of the sample plug is unchanged.

will stack, increasing the local concentration of analyte and creating a zone that is narrower than the original injection plug. This is illustrated in Fig. 7.

Because stacking is caused by a difference in conductivity between the buffer and the sample, it might be assumed that dissolving the sample in pure water would create the highest peak efficiencies. In practice, however, this is not usually the case. The resistance across a plug of nearly pure water can be so high that localized heating results. This heating causes convective mixing and de-stacking. There should be always be some buffer ions in the sample plug; keeping samples at about 1/10 the concentration of the running buffer is a good rule of thumb *(20)*.

One way to maximize stacking would be to increase the concentration of the buffer, particularly if the samples as received are high in salt. As stated in Section 1.1.2.2., EOF decreases with the square root of the buffer concentration. If EOF is to remain constant it will be necessary to increase it in some other way, such as a change in pH, temperature, or voltage. If desired, EOF can be reduced simply by increasing the buffer concentration. However, by increasing the buffer concentration the current that passes through the capillary will also increase. This in turn will increase the heat generated inside the capillary and, if not adequately dissipated, a variety of problems can result. Without adequate cooling the ability to exploit higher buffer concentrations is limited.

When trying to separate basic compounds or proteins that tend to interact with the capillary wall using bare silica capillaries, problems are frequently encountered. In extreme situations they may be totally adsorbed on the capillary wall and never pass the detector. In other cases the wall may provide a drag force that results in peak tailing, loss of resolution, and decreased signal-to-noise ratio. Although coated capillaries are one solution to this prob-

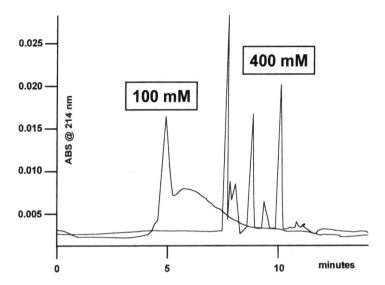

Fig. 8. Effect of buffer concentration on peak shape. The proteins in this sample interact strongly with the wall of the capillary. Increasing the buffer concentration can reduce this effect.

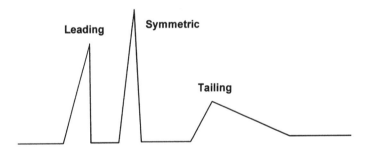

Fig. 9. Peak shape in CZE mode. The peaks shown here are indicative of variations between the mobility of the analytes and the mobility of the buffer ions. Peak shapes such as these do not necessarily indicate adsorption phenomena.

lem, merely increasing the concentration of the electrolyte can often reduce these interactions *(15,21)*. Figure 8 shows the effect on a protein separation of increasing the phosphate concentration.

Peak shape in many modes of CE differs from the bell shape that is commonly seen in HPLC and other chromatographic separations. In open capillary modes (such as capillary zone electrophoresis [CZE]), it is not uncommon to see peak shapes like those in Fig. 9. In CE the electrical field influences the buffer ions just as it does the analyte ions. The peak shape in these separations is due to the relative migration rates of the buffer ions and the analyte ions. The degree of asymmetry will increase with increased difference in mobility. Buffer mismatch can so distort the peak shape that analytes may be difficult to quantitate or may even be lost.

Because the buffer ions migrate in the electrical field, the concentration of the buffer ions in the inlet and outlet vials will change over time. Using buffer vials that are too small (i.e., do not contain an adequate volume of buffer) or running too many samples without replacing the buffer can result in ion depletion. This process can result in a change in the sample migration times or resolution.

1.2.2.4. ADDITIVES

Other reagents are frequently added to the buffer systems used in CE. The most common are detergents, such as sodium dodecyl sulfate (SDS) *(22)*, viscosity modifiers, such as linear polyacrylamide *(23)*, organic solvents, such as acetonitrile *(24)*, denaturants, such as urea *(25)*, or combinations of these additives.

The addition of detergent to a buffer used in CE can change dramatically the separation properties of the system. Detergents can aid in solubilizing analytes and in reducing analyte-wall interactions. They may also bind to the capillary wall, affecting the EOF. If the detergents are above their critical micellar concentrations (CMC), they can create a pseudostationary phase. Under these conditions the separation mechanism is referred to as micellar electrokinetic chromatography (MEKC), which is discussed in Section 2.5. Detergents for CE may be anionic, cationic, or nonionic. Protein separations can also be achieved with detergents. By titrating the concentration of SDS in the run buffer it is sometimes possible to achieve protein separations based on differential binding of the detergent to different proteins. This is not a separation by MEKC because the protein molecules are too large to be included in the micelle *(26)*.

Viscosity modifiers provide a physical retardation to the movement of molecules. Suitable viscosity modifiers include polymers, such as linear polyacrylamide or soluble cellulose derivatives, as well as small molecules like urea. By retarding large molecules more than they do small molecules the dimension of size separation is added to the electrophoretic separation. This is exploited fully in capillary gel electrophoresis (CGE) which is discussed in Section 2.2. At lower concentrations, viscosity modifiers can aid in the separation of very similar analytes. Viscosity modifiers can also have significant effects on EOF, both by the change in viscosity and by interacting with the capillary wall *(27)*.

Organic additives routinely used include acetonitrile, methanol, formamide, and dimethylformamide. These solvents improve the solubility of organic molecules that would otherwise be poorly soluble in an aqueous system. At sufficiently high concentrations, they can also reduce the degree of ionization of charged analytes. In MEKC they can alter the relative hydrophobicity of the micellar and non-micellar phases. Organic additives can also affect viscosity and wall charge (and hence EOF). The effect of solvents on viscosity can be complex. Acetonitrile has a lower viscosity than water, and any combination of water and acetonitrile will have a viscosity between that of water and acetonitrile. Methanol also has a lower viscosity than water, but combinations of water and methanol can be substantially more viscous than either solvent alone. In nonaqueous CE (described in Section 2.7.) organic solvent completely replaces water in the separation solution.

1.2.3. Temperature

Temperature control is crucial to reproducible separations in CE. However, temperature regulation is complicated by several factors. First is that the passage of electrical current through the buffer-filled capillary results in the production of heat. This self-heating effect is inherent in electrophoretic separations and is called Joule heating. Thus temperature control in CE is as much a task of removing heat as it is maintaining a constant temperature environment. Second is that the temperature of the contents inside the capillary is difficult to measure. A layer of silica and a layer of polyimide separate the small fluid volume inside the capillary from the thermostatted medium. Any heat must be transferred to and from the separation buffer through these layers.

Although the temperature inside the capillary cannot easily be measured it can be estimated. Equation 4 is used to estimate the Joule heating (Q). In this equation

$$Q = E^2 \Lambda c \qquad (4)$$

Q is the Joule heat generated (Ω/cm^3), E is the voltage gradient (V/cm), Λ is the molar conductivity of the electrolyte ($cm^2\,mol^{-1}\,W^{-1}$) and c is the concentration of the electrolyte (mol/L). Since the conductivity of the electrolyte will vary with temperature, a positive feedback mechanism occurs. In other words, as the temperature increases, the current will also increase. This in turn generates more heat thus generating more current. This feedback loop is moderated by the ability of the cooling system to remove heat and thus limit current. Because the cooling system must act at the surface of the capillary and not internally, a temperature gradient exists from the center of the capillary to the outside, which is illustrated in Fig. 10.

The temperature gradient within the capillary is parabolic. The difference in temperature between the center of the capillary and the wall will increase

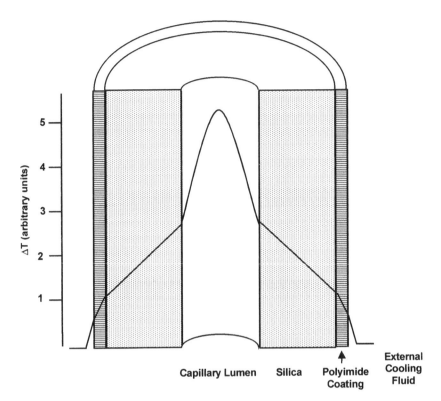

Fig. 10. Theoretical radial temperature profile. Joule heating occurs when current passes through the buffer-filled capillary. The temperature can be expected to be highest in the center of the capillary. Each layer through which the heat must pass will have its own thermal conductivity leading to a complex pattern such as that illustrated here. Adapted from Knox *(28).*

with increasing capillary internal diameter. Current will also increase as the diameter increases (current α radius^2). The combination of these two factors can lead to the conclusion that heating will cause band broadening and that the band broadening will increase as the internal capillary diameter increases. In systems with adequate temperature control, this thermal band broadening does not become a problem unless the capillary diameter is larger than about 100 µm. A more detailed discussion of heat transfer in CE can be found in an article by Knox *(28).*

A second temperature gradient can also exist in poorly designed systems if the entire length of the capillary is not maintained in the same thermal environment. The regions of the capillary that are in buffer vials, passing through cartridge walls, or in detector cells are frequently much less efficiently cooled than are other regions of the capillary. Depending on the system and the capillary length, this uncooled region can account for as much as 25% of the capillary's effective length and can account for much of the variation in performance seen between instruments of different design.

Dynamically cooled CE systems are conveniently divided into two groups: those employing gas and those employing liquid as a heat exchange medium. Liquid cooling is generally considered to be more efficient than gas cooling simply because the heat capacity of liquids exceed that of air. The most effective liquid coolant would be water because of its enormous heat capacity. However, when dealing with electrical equipment, the use of water as a heat exchange medium is not advisable. The requirements of safety has led to the use of perfluorinated organic molecules, having the general formula $(F_3C\text{-}[CF_2]_n\text{-}CF_3)$, because of their very low electrical conductivity. Because of their greater heat capacity, liquids tend to be slower to adjust to changes in temperature than gases. Liquid cooling also necessitates sealed recirculating systems, adding to the expense and complexity of the instrument. Whatever the cooling medium, most modern instrument systems use computer controlled Peltier devices to control the temperature of the cooling fluid. Peltier devices are semiconductor mechanisms that can be made to heat or cool by reversing the direction of current flow through them.

Changes in temperature can also impact other factors inside the capillary. For most liquids, an increase in temperature causes a decrease in viscosity. For example, water has a viscosity of 1.002 centipoise at 20°C. This drops to 0.798 centipoise at 30°C. In the absence of any other changes this change in viscosity will result in a substantial increase in EOF. In addition, the pH of a buffered solution may also change with temperature. A 10°C change in temperature will cause a 0.3 pH unit change in the pK_a of Tris. This may be sufficient to change both EOF and the charge on the analyte molecules.

A simple way to determine if a CE system is capable of coping with the heat that will be produced during separation is by creating an Ohm's Law plot. Ohm's Law states that $V = IR$. If we vary voltage (V), the current (I) should change in a linear manner so long as resistance (R) remains constant. An increase in temperature within the capillary generally results in a decrease in resistance (and hence an increase in current at constant voltage). By measuring the current at a variety of voltages a graph of current vs voltage can be created. Regardless of the type of cooling system the current will become nonlinear at some voltage. For the buffer system being considered the point at which the line deviates from linearity indicates the maximum voltage possible for that buffer system/capillary combination on that instrument. In practice it is possible to run at somewhat higher voltage if it is understood that the temperature within the capillary is higher than the thermostatted temperature under these conditions. It is good practice to monitor current during a run because an increasing current during a run may indicate that the heat dissipation capacity of the instrument is being exceeded. In the worst case the heat in the capillary may become sufficient to boil the buffer locally, usually at some poorly cooled location. This usually breaks the electrical circuit (and sometimes the capillary).

1.3. Volume Relationships

The dimensions employed in CE are much smaller than those with which most chemical analysts are accustomed to work. Capillary diameters typically are measured in microns and as such the entire volume of a capillary is usually a few microliters. Injected sample volumes are in nanoliters (10^{-9} L). At these scales the tolerances required of instrument systems are extremely small and difference of 1 μm in the diameter of a capillary can create very large differences in the results of an analysis.

1.3.1. Flow Dynamics

Most often the sample being analyzed by CE is injected into the capillary by pressure. To calculate the volume of liquid injected it is necessary to use the Poiseuille equation (Eq. 5), which estimates the flow of liquid through a cylinder.

$$V = (\Delta P d^4 \pi t)/(128\eta L) \tag{5}$$

In this equation, ΔP is the pressure drop down the length of the cylinder (Pascals), d is the cylinder's inside diameter (m), t is time the pressure is applied (s), η is the fluid viscosity (Pascal-seconds), and L is the total length of the cylinder (m). This equation has wide applicability in fluid dynamics and can be used to calculate fluid flow in CE capillaries, blood vessels, or a water main. It shows that the delivery of fluid into a capillary by pressure is directly proportional to the pressure that is applied and the length of time the pressure is applied. Fluid delivery is inversely proportional to the liquid viscosity and the length of the capillary, and proportional to the fourth power of the diameter. Temperature is indirectly involved in this relationship because the viscosities of most fluids change with temperature.

Table 1 exemplifies the volumes typically encountered in CE. This example assumes the viscosity of water at 25°C (1.000 centipoise). Typically injection and rinse pressures are 0.5 and 20 psi, respectively.

As predicted by Eq. 5, the volume of fluid delivered at a given pressure increases dramatically as the diameter of the capillary increases. Doubling the diameter of the capillary increases the delivered volume 16-fold. The implications of this are significant. As shown in Table 2, the volume injected under constant condition changes dramatically when the capillary diameter changes over a narrow range. Because tolerances of 1–2 μm are not uncom-

Table 1
Typical Volumes Encountered in Capillary Electrophoresis[a]

Diameter (μm)	Length (cm)	Capillary volume (nL)	Injected nL/s @ 0.5 psi	Injection plug (mm)	Rinse nL/s @ 20 psi
20	25	79	0.060	0.19	2.43
20	50	157	0.030	0.09	1.21
25	25	123	0.148	0.30	5.93
25	50	245	0.074	0.15	2.96
50	25	491	2.37	1.2	94.92
50	50	982	1.18	0.6	47.46
75	25	1104	12.0	2.71	480
75	50	2209	6.00	1.35	240
100	50	3927	18.9	2.41	759

[a]These values were calculated using Eq. 5.

Table 2
Injection Volume Variability with Capillary Internal Diameter[a]

Diameter (μm)	18	19	20	21	22
nL/s @0.5 psi	1.99	2.47	3.03	3.69	4.44

[a]Capillary for CE is typically manufactured to tolerances of +/- 2 μm.

mon in commercially available capillary, selecting different pieces of capillary nominally 20 μm in diameter could give peak areas that vary substantially. Cutting pieces from a large spool of capillary is no guarantee of uniformity because the diameter may vary along the length of the spool.

The injection plug length in Table 1 is the linear distance within the capillary that is occupied by the injected sample volume. An injection plug that is too long may result in wide bands and loss of resolution, particularly if the analytes cannot focus. Increasing the capillary diameter allows the injection of substantially larger volumes of sample without increasing the plug length. Because the volume of a cylinder increases with the square of the radius a doubling of the capillary diameter will allow the injection of four times as much sample without changing the plug length.

The viscosity of the fluid being delivered is the most difficult parameter to know with accuracy. The aforementioned examples have assumed the viscosity of water at 25°C. Within the range of temperatures typically used in CE separations (15–60°), the viscosity of water varies in a nonlinear manner from 1.138 to 0.467 centipoise. Almost anything added to the water will alter both the viscosity and the temperature-viscosity relationship. The additions of macromolecules, such as cellulose derivatives or acrylamide poly-mers, are extreme cases. These molecules display remarkable viscosity behavior with changes in flow rates. Linear polymers, for example, can extend and align themselves when forced through a capillary. They can show a reduction in viscosity with increased flow. Other systems may increase in viscosity with flow because of polymer entanglement. Even systems as simple as methanol-water can show complex behavior. For example, a 1:1 mix of methanol and water has a higher viscosity than either pure solvent. It is also important to remember that when calculating volumes injected into fluid-filled capillaries, the viscosity of the fluid in the capillary is usually more significant than the viscosity of the sample (unless one is analyzing highly viscous samples).

Entering the Poiseuille equation into a spreadsheet program simplifies fluid delivery calculations such as these. There is also a Windows*-compat-ible computer program called "CE Expert" that can perform these calcula-tions (this program is currently available at no cost directly from Beckman Coulter, Inc.).

1.3.2. Sample Handling

Four basic strategies are used to deliver these fluid volumes into capillar-ies: Positive pressure, vacuum, gravity, and electrophoresis. Positive pres-sure and vacuum have been the most common methods of filling and rinsing capillaries. Positive pressure up to 100 psi (7 bar) has been used for rinsing. This pressure is delivered either from a source of compressed gas, such as nitrogen, or from an on-board air pump that applies pressure to the headspace of a buffer reservoir. Vacuum delivery is limited to 10 psi or less but can be useful for drawing fluid from containers that cannot be made pressure tight.

Gravity and electrophoresis are not practical for filling and rinsing capil-laries, but they are used, along with pressure and vacuum, for injecting samples into capillaries. Gravity injection (sometimes called hydrostatic injection) is accomplished by inserting the inlet end of the capillary into the sample vial and raising the vial and capillary relative to the outlet end. Reproducible gravity injection requires that the vial be raised to the same height for the same duration of time at each injection (gravity itself being a fairly reliable source of motive power). Pressure and vacuum injections are more complicated. Regardless of how the pressure differential is created, a finite time is required for the pressure to reach a steady state. Changes in pressure on the order of 0.05 psi can be significant at the low pressures commonly employed (0.1–1 psi). Systems that rely on pressure or vacuum

---

*Windows is a trademark of Microsoft.

must have some sort of feedback mechanism to compensate for these variations. These systems either adjust the delivered pressure or the delivery time to maintain the desired product of pressure and time. In well-engineered systems a 3-s injection at 1 psi and a 10-s injection at 0.3 psi should give identical results, because both are 3 psi-second injections. In practice the longer, lower pressure injection usually gives better performance because it allows a longer time for the system to respond to variances.

Electrophoretic or electrokinetic injections do not conform to the Poiseuille equation. In this method of sample introduction, the inlet of the capillary is inserted into the sample and the outlet into a buffer vial. Voltage is briefly applied. Through a combination of electrophoresis and electroosmotic flow sample is drawn into the capillary. This technique is valuable when delivering sample to a gel-filled capillary or when pressure delivery is not possible. There is a possibility of bias when using this technique *(29)*. Components that migrate more rapidly in the electrical field will be over-represented in the sample compared to slower moving components. To maximize the volume injected, the sample should be at a considerably lower ionic strength than the run buffer. Subsequent injections will show reduced peak areas because each injection delivers salts from the capillary buffer into the sample vial, raising the ionic strength of the sample. This effect can be minimized (and injected quantity increased) by pre-injecting from pure water immediately prior to the sample injection.

Most commercial systems employ some sort of carousel or X-Y-Z robotic system to move the buffer and sample vials to the capillary. These systems may also provide refrigerated storage for labile samples. In this case the sample storage temperature should be regulated independently of the capillary thermostatting system.

1.4. Detection

In order to gain useful information from the separation technique, it is necessary to detect and measure the analytes. Detection may be qualitative and/or quantitative. Most CE detection is done on-capillary; that is, a section of the capillary is linked to the detection device and the capillary itself is the detection cell. It is also possible to couple to detectors that are outside of the separation capillary although this does require a specialized interface.

1.4.1. Geometry and Path-Length

The most frequently used method of detection involves absorbance of energy as the analytes move through a focused beam of light. The scale of the detection apparatus and of the signal produced has created some unique challenges for the instrument developer.

On-capillary detection eliminates the problems of coupling the capillary and its power supply to flow cells or other devices. However, detection through the capillary is complicated by the curvature of the capillary itself. The capillary and the fluid it contains make up a complex cylindrical lens. The curvature of this lens must be accounted for in order to gather the maximum amount of light and thereby maximize signal-to-noise ratio. The effective length of the light path through the capillary is actually about 63.5% the stated i.d. of the capillary. Thus a 50-μm capillary has an effective path length of only 32 μm. This can be compared to typical HPLC detectors that have detectors in the 5–10 mm range. Because of this very small light path, the absorbance signal obtained from a CE system is also correspondingly small. Therefore, a peak with an absorbance of 0.002 AU is a significant peak. Noise levels are correspondingly small and are usually measured in microabsorbance units. The maximum absorbance of typical CE detectors is 0.2 AU. The capillary lumen occupies only a small part of the diameter of the capillary; the remainder is transparent silica. This geometry allows for large amounts of stray light to enter the detector so that a fully opaque sample would not reduce the light passing through the capillary to zero. This factor must be considered in the design of effective CE detector hardware and software.

Several novel approaches have been taken to increase the path length (and the sensitivity) of CE detectors. One approach has been to use a specially constructed low-volume flow cell. These cells carry the analytes through two right-angle bends *(30)*. The segment between the bends, which may be over 1000 μm long, is thus at right angles to the direction of the capillary and parallel to the direction of the light beam. Properly designed, these cells can dramatically increase sensitivity but at the risk of some loss of resolution. Another approach has been to create a wide zone or "bubble" in the capillary at the window *(31)*. A 50-μm i.d. capillary may have a window that is 150 μm in diameter, giving a sensitivity increase of approximately threefold.

1.4.2. Absorbance

Absorbance detectors are the most commonly encountered types of detector in CE instrument systems. They rely on the absorbance of light energy by the analytes. This absorbance creates a shadow as the analytes pass between the light source and the light detector. The intensity of the shadow is proportional to amount of material present.

The simplest absorbance detector, shown in Fig. 11A uses only portion of the available energy. The broad-spectrum light from a source lamp is passed through a filter or diffracted by a grating so that a narrow range of the spectrum is used. In some cases lamps (such as hollow cathode types) are used, that produce light at only a few discrete wavelengths. Monochromatic

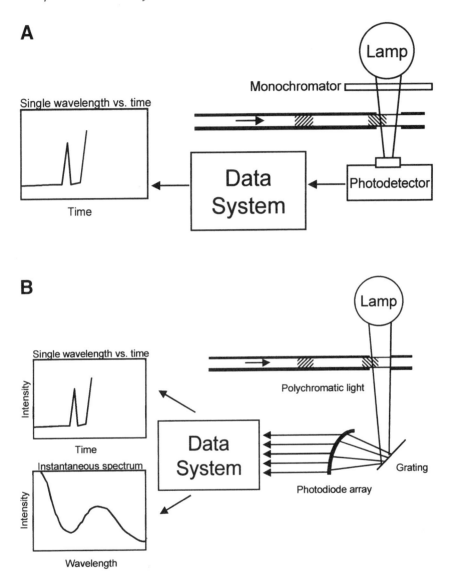

Fig. 11. Comparison of single wavelength **(A)** and photodiode array **(B)** absorbance detectors.

absorbance detectors are relatively inexpensive and rugged. However, because only a part of the spectrum is used, information may be lost from complex samples that have components with differing absorbance maxima.

Another type of absorbance detector looks at changes over a wide range of wavelengths simultaneously. The photodiode array detector (PDA) shown in Fig. 11B delivers the entire spectrum of light available from the source

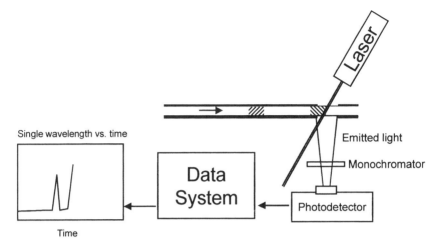

Fig. 12. Laser-induced fluorescence detector.

lamp to the capillary window. The light passing through the capillary is diffracted into a spectrum that is projected on a linear array of photodiodes. In this manner it is possible to record the entire absorbance spectrum of analytes as they pass by the detector window. PDA-type detectors are more expensive and less rugged than are monochromatic detectors. Because the spectrum can be divided into as many as 512 channels the amount of data acquired in a single run can be very large. The PDA type detector, however, is not suitable for all applications because nearly all the energy of the source lamp is focused onto a very small region of the capillary. Some capillary coatings and buffers will decompose under this onslaught of energy unless some of the energy is filtered out. Despite these limitations the information provided by the PDA detector can be valuable for confirming the identity of analytes. By comparing the change in spectral signature across a peak it is possible to estimate peak purity *(32)*.

1.4.3. Fluorescence

Fluorescence detectors do not rely on the measurement of shadows. These systems use an external energy source to excite the analyte molecules to a higher energy state. When these excited molecules return to the normal state they emit energy of a lower wavelength, which can be detected and recorded as evidence of the passage of the analytes. Fluorescent detectors in CE systems often use lasers as the source of the excitation energy (LIF detection, Fig. 12). Lasers have the advantage of producing intense light at a single wavelength. The intensity of the light contributes to good excitation efficiency. In addition, the monochromatic nature of the laser beam makes it easy to filter out any stray laser light to keep it from interfering with the detection of analytes. Analytes will vary in their excitation and absorbance wavelengths so that a fluorescent detector will not see all the components that may be in a sample. For analytes that are fluorescent or can be made fluorescent by a chemical reaction, the sensitivity of this type of detector can be 10–1000 times better than an absorbance detector *(33)*.

1.4.4. Amperometry and Conductivity

These two detection techniques potentially can offer a high degree of sensitivity and be applied to a wide variety of analytes, including those without appreciable UV absorption. Amperometry and conductivity are difficult to do in practice, and to date these devices are not commercially available. Both of these detection schemes require the use of sensing electrodes that are scaled to the dimensions of the electrophoresis capillary. In addition, these detectors place some limitations on the type of separation buffer employed.

In amperometric detection, an electroactive analyte undergoes an electrochemical reaction inside a detector cell *(34)*. The CE separation is generally carried out at microampere currents and kilovolt potentials, whereas the detection cell must operate at picoampere currents and millivolt potentials. The two circuits must therefore be isolated, usually by connecting the capillary to the high voltage at a point prior to the end of the capillary where the detection cell is located. This system depends on EOF to carry the analyte past the high voltage electrode to the detection cell. Amperometric detectors have been used successfully for the detection of biogenic amines at levels as low as 10^{-8} m *(35)*. With continued advances in microfabrication this type of detector should become routinely available.

There are two types of conductivity detector *(36,37)*. Both require that two electrodes be placed within the separation capillary. In the first type a short distance down the length of the capillary, separates the electrodes. Because there is a voltage gradient down the length of the capillary a portion of that voltage gradient can be measured between the two sensing electrodes. The presence of analyte zones will change the potential drop in the area of the zone. This change in potential will be sensed as the zone passes the electrodes. In the other arrangement the electrodes are placed opposite one another across the diameter of the capillary. In this case there is no voltage drop between the two electrodes. A circuit is constructed that passes a sensing voltage across the capillary diameter. If the conductivity of the system changes as analytes pass between the electrodes, there will be a change in the current in the sensing circuit. Conductivity detectors work best when there is a substantial difference between the conductivity of the analyte zones and the background buffer *(38)*. These conditions are not optimized for peak shape and lead to unacceptable peak asymmetry. Various schemes have been described for avoiding this problem. Conductivity detectors have been used for the measurement of inorganic ions and in isotachophoretic separations (Section 2.4.).

1.4.5. Capillary Electrophoresis-Mass Spectrometry

Hybrid systems such as CE-mass spectrometry (CE-MS) offer an additional dimension of analysis in addition to detection. CE data consists of migration time, quantity, and (using a PDA detector) spectral signature. MS adds the additional data of molecular weight and, using collision dissociation and MS-MS systems, structural information as well. This combination of techniques provides an orthogonal approach to analysis in a single analytical run.

The predominant form of MS that has been coupled to CE has been electrospray MS *(39)*. A more in-depth discussion of CE-MS can be found in Chapter 15. This section will focus on that technique. The outlet end of the CE capillary is inserted into the electrospray interface. Because the volume of liquid emerging from the capillary is very small, a make-up liquid is pumped through an axial needle. This sheath flow also provides a return connection to the high-voltage power supply of the CE system. The liquid is mixed with a flowing gas stream and nebulized into a spray. The spray vaporizes and the ionized analyte particles are carried into the MS detector. The MS system is usually set to scan across an expected range of mass values. Because the width of peaks in CE can be very small, the MS instrument must be able to scan across the desired mass range very rapidly or peaks may be missed.

Most mass spectroscopists prefer to use buffer systems that are volatile, such as ammonium formate, in order to reduce the accumulation of buffer salts inside the MS instrument. These buffers may not be optimized for the separation of the analyte mixture, although an incomplete separation can be acceptable in CE-MS because the MS systems provide an additional dimension of separation.

Many of the existing commercial CE systems have been interfaced to commercial MS systems. The design of these systems allows the use of UV or other detectors prior to the MS interface, but usually require quite long and awkward reaches of capillary to connect the two systems. Unlocking the true potential of this method will require the development of a CE system that is fully integrated with the MS system.

1.4.6. Indirect Detection

In the previous discussions it has been assumed that detection will be direct, that is, the presence of the sample in the detector cell or window will cause an increase in the output signal. This is not always the case. There are certain applications where the decrease of the background signal provides evidence of the passage of analytes through a detector. In some cases a detector that is useful for indirect detection would not detect the analytes in direct mode. An example of this is the detection of inorganic ions such as sodium or sulfate with a UV detector.

To detect such analytes, the capillary is filled with a buffer that has mobility close to that of the analytes and also has a significant UV absorbency. The buffer/chromophore must carry the same charge as the analyte. For the analysis of sulfate, a buffer containing sodium chromate is used *(40)*. In the area of the capillary occupied by the sulfate band the chromate is displaced, creating a chromate depleted region. Because chromate absorbs light at 254 nm, by monitoring background electrolyte absorbance at this wavelength the presence of sulfate will be indicated by a negative peak, with an area corresponding to the amount of chromate displaced and hence to the amount of sulfate present. Most CE data analysis packages can invert these negative peaks, producing a normal-appearing electropherogram.

1.4.7. Data Analysis

The collection and analysis of CE data has many characteristics in common with other chromatography-like analyses. Many analysts have utilized data systems developed for HPLC and GC systems. These data systems may not be optimal for CE for three reasons:

1. The signals obtained from CE are usually very small. A typical HPLC peak may have a maximum absorbance of 0.2 AU, whereas a CE detector may have a full range of 0.2 AU. A typical peak in CE may have a maximum absorbance of 0.002 AU.
2. CE peaks can be quite narrow with a width of only a few seconds. Some older data systems (particularly HPLC systems) cannot respond sufficiently fast to deal with this data. If data is to be collected digitally, it must be collected at a high data rate to define adequately the peak shape.
3. CE peaks are often non-Gaussian. Because of the low band broad spreading in CE and the effects of electrofocusing CE peaks tend to be more triangular and less bell-shaped than peaks in HPLC and GC. At times CE peaks may have one edge that is nearly vertical. Some data systems have difficulty locating the peak start and stop times for these shapes.

Two types of peak-detection methods dominate analytical data analysis: slope sensitive algorithm and the moving median filter algorithm. Slope sensitive algorithms look at the slope of the baseline over some interval of time. When the slope exceeds a pre-determined value, a peak is said to have begun. The point at which the slope goes to zero identifies the peak apex, and the point at which the slope returns to the starting value defines the peak end.

The slope-sensitive method looks for peaks independently of the baseline shape. Most commercial software packages use this method.

Moving median filter algorithms take a different approach. Peaks are relatively high frequency (impulse) events when compared to baseline drift. These algorithms seek to define how the baseline would look in the absence of peaks by filtering out all impulse events. Whatever differs from the baseline is defined as a peak. In practice, the algorithm makes several passes through the data set (iterations) to determine the best fit. This type of algorithm, commercially available as "Caesar," is more successful at dealing with the abrupt slope changes in CE data than are slope-sensitive algorithms *(41)*.

A data system for CE needs to include some calculations that can be deemed "CE specific." These include the calculation of mobility (a measure of the velocity of an analyte through the capillary) and corrected peak area. Corrected area is necessary because the peaks passing through a CE detector do not all pass through at the same velocity. Early eluting peaks move through more rapidly than do later eluting peaks. This is unlike the situation in HPLC where the velocity through the detector cell is dependent only on the flow rate and not on the retention time. Because later eluting peaks are moving more slowly, they appear to be larger relative to earlier eluting peaks. Corrected peak area normalizes peak area to unit migration time and allows accurate comparison of the components in a mixture.

1.4.8. Fraction Collection

Fraction collection is placed under the heading of detection under the assumption that fractions are being collected for analysis outside the CE instrument. At first glance, fraction collection in CE appears to be analogous to fraction collection in HPLC, but there are significant differences *(42)*.

The velocity of peaks through the HPLC detector is constant if the flow rate is constant. This is not true in CE where earlier eluting peaks are moving more rapidly than later eluting peaks. The delay time between peak detection and elution (the time for transit from the window to the capillary outlet) will therefore vary, becoming longer with each successive peak. This time can be quite long. Consider a capillary 60-cm long with the window located 10-cm from the outlet end. If a peak passes the detector at $t = 5$ min it will not emerge from the end of the capillary until $t = 6$ min. A peak detected at $t = 10$ min will emerge at $t = 12$ min. Peaks that pass the detector between 5 and 10 min will all be in the outlet segment of the capillary between $t = 6$ and $t = 12$ min. A further complication is that collection requires that the outlet of the capillary be moved to a new collection vial for each peak that is to be collected. At each move the circuit will be broken. The time needed for the power supply to ramp down and ramp up at each move, and the diminished peak velocities during the ramping segments cannot be disregarded. Complex algorithms are needed to do this process smoothly.

A more serious limitation to the collection of fractions from CE is the very small amount of sample that the fraction will contain. Consider a capillary 100 μm in diameter and 50 cm long, with the window located 10 cm from the end. A 5 psi-sec injection into this capillary will inject about 189 nL of sample (*see* Section 1.3.1.). If the analyte concentration is 1 mg/mL in the starting sample and the peak is collected with 100% efficiency, the recovered sample will be 189 ng. Repeating this run 10 times would yield less than a two micrograms of product. Although fraction collection in CE is possible, one must question whether it is worth the effort.

2. MODES OF SEPARATION IN CE

A CE system can be operated in several different modes. These modes offer the analyst a variety of ways to approach an analytical problem. The choice of mode will be based on the analytical problem under consideration. This section will describe the major modes of capillary electrophoretic separation that are currently in use and provide some applications for each.

2.1. Capillary Zone Electrophoresis (CZE)

2.1.1. Mechanism

Section 1 of this chapter dealt almost entirely with this form of CE. CZE is characterized by the use of open capillaries and relatively low viscosity buffer systems. Analyte molecules move from one end of the capillary to the other according to the vector sum of electrophoresis and electroosmotic mobility.

2.1.2. Applications

CZE is the most widespread mode of CE. It has been used for analytes as diverse as sodium ions, drugs, and protein molecules. Analyte species can be separated by CZE if they migrate at different velocities in the electrical field.

2.2. Capillary Gel Electrophoresis (CGE)

2.2.1. Mechanism

Capillary gel electrophoresis (CGE) is separation based on viscous drag. In this mode of CE the capillary is filled with a gel or viscous solution. EOF is often suppressed so that the migration of the analytes is solely by electrophoresis. Larger molecules tend to be retarded more by the viscous separation medium than are smaller molecules, so that the separation is effectively based on the molecular size.

2.2.2. Applications

This is the method of choice for molecules that differ in size but not in mass/charge ratio. DNA molecules, for example, can vary greatly in length, but the charge per unit length is quite constant. In a pure CZE separation, all the molecules move at very nearly the same velocity and no separation results. In a viscous medium, the longer molecules are retarded more than shorter molecules. Thus shorter pieces of DNA pass the detector sooner than do larger pieces of DNA. See Chapters 13 and 14 for a more detailed discussion of DNA separation by CE.

Protein molecules are composed of more complex subunits than DNA molecules. Even though proteins vary widely in their size, the wide range of charge states possible in a protein sequence complicates size separation. In order to separate proteins by size, it is necessary to mask the native charge and create a more nearly uniform charge-mass ratio. This is done by treating the proteins with the detergent SDS. Although there are exceptions, typically proteins bind to a constant number of SDS molecules per unit length. Because the SDS molecules are highly negatively charged the amino acid subunit charge contributes little to the mobility of the molecules and a separation based on chain length is possible. This technique of SDS-CGE is exactly analogous to SDS-polyacrylamide gel electrophoresis (SDS-PAGE).

2.3. Capillary Isoelectric Focusing (cIEF)

2.3.1. Mechanism

Molecules that carry both positively and negatively charged groups exhibit, at a specific pH, an equal number of positive and negative charges. At this pH, known as the isoelectric pH or pI, the molecule, although charged, behaves as if it is neutral because its positive and negative charges cancel each other. The molecule, therefore, has no tendency to migrate in an electrical field. In isoelectric focusing, special reagents called ampholytes are used to create a pH gradient within the capillary. These ampholytes are mixtures of buffers with a range of pK_a values. In an electrical field, ampholytes will arrange themselves in order of pK_a; this gradient is trapped between a strong acid and a strong base. Analytes introduced into this gradient will migrate to the point where the pH of the gradient equals their pI. At this point the analyte, having no net charge, ceases to migrate. It will remain at that position so long as the pH gradient is stable, typically as long as the voltage is applied.

2.3.2. Applications

Capillary isoelectric focusing (cIEF) is used almost exclusively for the separation of closely related protein species. Hemoglobin can be separated into several bands by this technique, whereas separation by SDS-CGE usually results in a single form being identified. In this application, the protein sample is mixed with the ampholyte solution and the mixture is pumped into the capillary. When voltage is applied, the proteins and the ampholytes migrate to their appropriate positions in the gradient. When focusing is complete, the proteins in the mixture are distributed throughout the length of the capillary. In order to detect the proteins it is necessary to mobilize them so that they pass by the detector in turn. There are two ways to accomplish this mobilization. Pressure mobilization utilizes positive pressure applied to one end of the capillary to drive the entire fluid column through the window. In order to prevent band distortion, this pressure must be applied carefully, preferably while the voltage is still being applied. Chemical mobilization requires that one end of the capillary be transferred to a salt solution after focusing has taken place. Upon application of voltage, salt will migrate into the capillary, disrupting the pH gradient and allowing the proteins to migrate past the detector by electrophoresis.

cIEF is also widely used for examining the distribution of carbohydrate isoforms of glycoproteins. In other techniques, such as SDS-CGE or CZE, these proteins tend to move as diffuse bands and to generate broad peaks. cIEF can often resolve these bands into peaks that differ by as little as one charged sugar group.

2.4. Capillary Isotachophoresis (cITP)

2.4.1. Mechanism

In this technique the sample plug is introduced between two different buffers. One of these, the leading electrolyte, has the highest mobility in the separation. The second, trailing electrolyte, has a mobility lower than anything else does. The sign of the charge on the analytes and the buffers must be the same. When the voltage is applied the ions in the sample form discrete zones that are not separated into peaks; one zone is adjacent to the next. The concentration of the analyte within a zone is constant within that zone and the length of the zone is proportional to the concentration within the zone. Because the voltage drop is uniform within a zone, isotachophoretic methods are quite compatible with conductance detectors (*see* Section 1.4.4.).

2.4.2. Applications

Capillary isotachophoresis (cITP) of peptides and proteins has been used with MS detection *(43)*. Since this mode of separation delivers zones of uniform concentration to the MS, it may be an ideal separation mechanism for this detection technique.

2.5. Micellar Electrophoresis

2.5.1. Mechanism

Electrophoresis is not possible for analytes that are not charged. In order to analyze such analytes, it is necessary to employ some agent in the separation buffer that will transport them through the capillary. The most commonly used mode of CE for these analytes is MEKC. In this technique a suitable charged detergent, such as SDS, is added to the separation buffer in a concentration sufficiently high to allow the formation of micelles. These micelles are arrangements of detergent molecules that have a hydrophobic inner core and a hydrophilic outer surface. Micelles are dynamic and constantly form and break apart. For any given analyte, there is a probability that the molecules of that analyte will associate within the micelle at any given time. This probability is the same as the partition coefficient in classical chromatography. When associated with the micelle, the analyte molecule will migrate at the velocity of the micelle. When not in the micelle, the analyte molecule will migrate with the EOF (if any). Differences in the time that analytes spend in the micellar phase will determine the separation.

2.5.2. Applications

MEKC is useful for a wide range of small molecules such as drugs, pesticides, and food additives that are not charged and are sufficiently hydrophobic to associate with the micelle. While SDS is probably the most widely used detergent for this purpose, cationic detergents such as TTAB can also be employed. Nonionic detergents by themselves do not provide mobility to uncharged analytes, but in combination with charged detergents they will modify the separation. Some detergents are useful in specific applications. For example, sodium cholate is useful in the separation and analysis of a variety of steroids. The micelles formed in this case are not the classical spherical shape but are probably sodium cholate molecules arranged on each other like a stack of coins. Different uncharged steroids differ in their tendencies to participate in these stacks.

2.6. Chiral Electrophoresis

2.6.1. Mechanism

Chiral molecules are molecules that can exist in two stereo-specific forms. These chiral forms or enantiomers are identical in molecular weight and chemical formula but differ in the arrangement of the atoms in space. Separation of these enatiomeric forms depends on the tendency to associate differentially with other chiral molecules known as chiral selectors. By incorporating a chiral selector into the CE buffer, it is often possible to separate enantiomers of a chiral molecule. This is analogous to MEKC described previously. The complex of the analyte and the selector will migrate at a different rate than will the analyte alone. Because one of the two enantiomers associates more strongly with the selector than does the other form a separation can be achieved.

2.6.2. Applications

The most commonly employed chiral selector in CE is cyclodextrin, ring shaped carbohydrates made up of 6, 7, or 8 D-glucose subunits. Cyclodextrins may be chemically modified to alter their hydrophobicity or charge. Uncharged cyclodextrins are not suitable for the analysis of uncharged analytes since the complex will move with the EOF. However, cyclodextrins modified to carry a charge by addition of sulfate groups, can serve both as chiral selectors and as carrier molecules (similar to the detergent in MEKC). Other molecules, such as the antibiotic vancomycin, have also been employed as chiral selectors.

Chiral CE can be used to separate the enantiomeric forms of pharmaceuticals as well as natural substances, such as amino acids. Impurities as small as 0.1% are easily detected by this method.

2.7. Nonaqueous Electrophoresis

2.7.1. Mechanism

Electrophoresis usually is considered to occur only in aqueous solutions. However, CE can be performed using nonaqueous systems based on such solvents as acetonitrile, methanol, formamide, and dimethylformamide, to which are added small amounts of anhydrous acid or buffer salts. The separation is by simple electrophoresis as EOF is very low under these conditions.

2.7.2. Applications

There are times when two analytes have the same charge to mass ratio and are not easily separated. In some cases this same analyte pair can be separated in a nonaqueous environment where they may have different pK_a values than those expressed in water. The degree of solvation, and hence the radius of the solvated species, may also differ in aqueous and nonaqueous environments. Hence, nonaqueous CE offers an alternative for analytes that are difficult to separate under aqueous conditions. In addition, some analytes are difficult to solubilize in aqueous systems but dissolve readily in organic solvents, thus nonaqueous CE offers an alternative to MEKC for these analytes. Separations by nonaqueous CE have been reported for drugs, dyes, preservatives, surfactants, and inorganic ions.

2.8. Capillary Electrochromatography

2.8.1. Mechanism

Capillary electrochromatography (CEC) is a hybrid technique between liquid chromatography and electrophoresis. It is a partitioning technique in which molecules distribute between a stationary and a moving phase. As described for MEKC, different analytes will tend to associate to a greater or lesser extent with the stationary phase, effecting a separation.

CEC capillaries are packed with particles like those used in HPLC columns. Unlike conventional LC techniques, CEC uses electroosmotic flow to drive the mobile phase down the column. The resulting plug flow improves the separation efficiency over that of the laminar flow of pressure driven systems.

2.8.2. Applications

As of this writing, most of the work done on CEC has used model systems, such as polyaromatic hydrocarbons. A great deal of effort is underway to identify applications where this technique can be the method of choice. Because the buffers used are typically high in organic content and hence volatile, CEC may be useful when coupled to mass spectroscopy (CEC-MS).

REFERENCES

1. Janini, G. M., and Issaq, H. J. (1993) The buffer in capillary zone electrophoresis, in Capillary Electrophoresis Technology, (Guzman, N.A., ed.), Marcel Dekker, Inc., New York, pp. 119–160.
2. Cifuentes, A. and Poppe, H. (1994) Rectangular capillary electrophoresis: some theoretical considerations. Chromatographia 39, 391–404.
3. Virtanen, R. and Kivalo, P. (1969) Quantitative high-voltage zone electrophoresis method. Suomen Kemistilehti B 42, 182.
4. Jorgensen, J. W. and Lukacs, K. D. (1981) Zone electrophoresis is open-tubular glass capillaries. Anal. Chem. 53, 1298–1302.
5. Smoluchowski, M. V. (1905) Elektrosche kataphorese. Physik. Z. 6, 529.
6. Lukacs, K. D. and Jorgensen, J. W. (1985) Capillary zone electrophoresis: effect of physical parameters on separation efficiency and quantitation J. High Resolut. Chromatogr. Chromatogr. Commun. 8, 407.
7. Kuhn, R. and Hoffstetter-Kuhn, S. (1993) Capillary Electrophoresis Principle and Practice. Springer Verlag, Berlin, p. 153.
8. Lambert, W. J. and Middleton, D. L. (1990) pH hysteresis effect with silica capillaries in capillary zone electrophoresis. Anal. Chem. 62, 1585–1587.
9. Cobb, K. A., Dolnik, V., and Novotny, M. (1990) Electrophoretic separations of proteins in capillaries with hydrodynamically stable surface structures. Anal. Chem. 61, 2478–2483.
10. Hjerten, S. (1988) High performance electrophoresis: elimination of electroendosmosis and solute absorption. J. Chromatogr. 347, 191–198.

11. Bruin, G. M., Chang, J. P., Kuhlmann, R. H., Zegers, K., Kraak, J. C., and Poppe, H. (1992) Capillary zone electrophoretic separations of proteins in polyethylene glycol-modified capillaries. J. Chromatogr. 471, 429–436.

12. McCormick, R. M. (1988) Capillary zone electrophoretic separation of peptides and proteins using low pH buffers in modified silica capillary. Anal. Chem. 60, 2322–2328.

13. Novotny, M. V., Cobb, K. A., and Liu, J. (1990) Recent advances in capillary electrophoresis of proteins, peptides, and amino acids. Electrophoresis 11, 735–749.

14. Wiktorowicz, J. E. and Colburn, J. C. (1990) Separation of proteins via charge reversal in capillary electrophoresis. Electrophoresis 11, 769–773.

15. Emmer, A, Jansson, M., and Roeraade, J. (1991) Improved capillary zone electrophoretic separation of basic proteins, using a fluorosurfactant buffer additive. J. Chromatogr. 547, 544–550.

16. VanOrman, B. B., Liversidge, G. G., and McIntire, G. L. (1991) Effects of buffer composition on electroosmotic flow in capillary electrophoresis. J. Microcol. Septo. 2, 176.

17. Ferguson, N. J., Braunschweiger, K. I., Braunschweiger, W. R., Smith, J. R., McCormick, J. J., Wasmann, C. C., et al. (1980) Hydrogen ion buffers for biological research. Anal. Biochem. 104, 300–310.

18. Vinther, A. and Soeberg, H. (1991) Temperature elevation of the sample zone in free solution capillary electrophoresis under stacking conditions. J. Chromatogr. 559, 3–26.

19. Vinther, A. and Soeberg, H. (1991) Mathematical model describing dispersion in free solution capillary electrophoresis under stacking conditions. J. Chromatogr. 559, 27–47.

20. Burgi, D. S. and Chien, R-L. (1991) Optimization in sample stacking for high-performance capillary electrophoresis. Anal. Chem. 63, 2042–2047.

21. Bullock, J. A. and Yuan, L. C. (1991) Free solution capillary electrophoresis of basic proteins in untreated fused silica capillary tubing. J. Microcol. Sep. 3, 241.

22. Terabe, S. (1989) Electrokinetic chromatography: an interface between electrophoresis and chromatography. Trends Anal. Chem. 8, 129.

23. Heiger, D. N., Cohen, A. S., and Karger, B. L. (1990) Separation of DNA restriction fragments by high performance capillary electrophoresis with low and zero crosslinked polyacrylamide using continuous and pulsed electric fields. J. Chromatogr. 516, 33–48.

24. Fujiwara, S. and Honda, S. (1987) Effect of addition of organic solvents on the separation of positional isomers in high-performance capillary electrophoresis. Anal. Chem. 59, 487–490.

25. Josic, D., Zeilinger, K., Reutter, W., Bottcher, A., and Schmitz, G. (1990) High performance capillary electrophoresis of hydrophobic membrane proteins. J. Chromatogr. 516, 89–98.

26. Harrington, S. J., Varro, R., and Li, T. M. (1992) High-performance capillary electrophoresis as a fast in-process control method for enzyme-labeled monoclonal antibodies. J. Chromatogr. 559, 385–390.

27. Reijenga, J. C., Aben, G. V. A., Verheggen, Th. P. E. M., and Everaerts, F. M. (1992) Effect of electroosmosis on detection in isotachophoresis. J. Chromatogr. 594, 317–324.

28. Knox, J. H. (1988) Thermal effects and band spreading in capillary electro-separation. Chromatographia 26, 329.
29. Jorgensen, J. W. and Lukacs, K. D. (1983) Capillary zone electrophoresis. Science 222, 266–272.
30. Chervet, J. P., van Soest, R. E. J., and Ursem, M. (1991) Z-shaped flow cell for UV detection in capillary electrophoresis. J. Chromatogr. 543, 439–449.
31. Gordon, G. B. (1991) Capillary zone electrophoresis cell system. United States Patent 5,061,361, October 29.
32. Kobayashi, S., Ueda, T., and Kikumoto, J. (1989) Photodiode array detection in high-performance capillary electrophoresis. J. Chromatogr. 480, 179–184.
33. Wu, S. and Dovichi, N. J. (1992) Capillary zone electrophoresis separation and laser-induced fluorescence detection of zeptomole quantities of fluorescein thiohydantoin derivatives of amino acids. Talanta 39, 173.
34. Wallingford, R. A. and Ewing, A. G. (1987) Characterization of a microinjector for capillary zone electrophoresis. Anal. Chem. 59, 678–681.
35. Wallingford, R. W. and Ewing, E. M. (1990) Separation of serotonin from catechols by capillary zone electrophoresis with electrochemical detection. Anal. Chem. 61, 98–100.
36. Huang, X., Pang, T. K., Gordon, M. J., and Zare, R. N. (1987) On column conductivity detector for capillary zone electrophoresis. Anal. Chem. 59, 2747–2749.
37. Huang, X., Zare, R. N., Sloss, S., and Ewing, A. G. (1991) End column detection for capillary zone electrophoresis. Anal. Chem. 63, 189–192.
38. Huang, X., Luckey, J. A., Gordon, M. J., and Zare, R. N. (1989) Quantitative analysis of low molecular weight carboxylic acids by capillary zone electro-phoresis/conductivity detection. Anal. Chem. 61, 766–770.
39. Banks, J. F. (1997) Recent advances in capillary electrophoresis/electrospray/mass spectrometry. Electrophoresis 18, 2255–2266.
40. Wildman, B. J., Jackson, P. E., Jones, W. R., and Alden, P. G. (1991) Analysis of anion constituents of urine by inorganic capillary electrophoresis. J. Chromatogr. 546, 459–466.
41. Wanders, B. J. (1997) Data analysis in CE, in Handbook of Capillary Electro-phoresis, 2nd ed. (Landers, J. P., ed.), CRC, Boca Raton, FL.
42. Kuhn, R. and Hoffstetter-Kuhn, S. (1993) Capillary Electrophoresis Principle and Practice. Springer Verlag, Berlin, p. 156.
43. Smith, R. D., Leo, J. A., Edmonds, C. G., Barinaga, C. J., and Usdeth, H. R. (1990) Sensitivity considerations for large molecule detection by capillary elec-trophoresis-electrospray ionization mass spectrometry. J. Chromatogr. 516, 157–165.

II
Protein Electrophoresis

3

Capillary Coatings for Protein Analysis

Kannan Srinivasan, Chris Pohl, and Nebojsa Avdalovic

1. INTRODUCTION

Protein analysis has become very important to the biotechnology, pharmaceutical, and food industries. Analytical techniques that provide fast, automated analysis, but still give high resolution separation of proteins derived from various sources, such as plasma, blood, and vaccine products, are in high demand. Chromatography and electrophoresis continue to be the preferred means for analyzing proteins. Capillary electrophoresis (CE), a micro-format of electrophoresis, has been successfully used for separating various proteins. A major problem encountered in CE analysis of proteins using a fused silica capillary is the interaction of basic analytes, such as proteins, with exposed surface silanol groups on the capillary wall. This interaction results in loss of efficiency and irreproducible separations. Several groups have worked on evaluating protein interactions with the silica surface and have reported mathematical models and computer simulations of these interactions *(1–3)*. Typical approaches in addressing the aforementioned problem include working at conditions where the silanol groups are either unionized *(4)* or fully ionized *(5)*. However, these conditions require working at extremes of pH and which may be unsuitable for many analytes. In addition, silica dissolves at extreme pHs, another limitation of this approach *(6)*. Other approaches in addressing the aforementioned problem include adding compounds *(7–9)* that compete with the analytes for the sites of interaction on the capillary wall. These additives, however, may adversely affect the separation of analytes.

Other researchers have worked with coatings that are either physically adsorbed or chemically attached to the capillary surface *(10–25)*. These coatings mask the presence of surface silanols, enhancing separation efficiency. The adsorbed coatings, however, suffer from limited stability and require repeated replenishment for effective operation *(10)*. Recently, Gilges et al.

From: *Clinical and Forensic Applications of Capillary Electrophoresis*
Edited by: J. R. Petersen and A. A. Mohammad © Humana Press Inc., Totowa, NJ

(10) showed excellent separation of basic proteins using a polyvinyl-alcohol (PVA) coated capillary. The PVA was immobilized on the capillary wall by a thermal treatment. Although this PVA coated capillary gave a low electroosmotic flow up to pH 9.0, only 40 runs were possible at pHs >8.5 without loss of efficiency. In addition, buffers such as borate, Tris-HCl, and Tris-phosphate did not provide good separation of proteins with this coated capillary, limiting its utility. A review of the literature on coatings for CE revealed numerous examples of chemically modified capillaries that were designed to minimize the effect of surface silanols and reduce analyte interactions. These modifications involve attaching or creating one or more polymeric layers on the capillary surface through various coupling chemistries *(11–25)*. In this chapter we will review some interesting developments in coated capillaries for CE and the potential utility for protein separations.

2. ELECTROOSMOTIC FLOW (EOF)

Electroosmotic flow (EOF) is a result of ionization of the surface groups on the fused silica capillary. Typically, this ionization begins above pH 2.0. The negatively charged surface silanols attract cations from the electrolyte and forms an electrical double layer. On applying a field (oriented from the positive to the negative electrode), the cations in solution start migrating toward the cathode, carrying the water of hydration. The resulting bulk flow is termed EOF and is similar to an *in situ* pump that allows fast separation of anions and cations in the same run (for many analytes). EOF also occurs in polymeric capillaries, as cited by Schutzner and Kenndler *(26)*. Here the EOF is thought to occur from surface-dissociative groups such as carboxyl or from adsorbed species on the capillary wall.

The EOF component is similar to an escalator, that carries passengers. In a manner similar to an escalator the velocity can be measured by measuring the time it takes a stationary passenger to move between two points. For a capillary, the EOF can be measured by injecting neutral molecules such as acetone or benzyl alcohol into the capillary and determining the migration time. Cationic analytes move faster than the EOF in the presence of the field, much like passengers who walk on the escalators and move faster. Anionic analytes move slower because they want to move backward towards the anode, but the EOF is stronger and keeps moving them forward. This scenario is similar to passengers who occasionally try to move in the direction opposite the escalator and, hence, move slower. If the anionic species moves faster than the EOF, it is not detected because it exits the capillary at the inlet side.

The apparent mobility of an analyte is described as the vector sum of the electrophoretic mobility of the analyte and the EOF mobility.

$$\overrightarrow{\mu app} = \overrightarrow{\mu} + \overrightarrow{\mu_{eo}} \tag{1}$$

In this case when μ_{eo} is very small (the case when the capillary surface is coated with a neutral polymer coating) then $\mu_{app} = \mu$, the true electrophoretic mobility of the analyte under the test conditions. The apparent mobility of a species is described by the following equation:

$$\mu = \frac{v}{E} \tag{2}$$

where μ is the mobility in units of $cm^2/V.s$, v is the velocity in units of cm/s, and E is the field strength in V/cm.

The velocity and field strength are experimentally derived or known from the CE run.

$$v = \frac{Id}{tm} \tag{3}$$

where I_d is the length of the capillary from the inlet to the detection point in cm and t_m is the migration time of the species in seconds.

$$E = \frac{V}{lt} \tag{4}$$

where V is the voltage applied across the entire capillary length in volts and lt is the total length of the capillary in cm.

The EOF mobility can be easily determined from Eq. 2–3 by plugging in the value for t_m, the migration time of a neutral marker such as benzyl alcohol. It is clear from the aforementioned expressions that CE separations can be optimized in terms of analysis time and resolution by varying the EOF mobility. Coating the capillary with a suitable (anionic, neutral, or cationic) coating, on the other hand, could modify the EOF mobility. A more in-depth discussion on EOF and mobility can be found in refs. *27–29*, in addition to Chapter 2 and will not be discussed here.

3. NEED FOR A COATING

As previously discussed, a fused silica capillary becomes ionized above pH 2.0, making it difficult to eliminate the undesirable interactions of the surface silanol groups with analytes, such as proteins. These undesirable interactions result in poor peak shapes, loss of efficiency, lack of resolution, and irreproducible separations. Since proteins, being made of amino acids, are amphoteric in nature and vary substantially in pI, it becomes difficult to tailor separations by optimizing only the pH. In addition, operating at extremes of pH is undesirable for many proteins. Another serious limitation of operating with uncoated fused silica capillaries is that the EOF is irreproducible. This limitation can be exaggerated when analyzing proteins, since they can interact with and modify the capillary surface and, consequently, the EOF properties. To overcome these limitations and allow operation under physiological pH, numerous researchers have investigated various coatings and chemistries *(11–25)*.

4. REVIEW OF COATINGS

It is well-established that covalently coated capillaries have a longer operational lifetime and are preferred to noncovalent methods for minimizing the effect of surface silanols. Typically, the coating protocol for covalently coated capillaries involves a step to activate the surface groups of the fused silica capillary. The goal of this activation is to make available a high density of surface silanols that are ionized. The activation step is followed by a silanization reaction that leaves reactive groups able to bind (react) with other monomers or polymers. The most popular silanization reagents are bifunctional silanes such as allyltrimethoxy silane, 3-aminopropyl-trimethoxysilane, γ-methacryloxypropyltrimethoxysilane, and 3-glycidoxy-propyltrimethoxysilane. Other suitable silanes are listed in refs. *(30)* and *(31)*.

In 1985, Hjerten *(11)* developed a two-step coating process, first by attaching a bifunctional silane to the surface of the capillary; this was then followed by *in situ* polymerization of monomer containing a vinyl group. The coating process involved activation of the surface groups prior to attachment after which the surface silanols were reacted with a bifunctional silane, such as 3-methacryloxy propyl trimethoxy silane in acetic acid. The reaction occurred between the surface silanols and one or more trimethoxy groups to yield a reactive 3-methacryloxy propyl layer attached through Si-O-Si linkages. Any residual unreacted trimethoxysilane groups were hydrolyzed to silanols. A dilute solution of suitable vinyl monomers such as acrylamide was then pumped into the capillary and polymerization initiated to yield a polymer coating of linear polyacrylamide on the capillary surface.

Although the aforementioned coating yielded capillaries with minimal EOF, some researchers found that the coating procedure was not optimal, particularly for protein separations. For example, Strege and Lagu *(12)* showed that although the aforementioned coating had a very low EOF, it did not give good separations of a mixture of proteins. The poor peak shapes obtained with this capillary were attributed to electrostatic or hydrogen bonding interactions of the proteins with either the capillary wall or coating. It was necessary to incorporate a surfactant in the CE run buffer in order to achieve good separations of the protein mixture. Similarly, a crosslinked *in situ* polymerized polyacrylamide coated capillary gave poor separation efficiencies for basic proteins when tested with no added cationic additives in the buffer *(13)*.

An alternative approach to *in situ* polymerized coatings is that obtained by reacting silanes having appropriate reactive groups with the reactive end groups on prederivatized polymers. Herren et al. *(14)* showed that these coatings minimized or reduced EOF. They discussed several synthetic procedures for creating various derivatives of dextran *(15)* and polyethyleneglycol (PEG) *(16)* and their utility in several applications. They showed that the EOF could be controlled by the size of the polymer chain attached to the capillary surface. The longer the polymer chain, the lower the EOF. However, data on the pH stability of this coating and its performance with proteins as test analytes were not shown. Using a similar approach, Hjerten and Kubo *(17)* discussed the attachment of several polymers (e.g., methylcellulose and dextran) after a pre-derivatization step. The polymer coupling process was dependent on a high yield of the pre-derivatization reaction.

Recently, Malik et al. *(18,19)* adapted a gas chromatography (GC)-type static coating procedure by depositing a mixture of polymer, initiators, and silane reagent on the capillary surface using a low boiling-point solvent. The capillary was then heat-treated to cross-link the surface film. They found that the coating thickness affected both the EOF and capillary performance. In comparing data from Malik et al. *(18,19)*, polymer coated capillaries tested under identical conditions gave different migration times and mobilities, indicating problems with the reproducibility of the coating process.

The aforementioned coatings were all attached through a Si-O-Si-C linkage. To overcome the limited pH stability of the Si-O-Si bond, several researchers attached polyacrylamide by *in situ* polymerization through a Si-C linkage *(20)* or a hydrolytically stable derivative of acrylamide by *in situ* polymerization *(21)*. These approaches enhanced the coating stability relative to Hjerten's original approach and provided better efficiencies for basic proteins. However, multiple reaction steps with stringent conditions were required during the coating process. For example, the approach by Cobb et al. *(20)* required anhydrous solvents and anhydrous conditions during the Grignard reaction step. Similarly, the work by Chiari et al. *(21)* required synthesis of a special monomer to achieve an acceptable coating. Other approaches involved cross-linking or attaching several polymeric layers on the capillary surface, which was expected to diminish interaction of the analytes with the exposed surface silanols. Smith et al. *(22)* showed separations of proteins in coated capillaries that had a primary silane layer with several polymeric layers adsorbed on top of the primary layer. Huang et al. *(23)* showed separation of proteins using a cross-linked, immobilized, hydrophilic polymer layer atop a hydrophobic, self-assembled, alkyl silane layer. Schmalzing et al. *(24)* showed excellent separations of basic proteins in a multilayered cross-linked coated capillary. *In situ* polymerization of a monomer on top of a crosslinked primary silane layer resulted in a hydrophilic polymeric layer that was subsequently crosslinked. All the above approaches were multistep processes and, in some cases, required additional crosslinking steps *(24)*.

A simple method for coupling pre-formed polymers on the surface of a fused silica capillary was recently disclosed by our group *(25)*. No additional derivatization of the polymer was required prior to coupling. The coating was achieved by the formation of polymer macro-radicals under polymeric crosslinking conditions. These macromolecules reacted with the surface of a silane treated capillary through a radical mechanism. Crosslinking between the polymer chains and coupling to the silane occurred simultaneously. The resulting coating was a highly cross-linked, stable layer on the capillary surface. The coating process was insensitive to the molecular weight change and concentration of the polymer. Separation of a variety of proteins with high efficiencies was demonstrated using neutral capillaries prepared by the previous approach. It was also possible to separate acidic proteins using a cationic polymer-coated capillary using reversed polarity *(27)*.

In the above coupling process, it was not necessary to have stringent control of reaction conditions for the reproducible generation of the coating layer, since the polymer was already formed *(30)*. *In situ* polymerized coatings, on the other hand, require stringent control of such variables as oxygen levels and temperature, because the polymerization has to occur at the capillary surface *(32)*.

4.1. Example of a Coating Procedure

The following is a capillary coating procedure that was adapted from a recent publication *(25)*

1. Activation: Fused silica capillaries (50-μm ID, 360-μm OD) were first rinsed with 1 M NaOH for 1 h, followed by rinsing with deionized water, and then with 1% (w/v) acetic acid in water for 2 h.
2. Silanization: The aforementioned treated capillary was filled with a 1% silane solution (e.g., 3-methacryloxypropyltrimethoxysilane) in 1% acetic acid (or 2% chlorodimethyloctylsilane in ethanol). The silane was allowed to react for 1 h with continual replenishment of solution under a pressure of 10 psi. The

capillary was stored in the silane solution for 24–48 h and then rinsed with deionized water.

3. Polymer bonding step: A polymer solution was prepared at the required concentration in water (e.g., 4% PVP in water) and 5 μL of TEMED and 50 μL of a 10% ammonium persulfate were added to 10 mL of the polymer solution. In place of the persulfate, a solution of 61.5 μL of a 10% solution (w/w) of 4,4'-Azo-bis-(4-cyano pentanoic acid) in methanol could also be used. The solution was then pressurized into the capillary, which was then sealed end-to-end with a Teflon tube (0.012" ID, 0.033" OD, Zeus Industrial Products, Inc., NJ) and placed in an oven at 80°C for 18 h. The unattached portion of the polymer solution was removed by rinsing with deionized water, leaving a cross-linked polymer layer covalently linked to the capillary wall.

4.3. Evaluating Capillary Coatings

A typical evaluation of a coated capillary involves measuring the EOF with a suitable flow marker. When evaluating capillaries with neutral coatings, we found that an EOF of $<2 \times 10^{-5}$ cm^2/V.s was acceptable. Because it is well known that a low EOF is not the only criteria to identify acceptable coated capillaries that are useful for protein separations, it is important to run a test mixture comprising standard proteins to verify the acceptability of the capillary coating. The CE electrolyte pH should be optimized to ensure that the proteins are charged under the test conditions to ensure efficient separations. Lower efficiencies can be obtained for proteins with pIs close to the pH of the electrolyte. This is because the proteins have no or minimal nets charge under these conditions and migrate with the EOF. Some researchers have also reported that electrophoretic runs were needed to ascertain pH stability of a coating, rather than mere contact of the coated surface with high pH electrolytes *(24,25)*.

5. APPLICATIONS OF COATED CAPILLARIES

Free solution separations of proteins remain the most widespread application of coated capillaries. A few examples are discussed later and also shown in Table 1. Basic protein separations (pI > 7) are typically done under acidic conditions because they carry a net positive charge. Under both high and minimal EOF conditions the applied polarity is positive. Figure 1 demonstrates a high-resolution, high-efficiency separation (500,000 plates/50 cm) of a mixture of five basic proteins using a preformed polymer-coated capillary. Acidic proteins (pI < 7) are typically run under basic conditions and carry a net negative charge. In neutral coated capillaries, where the EOF is minimized, these separations are normally done under negative or reversed polarity conditions. Mixtures of acidic and basic proteins are typically run under pH conditions that facilitate ionization of all the proteins while avoid-

Table 1
Protein Applications Using Various Coated Capillaries

Capillary coating	Proteins tested	Reference	Comments
Polyvinylpyrrollidone coated capillary	Standard proteins varying in pI from 4.5 to 11 and in size from 12–77 kDa	McCormick (1988); (4)	Electrolyte: 38.5 mM H_3PO_4, 20 mM NaH_2PO_4, pH 2.0
Epoxy-diol coating Maltose coating	Standard basic proteins at pH 4.0 Standard basic proteins at pH 4.0	Bruin et al. (1989); (33)	Electrolyte: phosphate buffer at pH 4.0; 35,000–50,000 plates achieved in a 52 cm capillary at an applied voltage of 20 kV Electrolyte: phosphate buffer at pH 4.0.; 25,000 plates in a 39.5 cm capillary at an applied voltage of 10 kV
Polyethyleneimine coating- (cationic coating)	Standard basic proteins at pH 7.0	Towns et al. (1990) (34)	Electrolyte: 20 mM hydroxylamine-HCl at pH 7.0
Polyacrylamide-coated capillary through Si-C bond	Model protein separations (mainly acidic) at pH 9.5 ranging in pI of 4.3–7.6; model protein separations (mainly basic) at pH 2.7 ranging in pI of 4.5–10.7.	Cobb et al. (1990) (20)	Electrolyte: 50 mM glutamine; triethylamine at pH 9.5: 30 mM citric acid (pH 2.7 adjusted with 1 M NaOH). (Note: Electrolyte at pH 9.5 has an amine additive that can potentially interact with residual unmasked silanol groups)
Alpha lactalbumin coated capillary	Model protein separations (mainly basic and myoglobin)	Maa et al. (1991) (35)	
Allyl-methyl cellulose coated capillary Allyl-dextran coated capillary	Model protein separations (acidic) at pH 9.8; Model protein separations (basic) at pH 7.0 stable coating	Hjerten and Kubo (1993) (17)	Electrolyte: 50 mM glycine-NaOH pH 9.8; 50 mM Tris-HCl pH 7.0. Cited to be pH and detergent

Coating	Application	Reference	Conditions
Crosslinked multilayer methylcellulose based coatings (neutral coating)	Model protein separations (basic proteins) at pH 3.0 and 4.5	Smith and Rassi (1993) (22)	Electrolyte: 100 mM Phosphate adjusted to pH 3.0 and 4.5. 400,000-550,000 plates/80 cm at an applied voltage of 18 kV
Multilayer PEG-based coating with anodal flow	Model protein separations— acidic proteins at pH 6.5 (crude trypsin inhibitor) and basic proteins at pH 3.0		Acidic proteins Electrolyte: 100 mM phosphate adjusted to pH 6.5; 80,000 plates/80 cm at an applied voltage of 18 kV. Basic proteins. Electrolyte: 100 mM phosphate adjusted to pH 3; 80,000 plates/80 cm at an applied voltage of 18kV
Hydrophilic-coated capillary (SGE, Milton Keynes, UK) or Celect P1 (Supelco, Belmont, PA)	Milk proteins – caseins (a$_{s1}$CN, a$_{s2}$CN, bCN, kCN); Serum proteins (β-lactoglobulin and α-lactalbumin)	Jong et al. (1993) (36)	Electrolyte: 10 mM sodium phosphate containing 6 M urea and 0.05% methylhyroxyethyl cellulose (pH 2.0–3.0).
Hydroxypropyl cellulose based coating	1. Tryptic digests of cytochrome c 2. RNase A and RNase B glycoform separations 3. Horseradish peroxidase isoenzymes 4. Ovlabumin glycoforms	Huang et al. (1995) (23)	1. Electrolyte: 25 mM Tris-HCl, 1-propanol. 2. Electrolyte: 25 mM Tris-HCl, pH 3.0, by addition of 2% (v/v) 1-propanol 3. Electrolyte: 50 mM Tris-HCl, pH 2.8, by addition of 2% (v/v) 1-propanol 4. Electrolyte: 50 mM AMPD/H$_3$PO$_4$ pH 9.1.

(continued)

Table 1 (*continued*)
Protein Applications Using Various Coated Capillaries

Capillary coating	Proteins tested	Reference	Comments
Polyacrylamide coated capillary, Fluorocarbon capillary, J&W Scientific (Folsom, CA)	Hemoglobin variants; Antibodies-anti-α_1-antitrypsin; Human IgG	Wu et al. (1998) (37)	Capillary isoelectric focusing separations
C18-coated capillary, Supelco; ISCO (Lincoln, NE).	Human growth hormone precursor Pre-bhGH of less than 2% was demonstrated for runs done with 5 coated capillaries.	Jorgensen et al. (1998) (38)	Electrolyte: 150 mM Tricine, 7.5% (v/v), methanol, pH 7.55. Precision
Polyacrylamide polymer coated capillary, Polyvinylpyrollidone polymer coated capillary	Model protein separations (basic proteins); Hemoglobin variants; Milk proteins (acidic proteins)	Srinivasan et al. (1997) (25)	Electrolyte: 50 mM sodium acetate, pH 4.5. 500,000 plates/ 50 cm at an applied voltage of 20 kV; 650,000 plates /65 cm at an applied voltage of 20 kV for hemoglobin variants separations
Polyacrylamide polymer coated capillary. Poly(ethylene) oxide polymer coated capillary	Model protein separations (basic proteins); Acidic proteins		Eluent: 100 mM Sodium phosphate, pH 8.4, with 6 M urea
Copolymer of acrylamide and (methacrylamidopropyl) trimethylammonium chloride polymer coated capillary.			Electrolyte: 50 mM sodium acetate, pH 4.5; 300,000 plates/ 50 cm capillary for basic proteins at an applied voltage of 20 kV
			Electrolyte: 25 mM phosphate buffer at pH 7.0>200,000 plates/50 cm at an applied voltage of 20 kV

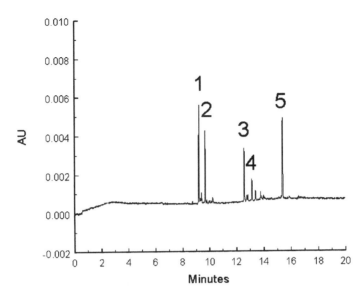

Fig. 1. Separation of basic proteins using a polymer coated capillary. Conditions: 50-cm total length; 45 cm to detector; 50 µm i.d.; Electrolyte: 50 m*M* sodium acetate, pH 4.5; 20 kV (400 V/cm); gravity injection 50 mm × 10 s; detection UV 210 nm; sample concentration, 100 µg/mL. Peak identification: (1) lysozyme (chicken egg white) (2) cytochrome c (bovine heart) (3) ribonuclease A (bovine pancreas), (4) myoglobin (horse skeletal muscle) and (5) α-chymotrypsinogen A (bovine pancreas).

ing extremes of pH, because this can denature the proteins. Several coated capillaries have been employed for protein separations with mixed success. Table 1 cites some examples of protein separations done using coated capillaries.

5.1. Separations of Hemoglobin Variants

Literature shows several examples of separations of hemoglobin variants using capillary isoelectric focusing (cIEF) with coated capillaries *(32,39)* or capillary zone electrophoresis with coated capillaries *(25,32)* (*see* Fig. 2). An additional mobilization step is required when using cIEF, adding another step to the process and increasing the analysis time. Some researchers have also reported problems in the reproducibility of the mobilization process *(32)*. The aforementioned technique is also sensitive to the presence of salt in the samples. In some instances, prior knowledge of the salt concentration in the sample is required for optimizing the focusing conditions. A recently developed whole-column detection scheme overcomes some of the afore-

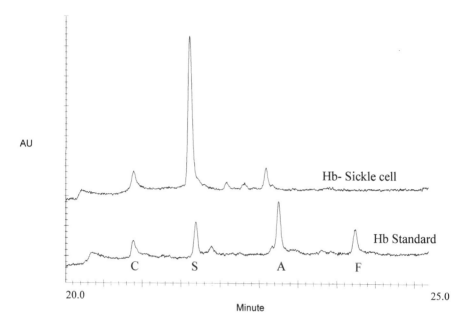

Fig. 2. Separation of four commonly occurring hemoglobin variants using a polymer coated capillary. CE conditions were same as in Fig. 1.

mentioned problems and has shown to detect proteins without the mobilization step *(32)*. However, this approach is complicated in terms of instrumentation. Capillary zone electrophoresis (CZE), on the other hand, offers a simpler means of achieving the same separations without the limitations noted. Separation of hemoglobin variants in single human erythrocytes was shown using a fluorocarbon-coated capillary and fluorocarbon surfactant added to the CE buffer *(32)*. This approach, however, suffered from lack of reproducibility due to coating deterioration over time. In a recent publication, a PVP polymer-coated capillary and 50 m*M* sodium acetate electrolyte at pH 4.5, showed efficiencies of >650,000 plates/65 cm for the separation of the four common variants of hemoglobin *(25)*. The high efficiencies observed in the above approach demonstrate that there was minimal interaction of the analytes with the surface of the capillary.

5.2. Transferrin Isoforms

Using CE along with coated capillaries, it has been possible to monitor changes in the structures of the isoforms of transferrin (*see* Fig. 3). By gel electrophoresis it is not possible to resolve the isoforms of transferrin *(32)*, however, using CE separation of the isoforms is possible *(32,39)*. CE has

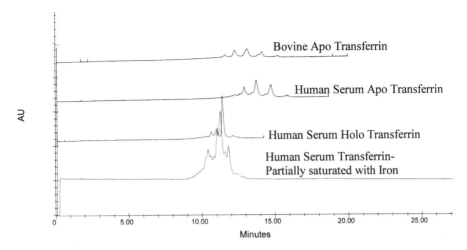

Fig. 3. Separation of transferrin isoforms using a polymer coated capillary. CE conditions were same as in Fig. 1 except the applied voltage was –30 kV (600 V/cm). Electrolyte: 10 m*M* borate, pH 9.0.

also been used to monitor the unfolding of human serum transferrin using a denaturing buffer and a coated capillary *(32)*. Under free solution conditions, Srinivasan and Avdalovic *(40)* have shown that iron-free "Apo" transferrin migrated slower than the iron-rich "Holo" transferrin. The " Holo" and partially saturated samples migrated almost identically, although the number of isoforms were different. The difference in migration was attributed to the difference in sialic acid/sialylated oligosaccharide content. These separations were done using a proprietary neutral polymer-coated capillary with 10 m*M* borate buffer at pH 9.0.

5.3. Milk Proteins

Excellent separations of milk proteins (serum proteins and caseins) were demonstrated using a coated capillary and a sodium phosphate or sodium citrate buffer in the presence of a cellulose additive and urea *(32)* (*see* Fig. 4). Separation and identification of the genetic variants of casein and β–lactoglobulin has also been done with various types of bovine milk. Using this method it has also been possible to identify the possible adulteration of bovine milk with milk from other species, such as goat or sheep. Recently, we demonstrated excellent separations of milk proteins using a PVP polymer-coated capillary without adding any polymer additives to the run buffer. The effect of heat treatment on milk proteins was also studied *(40)*. In some instances polymer additives may be needed in some applications to reduce

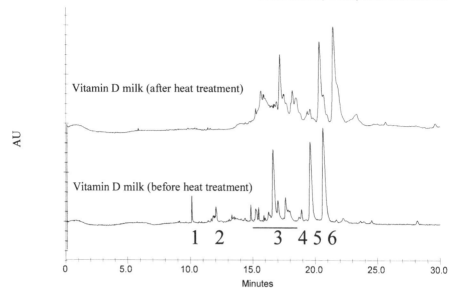

Fig. 4. Separation of milk proteins using a polymer-coated capillary. Conditions: 50-cm total length; 45 cm to detector; 50 µm i.d.; Electrolyte: 100 mM sodium phosphate, pH 8.4, with 6 M urea; –30 kV (600 V/cm); gravity injection 150 mm × 30 s, detection, UV, 210 nm. Peak identification (1) α-lactalbumin, (2) β-lactoglobin A and B, (3) α-caseins (4) κ-caseins, and (5/6) β-caseins.

further the EOF or to re-coat the surface to compensate for the lack of coating homogeneity.

5.4. Miscellaneous Applications

In addition to being useful for the free solution separation of proteins, peptides, and a number of amino acids, coated capillaries are also useful in size-based separations of proteins. In this application, a sieving or sizing medium in combination with SDS is used similar to SDS-PAGE. Several examples of size-based separations of proteins have been shown in literature *(32,33)*. In these applications the polymer solution is viscous, and thus to some extent it inhibits EOF. The use of a coated capillary in these applications improves peak shapes and the reproducibility of the separations. Again, the role of the capillary coating was to provide a noninteracting environment for the separations.

A number of papers have discussed the utility of CE with coated capillaries in peptide-mapping applications *(32,33)*, where the protein samples were enzymatically or chemically digested to generate representative peptide maps. The utility of CE in combination with coated capillaries in looking for subtle structural changes in synthetic peptides and proteins, such as deamidation, dephosphorylation, and acetylation is also anticipated.

6. CONCLUSIONS

CE has made significant progress in the field of bioseparations. With the recent advances in coating chemistries and capillaries the technique has become more robust, particularly for protein analysis. The benefit of improved separation efficiencies, recovery, and reproducibility of protein separations using coated capillaries translates into wider acceptability of CE. As the demand for recombinant drugs increases, the need for analytical techniques that give complementary results increases and the utility of CE in this area is anticipated.

REFERENCES

1. Stedry, M., Gas, B., and Kenndler, E. (1995) Dynamics of peak dispersion in capillary zone electrophoresis including wall adsorption II. Exact analysis of unsteady linear adsorptive dispersion. Electrophoresis 16, 2027–2033.
2. Minarik, M., Gas, B., Rizzi, A., and Kenndler, E. (1995) Plate hieght contribution from wall adsorption in capillary zone electrophoresis of proteins. J. Capillary Electrophor. 2, 89–96.
3. Zhukov, M. Y., Ermakov, S. V., and Righetti, P. G. (1997) Simplified mathematical model of irreversible sample adsorption in capillary zone electrophoresis. J. Chromatogr. A, 766, 171–185.
4. McCormick, R. M. (1988) Capillary zone electrophoretic separation of peptides and proteins using low pH buffers in modified silica capillaries. Anal. Chem. 60, 2322–2328.
5. Lauer, H. H. and McManigill, D. (1986) Capillary zone electrophoresis of proteins in untreated fused silica tubing. Anal. Chem. 58, 166–170.
6. Encyclopedia of Polymer Science and Engineering, John Wiley & Sons, New York, NY, 1990, p. 183.
7. Gordon, M. J., Lee, K. J., Arias, A. A., and Zare, R. N. (1991) Protocol for resolving protein mixtures in capillary zone electrophoresis. Anal. Chem. 63, 69–72.
8. Bushey, M. M. and Jorgenson, J. W. (1989) Capillary electrophoresis of proteins in buffers containing high concentrations of zwitterionic salts. J. Chromatogr. 480, 301–310.
9. Stover, F. S., Haymore, B. L., and McBeth, R. J. (1989) Capillary zone electrophoresis of histidine-containing compounds. J. Chromatogr. 470, 241–250.
10. Gilges, M., Kleemiss, M. H., and Schomburg, G. (1994) Capillary zone electrophoresis separations of basic and acidic proteins using poly(vinyl alcohol) coatings in fused silica capillaries. Anal. Chem. 66, 2038–2046.
11. Hjerten, S. (1985) High performance electrophoresis—elimination of electroendosmosis and solute adsorption. J. Chromatogr. 347, 191–198.

12. Strege. M. A. and Lagu, A. L. (1993) Capillary electrophoretic protein separations in polyacrylamide-coated silica capillaries and buffers containing ionic surfactants. J. Chromatogr. 630, 337–344.
13. Cifuentes, A., de Frutos, M., Santos, J. M., and Diez-Masa J. C. (1993) Separation of basic proteins by capillary electrophoresis using cross-linked polyacrylamide-coated capillaries and cationic buffer additives. J. Chromatogr. 655, 63–72.
14. Herren, B. J., Shafer. S. G., Van Alstine, J., Harris, J. M., and Snyder, R. S. (1987) Control of electroosmosis in quartz capillaries. J. Colloid Interface Sci. 115, 46–55.
15. Yalpani, M. and Brooks, D. E. (1985) Selective chemical modifications of dextran. J. Polymer Sci. 23, 1395–1405.
16. Harris, J. M., Struck, E. C., Case, M. G., Paley, S., Yalpani, M., Van Alstine, J. M., and Brooks, D. E. (1984) Synthesis and characterization of poly(ethylene glyclol) derivatives. J. Polymer Sci. 22, 341–352.
17. Hjerten, S. and Kubo, K. (1993) A new type of pH-and detergent-stable coating for elimination of electroendosmosis and adsorption in (capillary) electrophoresis. Electrophoresis, 14, 390–395.
18. Malik, A., Zhao, Z., and Lee, M. L. (1993) Simple method for the preparation of highly efficient polymer coated capillary electrophoresis columns. J. Microcol. 5, 119–125.
19. Zhao, Z., Malik, A., and Lee, M. L. (1993) Solute adsorption on polymer-coated fused silica capillary electrophoresis column using selected protein and peptide standards. Anal. Chem. 65, 2747–2752.
20. Cobb, K. A., Dolnik, V., and Novotny, M. (1990) Electrophoretic separations of proteins in capillaries with hydrolytically stable surface structures. Anal. Chem. 62, 2478–2483.
21. Chiari, M., Nesi, M., Sandoval, J. E., and Pesek, J. J. (1995) Capillary electrophoretic separation of proteins using stable, hydrophilic poly(acryloylaminoethoxyethanol)-coated columns. J. Chromatogr. 717, 1–13.
22. Smith, J. T. and Rassi, Z. E. (1993) Capillary zone electrophoresis of biological substances with fused silica capillaries having zero or constant electroosmotic flow. Electrophoresis, 14, 396–406.
23. Huang, M., Plocek, J., and Novotny, M. V. (1995) Hydrolytically stable cellulose-derivative coatings for capillary electrophoresis of peptides, proteins and glycoconjugates. Electrophoresis, 16, 396–401.
24. Schmalzing, D., Piggee, C. A., Foret, F., Carrilho, E., and Karger, B. L. (1993) Characterization and performance of a neutral hydrophilic coating for the capillary electrophoretic separation of biopolymers. J. Chromatogr. A 652, 149–159.
25. Srinivasan, K., Pohl, C., and Avdalovic, N. (1997) Cross-linked polymer coatings for capillary electrophoresis and application to analysis of basic proteins, acidic proteins, and inorganic ions. Anal. Chem. 69, 2798–2805.
26. Schutzner, W. and Kenndler, E. Electrophoresis in synthetic organic polymer capillaries: Variation of electroosmotic velocity and x potential with pH and solvent composition. Anal. Chem. 64, 1991–1995.

27. Hjerten, S. (1967) Free zone electrophoresis. Chromatogr. Rev. 9, 122.
28. Pretorius, V., Hopkins, B. J., and Schieke, J. D. (1974) Electroosmosis—new concept for high speed liquid chromatography. Chromatogr. 99, 23–30.
29. Ewing, A. G., Wallingford, R. A., and Olefirowicz, T. M. (1989) Capillary electrophoresis. Anal. Chem. 61, 292A–303A.
30. Silicon Compounds: Register and Review," United Technologies, 5th ed., (1991).
31. Tailoring Surfaces with Silanes. Chemtech (1977) 7, 766.
32. Acrylamide Polymerization: A Practical Approach, BioRad, Bulletin 1156, (1987) p. 3.
33. Zhu, M., Rodriguez, R., Wehr, T., and Siebert, C. (1992) Capillary electrophoresis of hemoglobin and globin chains. J. Chromatogr. 608, 225–237.
34. Molteni, S., Frischknecht, H., and Thormann, W. (1994) Application of dynamic capillary isoelectric focusing to the analysis of human hemoglobin variants. Electrophoresis, 15, 22–30.
35. Huang, T. L., Shieh, P. C. H., and Cooke, N. (1994) The separation of hemoglobin variants by capillary zone electrophoresis. J. High Resolut. Chromatogr. 17, 676–678.
36. Pritchett, T. J. (1996) Capillary isoelectric focusing of proteins (review). Electrophoresis, 17, 1195–1199.
37. Wu, J., Li, S. C, and Watson, A. (1998) Optimizing separation conditions for proteins and peptides using imaged capillary isoelectric focusing. J. Chromatogr. A, 817, 163–171.
38. Lillard, S. J., Yeung, E. S., Lautamo, R. M. A., and Mao, D. T. (1995) Separation of hemoglobin variants in single human erthrocytes by capillary electrophoresis with laser-induced native fluorescence detection. J. Chromatogr. A, 718, 397–404.
39. Chasteen, N. D. and Williams, J. (1981) The influence of pH on the equilibrium distribution of iron between the metal binding sites of human transferrin. J. Biochem. 193, 717.
40. Kilar, F. and Hjerten, S. (1989) Separation of the human transferrin isoforms by carrier free high performance zone electrophoresis and isoelectric focusing. J. Chromatogr. 480, 351.
41. Srinivasan, K. and Avdalovic, N. Eighth International Symposium on High Performance Capillary Electrophoresis, Poster P153, January 1996.
42. Kilar, F. and Hjerten, S. (1993) Unfolding of human serum transferrin in urea studied by high-performance capillary electrophoresis. J. Chromatogr. 638, 269–276.
43. Jong, N., Visser, S., and Oliemann, C. (1993) Determination of milk proteins by capillary electrophoresis. J. Chromatogr. A652, 207–213.
44. Werner, W. E., Demorest, D. M., Stevens, J. and Wiktorowicz, J. E. (1993) Size-dependent separation of proteins denatured in SDS by capillary electrophoresis using a replacable sieving matrix. Anal. Biochem. 212, 253.
45. Ganzler, K., Greve, K. S., Cohen, A. S., and Karger, B. L. (1992) High performance capillary electrophoresis of SDS-protein complexes using UV-transparent polymer networks. Anal. Chem. 64, 2665.

46. Zhu, M. D., Rodriguez, R., Hansen, D. L., and Wehr, T. (1990) Capillary electrophoresis of proteins under alkaline conditions. J. Chromatogr. 516, 123–131.
47. Frenz, J., Wu, S. L., and Hancock, W. S. (1989) Characterization of human growth hormone by capillary electrophoresis. J. Chromatogr. 480, 379–391.
48. Bruin G. J. M., Huisden, R., Kraak, J. C., and Poppe, H. (1989) Performance of carbohydrate-modified fused silica capillaries for the separation of proteins by zone electrophoresis. J. Chromatogr. 480, 339–349.
49. Towns, J. K. and Regnier, F. E. (1990) Polyethyleneimine-bonded phases in the separation of proteins by capillary electrophoresis. J. Chromatogr. 516, 69–78.
50. Maa, Y. F., Hvyer, K. J., and Swedberg, S. A. (1991) Impact of wall modification on protein elution in high performance capillary zone electrophoresis. J. High Resolution Chromatogr. 14, p. 65–67.
51. Jorgensen, T. K., Bagger, L. H., Christiansen, J., Johnsen, G. H., Faarbaek, J. R., and Welinder, B. S. (1998) Quantifying biosynthetic human growth hormone in Escherichia coli with capillary electrophoresis under hydrophobic conditions. J. Chromatogr. A, 817, 205–214.

4

Clinical Serum Protein
Capillary Zone Electrophoresis

Carl R. Jolliff

1. HISTORICAL PERSPECTIVE

In 1937 Tiselius *(1)* reported on a methodology that was to become one of the most novel ways by which proteins could be separated from one another. His apparatus, although large in size relative to current systems, established the serum protein profile still used today. The apparatus, a U-tube, separated the serum proteins in the liquid phase into five fractions, albumin, α-1, α-2, β, and γ globulins. Through the years chemical pathologists and clinical chemists have refined both the methodology and the apparatus. The driving forces behind the development of newer modifications and innovations to his methodology was dependent on:

1. Building a more compact and less expensive form of instrument.
2. Recording the resultant separation, on solid, visible media that could be stored, and that was capable of visual interpretation.
3. Densitometric scanning, so that semi-quantitative values might be assigned to the separated components.
4. Making the apparatus available through commercial channels to make it widely available.

Later, Kunkel and Tiselius *(2)* described the first separation on solid media using buffer-saturated filter paper strips. This method was replaced when cellulose acetate strips were used by Kohn *(3)* and then subsequently miniaturized by Grunbaum (Microzone System®) *(4)*. Johansson *(5)* later developed a system using agarose and ionagar, resolving additional protein bands. Starch gel electrophoresis was developed by Smithies *(6)* and modified by Marsh *(7)* allowing further improved separation. Starch gel electrophoresis, however, was very time consuming. Finally, in 1966 Elevitch *(8)* proposed

From: *Clinical and Forensic Applications of Capillary Electrophoresis*
Edited by: J. R. Petersen and A. A. Mohammad © Humana Press Inc., Totowa, NJ

a thin layer agarose method that is the basis of the serum protein electro-phoresis procedure used in most clinical laboratories today.

In the early 1980's Hjerten (9) and Jorgenson (10) established the useful-ness of microcapillary electrophoresis for protein separation, returning to the use of a liquid phase during separation. In essence, the U-tube was inverted, its surface components changed, and the tube miniaturized. Instead of protein bands being detected because of changes in diffraction of the liq-uid phase, peaks are detected by the change in absorbance at 214 nm. It is critical to remember that no matter what apparatus or separation media is used, a person is ultimately charged with the interpretation of the resulting serum protein pattern. This interpretation is based on changes from the "ref-erence control" pattern, which one must use to access either visually or quan-titatively a dysproteinemia.

A number of papers have been written on the comparison of the separa-tion of serum proteins by high resolution agarose gel electrophoresis (HRAGE) with various capillary zone electrophoresis (CZE) instruments (11–28). My experience has been with both a single-capillary instrument as well as a fully automated seven-capillary system. In the original report, my group confirmed that CZE worked well for the elucidation of serum proteins on a single-capillary system (11). In 1997 our findings were reported using a multi-channel instrument (12). Both reports found that either instrument was capable of giving serum protein separation patterns comparable to HRAGE. These findings have also been confirmed in reports from other investigators (13–28).

Various techniques and instrumentation are available for separation of serum proteins by CZE. Instrument manufacturers have developed sys-tems sold as kits that contain all necessary components to separate serum proteins, such as ready-to-use buffer and capillary wash solutions. As of this writing there are only two manufacturers that make CZE instruments dedicated to the separation of serum proteins. They are the Bio-Rad BIOFOCUS 2000™ (Fig. 1) and the Beckman Coulter Paragon CZE® 2000 (Fig. 2) systems. However, research platforms have also been used and are included in Table 1 with the particulars of each method. The Beckman Coulter Paragon 2000® Clinical Capillary Electrophoresis instrument is currently the only available commercial instrument that is fully automated and is capable of producing 48 serum electrophoretic pat-terns per hour. It also has the capability of generating a report form that can be sent to the chart for later review by the clinician. This is extremely helpful to those institutions that must process a large daily serum protein electrophoresis (SPE) workload.

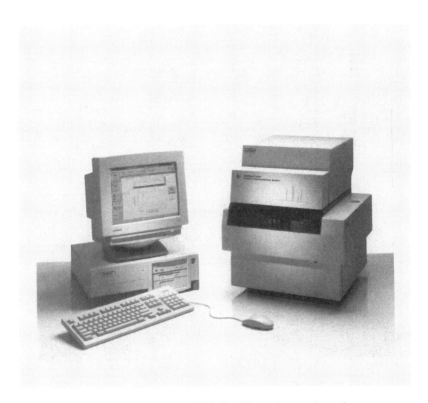

Fig. 1. Bio-Rad BIOFOCUS 2000 Capillary electrophoresis system.

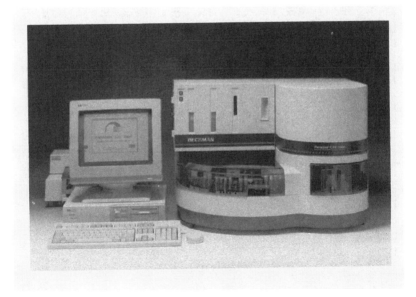

Fig. 2. Beckman Coulter Paragon CZE® 2000 Clinical Capillary electrophoresis system.

Table 1
Chronological List of Serum Protein Studies by Capillary Electrophoresis

Year	Author	Instrumentation	Capillary	Buffer	Sample	Detection voltage	Absorbance
1990	Chen et al.	Research platform Beckman Coulter (Fullerton, CA)	Single fused silica 100 cm L 25 µm I.D. 360 µm O.D.	pH 10.0 Proprietary buffer	Serum N.G.	200 kV/cm	214 nm
1991	Kim et al.	Research platform Beckman Coulter	Single fused silica 100 cm L 50 mm I.D. 360 mm O.D.	30 mM/L sodium borate	Serum Sodium borate	30 kV CV	200 nm
1994	Klein et al.	P/ACE 2100 Beckman Coulter	Single fused silica 20 cm L 75 µm I.D. 365 µm O.D.	Borate	Serum Dil 1:20 PBS	6 min 10 kV	214 nm
1994	Chen et al.	P/ACE 2100 Beckman Coulter	Single fused silica 25 cm L 20 µm I.D.	Borate	N.G.	800 v/cm	214 nm
1994	Reif et al.	P/ACE 2000 Beckman Coulter	Single fused silica 27 cm L 50 µm I.D.	40 mM Borate, pH 10.0	N.G.	15 kV	214 nm
1995	Jenkins et al.	Applied Biosystems Model 270A HT (Foster City, CA)	Single fused silica 75 cm L 50 µm I.D.	Borate	Serum Dil 1:49 Borate buffer	18 kV 15 min	200 nm
1995	Dolnik et al.	Crystal C.E. System Model 310 ATI UNICAM (Cambridge, UK)	Single fused silica 55 cm L 75 µm I.D. 360 µm O.D.	Single fused silica	10 mM Methyl glucamine 5 mM Lauric acid	30 kV	200 nm

Year	Author	Instrument / Capillary	Buffer	Sample	Conditions	Wavelength
1995	Jenkins et al.	Applied Biosystems Model 720A HT; Single fused silica	50 mM Borate, with 1 mM Calcium	Serum Dil 1:49 with buffer	18 kV 15 min	200 nm
1995	Lehman et al.	Bio-Focus 3000 Bio-Rad CE (Hercules, CA); Single fused silica 50 cm L 50 µm I.D.	30 mM Borate, pH 10.0	Dil 1:30	20 kV 15 min	220 nm
1995	Landers et. al.	Research platform Beckman Coulter; Single fused silica 20 cm L 25 µm I.D.	Borate, pH 8.3	Dil 1:9 P.B.S.	10 kV 24°C	214 nm
1996	Lehmann et al.	Dionex CES I Iastein, Germany 50 µm I.D.; Single fused silica 50 cm L	N.G.	N.G.	18 min	195 nm
1996	Wijnen et al.	P/ACE 5500 Beckman Coulter; Single fused silica 20 cm L 50 µm I.D.	100 mM Borate, pH 10.2	Serum PBS Dil 1:39 1/2 ionic strength	10 kV 10 min	200 nm
1996	Clark et al.	P/ACE 5510 Beckman Coulter; Single fused silica 27 cm L 20 µm ID	Borate	1:10 PBS	20 kV	2114 nm
1997	Doelman et al.	P/ACE 5000 27 cm L 25 µm ID; Single fused silica	150 mM/L Sodium borate, pH 10.1	1:4 PBS	12.5 kV 20C	214 nm
1997	Jellum et al.	Paragon CZE 2000 Beckman Coulter; Seven fused silica 20 cm L 25 µm ID	5% Sodium borate	Serum Dil 1:7 and 1:20 Buffer	9 kV 24°C 4.3 min	214 nm
1997	Jolliff et al.	Paragon CZE 2000 Beckman Coulter; Seven fused silica 20 cm L 25 µm ID	Borate	Serum Dil 1:7 and 1:20 Buffer	9 kV 24°C 4.3 min	214 nm
1998	Bossuyt et al.	Paragon CZE 2000 Beckman Coulter; Seven fused silica 20 cm L 25 µm ID	Borate	Serum Dil 1:20 <1 nL	9 kV 24°C 4.3 min	214 nm
1998	Bienvenu et al.	Paragon CZE 2000; Seven fused silica 20 cm L 25 µm ID	Borate	Serum Dil 1:20 <1 nL	9 kV 24°C 4.3 mm	214 nm

Table 2
Normal Ranges: HRAGE and CZE Compared

Serum fraction	Paragon® HRAGE (2 SD)* Relative percent (%)	Paragon CZE® 2000 (2 SD) Relative percent (%)
Albumin	56.0–72.0	52.0–67.0
α-1	1.8–4.5	3.8–8.3
α-2	7.3–15.0	5.0–12.4
β	6.1–11.5	9.8–13.0
γ	7.8–18.2	9.3–20.4

*Standard deviation.

2. COMPARSION OF CZE AND HRAGE

The investigators listed in Table 1 have all determined that CZE will give results comparable to HRAGE for routine the electrophoretic separation of serum proteins in the clinical laboratory. However, as with any procedure, correlation between methods depends on many factors. As such, normal ranges should be established in each individual laboratory. As a comparison, normal values obtained by CZE vs HRAGE in my laboratory are given Table 2.

We found that for the five standard fractions of a normal serum control the within-capillary precision (coefficient of variation or CV) over 10 runs ranged from 0.6 to 3.4%. As expected, this was dependent upon the fraction analyzed. This can be compared to the between-run precision for HRAGE that had CVs in a range of 3.8–8.0% *(12)*. In addition, Petall et al. *(23)* found the between individual variations of the protein bands, albumin, α1, α2, β, and γ, were similar being 6, 21, 19, 14, and 18%, respectively, by the CZE 2000 and 5, 10, 17, 18, and 22%, respectively, for Paragon HRAGE.

3. DYSPROTEINEMIAS

Serum protein patterns reflect many categories of dysproteinemia. What is disturbing is the apparent disregard by many that are charged with the interpretation SPE patterns to report only changes in the peak values of the electrophoretic pattern. In many instances interpretation of SPE patterns have been reported as "no gamma globulin spike detected" or in some instances no interpretation is given at all, leaving the physician to try to interpret the pattern without the experience to do so.

Interpretation of patterns comes with experience gained over years of correlating patterns with the pathophysiology. Electrophoresis, especially on agarose, is not a quantitative procedure. First the pattern on the gel is visually compared with a "normal" control gel. It is then necessary to look at the densitometric tracing and be certain that the percentages of the separated proteins are within the limits established by the laboratory. Reporting the individual peaks (albumin, and so forth) in g/L is not necessary. It is adequate to report as a percentage of the total protein. When a case of paraproteinemia is found, reporting the peak in g/L serves to help the physician when treating the monoclonal gammopathy. Quantitation of monoclonal proteins by nephelometry should not be done, as it is inaccurate *(29)* possibly giving the physician a false sense of the patient's condition.

Dysproteinemia identification, in many instances, may be a clue for the physician of some previously undiagnosed condition, or at least verify his diagnosis *(30)*. Some years ago, I prepared a classification system of dysproteinemia *(31)* to help those who are starting interpretation of SPE patterns. This classification will help the beginner; however, the best way to learn to interpret SPE is still to run serum samples on patients with known clinical conditions to see how the condition affects the SPE pattern.

CZE, when compared with HRAGE, showed a 96% concordance in the study of 240 patients with dysproteinemia *(12)*. Because CZE does not detect the β-lipoprotein band, conditions such as hyperlipidemia, diabetes mellitus, and nephrotic syndromes may not be detected. Paraprotein concordance between CZE and HRAGE was also 100% when the paraprotein was in the detectable concentration range (*see* Chapter 5).

The CZE separation pattern of serum proteins is shown in Fig. 3. Although CZE compares very well with HRAGE *(12)*, it was still necessary to identify the proteins in the various peaks. Attempts at identification by adding purified proteins were useless due to the impurities in these preparations. Thus, it was necessary to identify the proteins found in each peak by using the technique immunosubtraction *(32–34)*.

Figure 4A–F shows examples of various dysproteinemias as compared to those obtained by HRAGE. Examples of paraprotein specimens are shown in Chapter 5. Since the data collection for the CZE method is computer controlled, it is possible to superimpose the patient's pattern over a normal serum pattern for a better visualization of increases or decreases in the various peaks. Also when doing an SPE on children, age related "normal" serum must be used. An additional advantage of the Beckman Coulter CZE 2000 system is the ability to generate a computer-derived simulated gel on the screen, which can aid in the interpretation process.

Protein dye binding in HRAGE is not equal for all of the separated proteins. This can mean inconsistency in staining of the proteins if times in the staining procedure are compromised. In CZE the proteins separated in the liquid phase are detected at 214 nm (absorbance maximum of the amide bond). From this

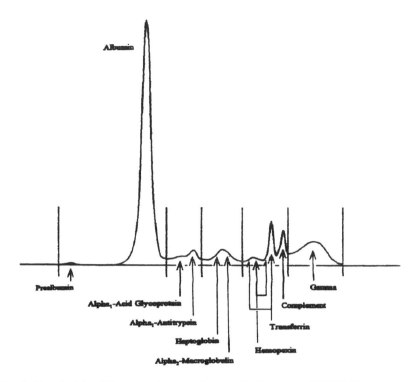

Fig. 3. Protein identification of separation on the Paragon CZE 2000 instrument.

absorbance the protein concentration can be estimated ensuring consistency within a run as well as between runs. Time, temperature, dye content, washing, drying, and destaining are parameters in the HRAGE procedure that are no longer a factor for error in the CZE procedure. However, unlike HRAGE, β-lipoprotein and fibrinogen do not appear on the CZE serum or plasma patterns. In addition, if the serum is highly lipemic and liposol (lipid removing reagent) is used to clarify the serum it is important to remember that the α-1 fraction will also be removed. Also the major bands in a fresh serum in the β-globulin region are transferrin and C3. In older specimens, the C3 band will disapear because of activation by endogenous serum enzymes. It is also important to remember that α-2 macroglobulin is more anodic than haptoglobin, thus in elevations of α-2 macroglobulin the α-2 band may well be skewed towards the anode.

4. CZE INSTRUMENTATION

4.1. Advantages

CZE instrumentation offers a semi-automated (Bio-Focus 2000) or completely automated (Paragon CZE 2000) system. These instruments elimi-

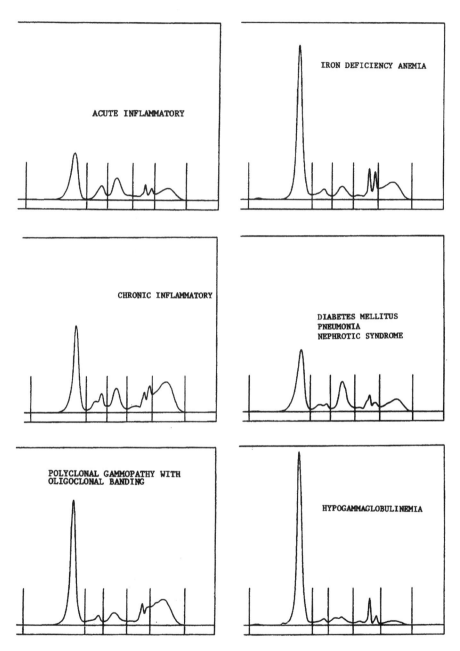

Fig. 4. Dysproteinemias as identified by CE.

nate many of the errors mentioned in the previous section that are associated with conventional HRAGE methods. Labor costs are also decreased with

CZE since there is no time spent in specimen application, fixing, staining, washing, and drying of the gels. Both methods, however, require visual and densitometric, as well as interpretation of the patterns.

Sample throughput for CZE is also higher than for HRAGE being able do 40–50 samples per hour. In addition, scan patterns for CZE can be enlarged to better study the peaks and delimit them if necessary. The ability to overlay a simulated normal gel on that of the patient's also makes pattern interpretation easier.

4.2. Disadvantages

Because β-lipoproteins and fibrinogen cannot be seen with the CZE method, the interpretative clues to hyperlipidemia, diabetes mellitus, nephrosis and some coagulinopathies are not as clear. Also due to the short separation time the gamma globulin area may be somewhat narrower than on HRAGE, making it more difficult to recognize and interpret the β-γ bridging normally seen in cirrhosis. In addition certain amino acids and contrast dyes that may absorb at 214 nm can interfere, resulting in poor scans *(27)*.

From my experience, it may be necessary to delimit peaks more often than seems necessary. However, with new software that allows multitasking or the bidirectional relay of the information to another stand-alone computer, pattern interpretation should not interfere with the operation of the instrument.

Currently the Beckman Coulter Paragon CZE 2000 instrument has been designed to evaluate only serum protein and immunosubtraction results. Urine proteins must still be performed on HRAGE or on an instrument with the capability to accomplish this task. Additionally, hemoglobin electrophoresis also must be performed on an instrument that has the capability of detection at 415 nm.

5. CZE IMPLEMENTATION

When instituting any new procedure in the clinical laboratory, comparative studies between the old and new methodology must be run. When comparing HRAGE and CZE, one should not expect separation of proteins on instrumentation as different as these two methods to give identical results. Because of the difference of detection methods of HRAGE and CZE (dye binding vs absorbance at 214 nm), the inter-individual variations by CZE were less than HRAGE *(23)*. However, variations in patient populations do occur and each laboratory should establish reference ranges. As a point of reference, normal ranges for adult serum protein electrophoresis (CZE) in various laboratories are shown in Table 3.

For the laboratories having a high volume of protein electrophoresis, CZE can offer a welcome change. If analyses other than serum protein or immunosubstraction are desired then a smaller unit might be needed.

Table 3
Adult Reference Ranges for Serum Protein Electrophoresis
on Capillary Instruments (CZE)

Author	Ref.	Albumin %	α-1 %	α-2 %	β %	γ %
Jellum	(26)	54.7–68.7	3.7–7.8	5.2–10.7	8.6–13.7	10.7–19.2
Klein	(11)	51.2–63.2	2.7–5.1	6.5–12.7	Trf[a] 7.7–9.8	9.3–20.4
and Jolliff					C3[b] 3.8–7.0	
Jolliff	(12)	52.0–67.0	3.8–8.3	5.8–12.4	9.8–13.0	9.3–20.4
and Blessum						
Petal	(23)	38.1–68.1	3.24–8.01	5.53–12.1	11.1–19.5	9.08–19.7
Bossnyt	(27)	[c]M 41.7–52.3	2.6–4.5	3.4–6.4	5.8–9.5	5.3–13.2
		[d]F 37.4–49.8	2.6–5.1	3.9 – 6.4	5.5–8.7	
Bio-Rad	(33)	51.3–66.6	3.8–6.6	6.8–13.0	8.8–15.7	9.4–19.5

[c]M, Male.
[d]F, Female.
[a]Trf, Transferrin.
[b]C3, C3 Component of complement,

Although it will have a slower output, the smaller unit will have the capability to change times, temperature, capillary sizes, and detection parameters, making the instrument more versatile.

6. CONCLUSION

The CZE procedure offers many advantages in labor saving, cost per test, and reproducibility compared to the HRAGE procedure. The literature on this procedure, in which comparative studies with HRGE have been reported, have been extremely favorable for its adaptation in the clinical laboratory for serum protein separation. Although it may make sense to replace HRAGE with CZE, the laboratory should not totally discard HRAGE because it will be useful as a backup confirmation method when patterns difficult to interpret occur.

REFERENCES

1. Tiselius, A. (1937) A new apparatus for electrophoresis of collodial mixtures. Transcripts. Faraday Soc. 33, 524–531.
2. Kunkel, H. C. and Tiselius, A. (1951) Electrophoresis of proteins on filter paper. Gen. Physiol. 35, 1189–1193.
3. Kohn, J. (1957) A new supporting medium for zone electrophoresis. Biochem. J. 65, 9.
4. Grunbaum, B. W. (1960) Microelectrophesis on cellulose acetate membranes. Anal. Chem. 32, 1361–1362.

5. Johansson, B. G. (1972) Agarose gel electrophoresis. Scand. J. Clin. Lab. Invest. 29, 7–21.
6. Smithies, O. (1955) Biochem. J. 62, 61–629.
7. Marsh, C., Jolliff, C., and Payne, L. (1964) Amer. J. Clin. Path. 41, 217.
8. Elevitch F. R., Aronson S. B., Feichtmeir T. V., and Enterline, M. L. (1966) Thin gel electrophoresis in agarose. Amer. J. Clin. Path. 46, 692–697.
9. Hjerten, S. (1967) Free zone electrophoresis. Chromatogr. Rev. 9, 122.
10. Jorgenson, J. W. and Lukacs K. D. (1981) Free zone electrophoresis in glass capillaries. Clin. Chem. 27, 151–153.
11. Klein, G. and Jolliff, C. (1994) Capillary electrophoresis for the routine clinical laboratory, in Landers, J. P. (ed.), CRC Press, Boca Raton, FL, pp. 420–457.
12. Jolliff, C. R. and Blessum, C. R. (1997) Comparison of serum protein electrophoresis by agarose gel and capillary zone electrophoresis in a clinical setting electrophoresis. Clin. Chem. 18, 1781–1784.
13. Chen, F. A., Lui, C. M., Hsieh, Y. Z., and Sternberg, J. C. (1991) Capillary electrophoresis: a new clinical tool. Clin. Chem. 37, 14–18.
14. Kim, J. W., Park, J. H., Park, J. W., Doh, H. J. Heo, G. S., and Lee, K. J. (1993) Quantitative analysis of serum proteins separated by capillary electrophoresis. Clin. Chem. 39, 689–692.
15. Chen, F. A. (1991) Rapid protein analysis by capillary electrophoresis. J. Chromatog. 559, 445–453.
16. Reif, O. W., Lausch, R., and Freitag, R. (1994) Application of CE to the quantitative analysis of serum proteins. International Laboratory 10, 11–14.
17. Jenkins, M. A. and Guerin, M. D. (1985) Quantification of serum proteins using capillary electrophoresis. Ann. Clin. Biochem. 32, 493–497.
18. Dolnik, V. (1995) Capillary zone electrophoresis of serum proteins: study of separation variables. J. Chromatogr. A 709, 99–110.
19. Jenkins, M. A., Kulinskaya, E., Martin, H. D., and Guerin, H. (1995) Evaluation of serum protein separation by capillary electrophoresis: prospective analysis 1000 specimens. J. Chrom. B 672, 241–251.
20. Lehmann, R., Liebich, H., Grubler, G., and Voelter, W. (1995) Capillary electrophoresis of human serum proteins and apolipoproteins. Electrophoresis 16, 998–1001.
21. Landers, J. P. (1995) Clinical capillary electrophoresis. Clin. Chem. 41, 495–509.
22. Lehmann, R., Koch, M., Voelter, W., Haring, H. U., and Liebich, H. M. (1997) Routine serum protein analysis by capillary zone electrophoresis: a clinical evaluation. Chromatographia 45, 390–395.
23. Petal, A. H. M., Wijnen, V. D., and Visser, M. (1996) Capillary Electrophoresis of serum proteins. Reproducibility, comparison with agarose gel electrophoresis and a review of the literature. Eur. J. Clin. Chem. Clin. Biochem. 34, 535–545.
24. Clark, R., Katzman, J. A., Wiegert, E., Namyst-Goldberg, C., Sanders, L., Oda, R. P., et al. (1996) J. Chromatogr. 744, 205–213.
25. Doelman, C. J. A., Siebelder, C. W. M., and Penders, T. (1997) Routine serum protein analysis using capillary electrophoresis. Eur. J. Clin. Chem. Clim. Biochem. 35, 393,394.

26. Jellum, E., DolleKamp, H., Brunsvig, A., and Foss, R. (1997) Diagnostic Applications of chromatography and capillary electrophoresis. J. Chromatogr. B 689, 155–164.

27. Bossuyt, X., Schiettekatte, G., Bogaerts, A., and Blanckaert, N. (1998) Serum protein electrophoresis by CZE 2000 clinical capillary electrophoresis system. Clin. Chem. 44, 749–759.

28. Bienvenu, J., Graziani, M. S., Arrin, F., Bernon, H., Blessum, C., Marchett, C., et al. (1998) Multicenter evaluation of the Paragon CZE™ 2000 capillary zone system for serum protein electrophoresis and monoclonal component typing. Clin. Chem. 44, 599–605.

29. Aguzzi, F., Merlini, G., and Whicher, M. A. (1996) Serum Monoclonal Components in Serum Proteins in Clinical Medicine. Blood Research, Scarborough, ME, pp. 11.03–11.08.

30. Laurell, C-B. (1996) Serum proteins in clinical medicine, in Perspective, vol. 1, Ritchie, R. F. (ed.) Blood Research, Scarborough, ME, pp. 11.1–11.3.

31. Jollif, C. R. (1991) Classification and interperation of Paragon® serum protein electrophoresis. Beckman Instruments, Inc., Brea, CA.

32. Aguzzi, F. and Boggi, N. (1997) Immunosubtraction electrophoresis: A simple method for identifying specific proteins producing the cellulose acetate electropherograms. Ann. Clin. Biochem. 32, 493–499.

33. Keren, D. L. (1998) Personal communication.

34. Bio-Rad Laboratories. (1997) Serum Proteins by Capillary Electrophoresis: Instruction Manual for Bio-Focus™ Capillary Electrophoresis Unit. Hercules, CA.

5

Serum and Urine Paraprotein Capillary Electrophoresis

Carl R. Jolliff

1. INTRODUCTION

Most requests for serum and urine electrophoresis occur because of the reversal of albumin/globulin ratios in the general chemistry profile or the presence of protein in the urine. The suspicion of possible myelomatosis by the physician also alerts him/her to rule out the presence of a monoclonal gammopathy in the serum or light chain in the urine. Because of the increased sensitivity afforded by the newer electrophoresis systems, paraproteins are found more often. Their appearance in a number of conditions exhibiting a B-cell lymphoproliferative response has renewed the interest of oncologists, hematologists, nephrologists, rheumatologists, internists, and neurologists.

Historically, the procedures for clinical electrophoresis have progressed through the techniques discussed in Chapter 4. To date, the most commonly used method is thin layer agarose electrophoresis to identify the presence of proteins of restricted mobility. Once identified, more definitive techniques, such as immunofixation electrophoresis, are used to classify the proteins involved.

2. IDENIFICATION OF PARAPROTEINS BY CAPILLARY ZONE ELECTROPHORESIS (CZE)

Capillary zone electrophoresis (CZE) has the potential to replace agarose electrophoresis in the identification of paraproteinemia. However, it was first necessary to determine whether this procedure would be able to detect paraproteinemia and paraproteinuria with the sensitivity of high-resolution agarose gel electrophoresis (HRAGE). In addition, it was critical to find out whether CZE or a modification thereof could be used to replace the agarose

From: *Clinical and Forensic Applications of Capillary Electrophoresis*
Edited by: J. R. Petersen and A. A. Mohammad © Humana Press Inc., Totowa, NJ

immunofixation method used in the identification of paraproteins. It was also important to determine if CZE could be used to detect the presence of protein in urine, especially free-light chain or Bence Jones protein (BJP).

The answer to these questions came after considerable research was done in the academic as well as commercial environment. To date there are two instruments on the market that have been approved by the United States Food and Drug Administration (FDA) for the separation of serum proteins, the Bio-Rad Bio-Focus 2000™ and Beckman Coulter's Paragon CZE 2000. Only one, the Beckman Coulter Paragon CZE(2000, is approved for the identification of paraproteins. To date neither instrument has been approved for the identification of protein in urine or other body fluids (e.g., cerebrospinal fluid). Various authors, however, have reported methods on research platforms that can measure urine proteins as well as cerebrospinal fluid proteins.

Monoclonal gammopathies (MG) are seen as bands of restricted mobility after separation of serum has been completed. However, not all proteins of restricted mobility (PRM) are MGs. MGs are produced when a single clone of a cell proliferates producing an immunoglobulin molecule, or portion thereof. These proteins are also known as paraproteins, monoclonal (MC) proteins or simply (M) proteins.

If seen in the serum MGs are an indication of "B" lymphocyte expansion, which may indicate monoclonal gammopathy of undetermined significance (MGUS), multiple myeloma (MM), Waldenstrom's disease, plasmacytoma, heavy chain disease, light chain disease, lymphoproliferative disorders, or primary amyloidosis. They may be also related to immune complexes such as seen in cryoglobulinemia, pyroglobulinemia, and various antigen/antibody complexes.

With the increased sensitivity of the new electrophoretic methods, small PRMs are being found more often. Often the question is asked, "Are these small PRMs seen in the gamma or near gamma gobulin region important enough to alert the clinician of their presence?" The answer to this question is always yes. In most instances the patient history or symptomology is not available to the laboratorian, nor is it known if a condition that could be just starting has been found. If this condition has just started it needs to be followed over subsequent months/years. Small PRMs may also be an indication of "B" cell lymphoproliferative disease, primary amyloidosis, light-chain disease, or other previously undiagnosed disease. When a PRM is found,the laboratorian should follow up with some type of identification procedure. The incidence of the PRMs, which is usually a MGUS, is approx 1% of people over 50 yr of age and 3% in those over 70.

Kyle *(1)* has reported that 20–25% of MGUS patients will develop some type of malignant disease within a 24–35 yr time-span. Once identified follow-up studies should be performed every 3 mo for the first year. If no change has occurred during that period, tests should be repeated every year or else left up to the discretion of the physician. The important consideration is that the monoclonal protein has not increased over 5 g/L between studies. Treatment of the patient is usually not instituted unless this elevation occurs because of the possibility of exacerbating the clonal expansion.

The measurement of MC proteins is best done by serum protein electrophoresis (SPE) and not by immunoassay, for the reasons mentioned in Chapter 4. This is because immunoassay may not give an accurate measurement of the levels of MC. Also, because of problems with immunoassay, comparison of the levels of the MC by SPE and immunoassay should not be made, because the levels may not correlate. In addition, MC over 50 g/L should be diluted 1:2 *(2)*.

The evaluation of urine for MC is also mandated when the SPE pattern exhibits hypogammaglobulinemia, that may signal light-chain disease. In this situation, it is necessary to obtain a 24-h specimen or at least a first morning specimen for urine electrophoresis. If the electrophoresis is negative for a peak in the gamma or beta region, immunofixation to look for free kappa and lambda light chains is indicated. This is because free light chains may not be seen by electrophoresis alone.

3. COMPARISON OF CZE WITH HRAGE

Chapter 4 discussed the classification of serum protein dyscrasias using CZE and HRAGE. This chapter covers paraproteinemia and the comparison of CZE vs HRAGE. CZE appears to offer an alternative to HRAGE for the detection of paraproteinemias in serum. When we used the Paragon CZE 2000, we obtained a 100% concordance between CZE and HRAGE in the detection of monoclonal gammopathies *(3)*. However this was only when the paraproteins were within the detection limits of HRAGE: IgG 0.5 g/L, IgA 0.75 g/L, and IgM 0.75 g. In instances when the paraprotein band falls within the transferrin band it is sometimes difficult to identify by HRAGE. However, with CZE it is usually obvious due to a separate peak being seen along side the transferrin band. As discussed in Chapter 4, with computer accusation of the data it is possible to magnify specific areas in the electropheorgram making it is possible to see the separate banding. (Fig. 1A–E)

In a recent study of 1,518 serum samples CZE detected a MC protein in 204 CZE patterns vs 195 by HRAGE *(4)*. It was reported that the increased sensitivity of CZE as a screening test was due to the detection of 3 IgA M

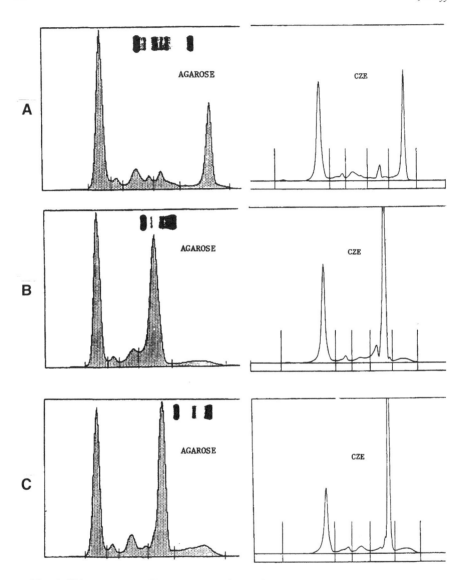

Fig. 1. (A) Agarose vs CZE patterns of an IgG lambda monoclonal gammopathy. **(B)** Agarose vs CZE patterns of an IgA kappa monoclonal gammopathy. **(C)** Agarose vs CZE patterns of an IgM kappa monoclonal gammopathy.

proteins in the beta region, 4 small monoclonal free light chains and 4 small M proteins superimposed on a polyclonal background. None of these were seen on HRAGE, giving sensitivities for CZE and HRAGE of 95% and 91%, respectively.

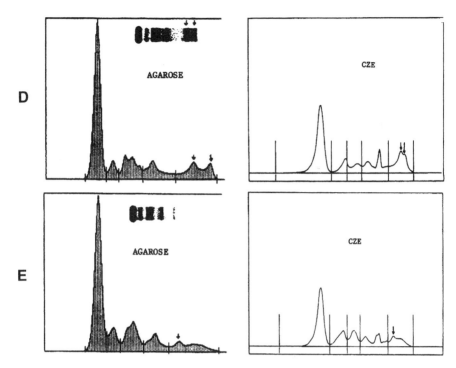

Fig. 1. *(continued)* **(D)** Agarose vs CZE patterns of a biclonal IgG kappa gammopathy. **(E)** Agarose vs. CZE of an acute inflammatory pattern with a pseudomonoclonal gammopathy that is identified as C-reactive protein.

Heskens et al. *(5)* used the Beckman Coulter P/ACE 5000 system to detect 70 of 74 MC proteins as detected by agarose gel electrophoresis. Similar results were seen by Bossuyt et al. *(6)* who looked at 58 serums that had been previously identified as having an M component. They detected MC proteins in 93% of the serums using Beckman Coulter's Paragon CZE 2000 unit compared to 74% by cellulose acetate electrophoresis and 86% by HRAGE. Clark et al. *(7)* also examined 305 serum samples for the presence of a monoclonal gammopathy using the Beckman P/ACE 5510 unit and compared the results with those found by HRAGE. They found that CZE detected 100% of the paraproteins detected by HRAGE.

Jenkins et al. *(7)* were able to correctly identify all 76 paraproteinemic samples, previously identified by HRAGE, using an Applied BioSystems CZE unit. They claimed that the CZE procedure was more sensitive in the detection of IgA paraproteins in the beta region. However, two cases of an IgM paraproteinemia were not detected by their procedure that were identified by HRAGE. In another report by Jenkins et al. *(9)* the results obtained by CZE and HRAGE were compared for 1000 clinical specimens that contained 362 specimens containing monoclonal proteins whose concentrations ranged from 1 to 71 g/L. They found a correlation of 0.96 between HRAGE and CZE. In this case three IgA M proteins were detected by CZE but not by HRAGE because of their presence in the transferrin band. However, two IgM monoclonal bands were detected by HRAGE but not by CZE. In addition, one of 11 light chains was not detected by CZE.

Doleman et al. *(10)* in a study of 250 outpatients reported excellent concordance between HRAGE and CZE. However, 19 patients had an IgM paraprotein that was not detected by CZE. Once identified by HRAGE, however, the paraproteins were visible on the CZE electrophorogram. This implies that there is a steep learning curve in CZE interpretation that must occur before it can be used as an alternative to HRAGE in the clinical laboratory.

It is evident from the published data that CZE offers an excellent alternative to HRAGE for the screening of serum samples to detect paraproteinemia. However, one must realize that any one method may not be acceptable as a final interpretative procedure for paraproteinemia. Reliance on a back-up procedure, such as immunofixation electrophoresis, HRAGE, polyacrylamide gel electrophoresis, and two-dimensional electrophoresis, may be necessary for the study of any paraprotein.

4. IMMUNOFIXATION ELECTROPHORESIS VS IMMUNOSUBTRACTION

Immunofixation electrophoresis (IFE) is in all probability the "gold standard" for the detection of monoclonal gammopathies in the clinical laboratory and to identify the type as well as the heavy- and light-chain class. It has also replaced the classical immunoelectrophoresis because of its simplicity of interpretation. In addition, it is also an extremely sensitive procedure because of the combination of two proteins, antigen and antibody, which increases the amount of dye uptake almost 10-fold. Such sensitivity must be utilized when looking at an extremely small amount of protein or one hidden in an otherwise heterogeneous amount of background immunoglobulin. However, as with any immunologic method, attention to the Heidelberger equivalency curve of antigen or antibody excess must be considered when interpreting the procedure. Either antigen or antibody excess may render the precipitin band unreadable. This is especially true with Bence Jones proteins in urine IFE studies.

In capillary electrophoresis (CE), the technique of simple IFE was not practical. However, modification of the immunosubtraction electrophoresis method of Aguzzi et al. *(11)* by Klein et al. *(12)* allowed specific protein

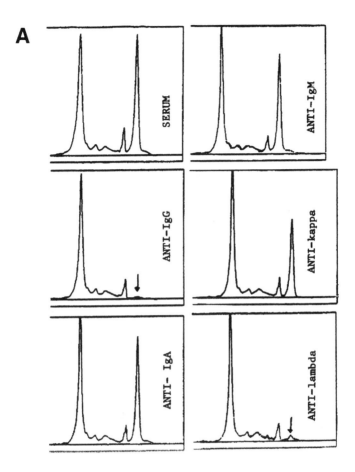

Fig. 2. (A) Immunosubtraction patterns of an IgG lambda monoclonal gammopathy.

identification by CZE. This method of immunosubtraction uses IgG, IgA, IgM, kappa- and lambda-specific antibodies attached to sepharose beads. The serum is mixed and incubated with sepharose beads coated with antiserum to specific proteins. After removal of the sepharose beads along with the specific protein attached to the beads, the remaining serum proteins are separated by CZE. The absence of the specific protein identifies the protein of restricted mobility when compared to the original CZE pattern (*see* Fig. 2A–C).

Using this technique for identification of monoclonal peaks has also allowed for the possibility of automation. This time-saving addition was welcome in laboratories performing large numbers of these procedures. IFE,

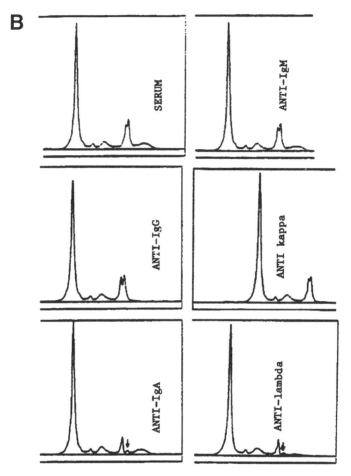

Fig. 2. (B) Immunosubtraction patterns of an IgA lambda monoclonal gammopathy.

however, still remains as a necessary back up if the MC protein falls below the detection limit of the CZE.

5. URINE PROTEINS

Currently, no CZE methods have been approved for the separation of urine proteins by the FDA. Various authors, however, have developed techniques that have used CZE to separate urine proteins. These reports may well help in the eventual introduction of such methods. A limiting factor appears to be salt concentration of urine as well as degraded protein fragments, which can present a very confusing picture.

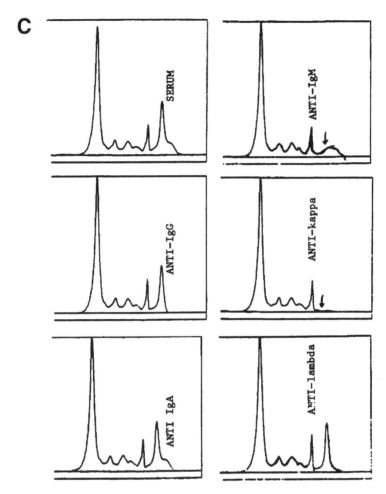

Fig. 2. (C) Immunosubtraction patterns of an IgM kappa monoclonal gammopathy.

Jellum et al. *(13)* used a Hewlett-Packard HP 3D CZE unit with a built-in diode array detector to analyze urine. The capillary had an effective length of 56 cm (injector to detector) with an internal diameter of 50 µm. The light path was 150 µm using a bubble cell at the detector site. The buffer used was 300 mM borate, pH 8.3, and a potential of 30 kV employed. The urine was injected into the capillary without preconcentration or pretreatment. Because there was no preconcentration the method did not detect albumin, transferrin or other proteins that are usually observed in glomerular or tubular proteinemia. Rather, only metabolites that are found in various metabolic disorders were detected.

The most promising work in the detection of urine proteins by CZE has been by Jenkins et al. *(14)* who identified albumin and Bence Jones protein in urine. The results were compared to HRAGE with correlation coefficients of 0.93 and 0.95, respectively. A BioSystems CZE model 2027A HT was used and urine concentrated 100× in a Minicon B-15 concentrator, after which it was diluted 1:50 in the assay buffer. Anionic species were then removed from the specimens with Dowex 2 ion-exchange resin obtained from Sigma (St. Louis, MO) (1 g in 1 mL of deionized water). A 1:1 mixture of urine and Dowex is prepared and allowed to stand for 30 min. After centrifugation at 9500g for 2 min, 20 µL of supernatant is mixed with 60 µL assay buffer. Separation time was 18 min at 18 kV in a fused silica capillary, 72 cm × 50 µm I.D with detection was at 200 nm. The buffer was 150 mM boric acid and 1 mM calcium lactate at pH 9.7. This method is used routinely in their laboratory for the quantitative analysis of urinary proteins.

6. ADVANTAGES AND DISADVANTAGES OF CZE

For the separation of paraproteins in serum, CZE is comparable to HRAGE. The separations obtained by CE in the beta globulin region where transferrin can potentially interfere with IgA MC proteins appear to be superior to HRAGE. This also appears to be true for IgM MC proteins.

No application artifacts are seen with the CZE procedure and the concentrations of the proteins in the individual peaks are not dependent on staining differences for the individual proteins. This is particularly important in following patients with monoclonal disorders. Coefficients of variation within capillaries and between capillaries are low and well within acceptable limits. In addition, the ability to overlay a normal serum and to generate a gel-simulated pattern on the Beckman system, as well as being able to magnify an area, is especially helpful in examination for paraproteinemia.

The immunosubtraction procedure is excellent and compared well with immunofixation on agarose. However, the agarose IFE will detect smaller amounts of protein and is superior for the detection of small amounts of Bence Jones protein in urine or serum. Small monoclonal bands in the IgM region are also been best seen by immunofixation on agarose.

MC arising in the very cathodic portion of the HRAGE patterns may not be detectable on CZE *(15)*. This may be a phenomenon of lipoprotein binding to the MC protein because these particular proteins stain with lipid dyes on agarose gels *(16)*. This can be circumvented as indicated by Jenkins et al. *(15)*. Also there are no commercial kits available that can check for IgD and IgE MC proteins if only a light chain is seen on the serum CZE pattern. This is not too important in that such conditions are rare and can be ruled out by immunofixation on agarose with the specific antiserum.

Finally, identification of urinary paraproteinuria is at the present time not available on existing CZE units in the United States. This can be a disadvantage with the specifically dedicated serum protein units since another smaller unit would be needed in investigate the urine.

7. CONCLUSION

CZE offers an alternative way of evaluating serum samples for paraproteinemias. The two automated instruments available and approved by the FDA offer a time saving and labor saving approach to these assays. There are a number of other instruments that have greater flexibility with regard to various parameters such as temperature, time of separation, changes in buffer, and capillary size. However, these instruments are considered research platforms and as such can offer a great number of methods, examining such analytes as hemoglobin, amino acids, drugs, and other clinically important substances.

The main advantage of CZE is its ability to screen large numbers of specimens with very little hands-on time at a relatively low cost per test. This is because only buffer and rinse solutions are needed to separate proteins. IFE/immunosubtraction on the other hand, requires the use of anti-immunoglobulin sepharose bead units and increases the time necessary to produce a result. However, immunosubstration CZE can still produce results faster than the current IFE used in the clinical laboratory.

Not only is the detection of the paraproteinemias automated by the Beckman Coulter Paragon CZE 2000 instrument, but also their classification. In our hands, as well as in others, excellent correlation with the HRAGE is obtained. Instruments for urine, cerebrospinal fluid, and other body fluids will no doubt be forthcoming in the future on the two available clinical models, which will further aid in the detection and classification of the paraproteinemias.

REFERENCES

1. Kyle, R. A. (1993) Benign monoclonal gammopathy: after 20–35 years of follow up. Mayo Clin. Proc. 68, 26–36.
2. Chang, C.-Y., Fritsche, H. A., Classman, A. B., Mc Clure, K. C., and Liu, F. J. (1997) Underestimation of monoclonal proteins by agarose gel serum protein electrophoresis. Ann. Clin. Lab. Sci. 27, 123–129.
3. Jolliff, C. R. and Blessum, C. R. (1997) Comparison of serum protein electrophoresis by agarose gel and capillary zone electrophoresis in a clinical setting. Electrophoresis 18, 1781–1784.
4. Katzmann, J. A., Clark, R., Sanders, E., Landers, J. P., and Kyle, R. A. (1998) Prospective study of serum protein capillary electrophoresis immunotyping of monoclonal proteins by immuno-sutraction. Amer. J. Clin. Path. 110, 503–509.

5. Henskens, Y., DeWinter, J., Pekelharing, M., and Ponjee, G. (1998) Detection and identification monoclonal gammopathies by capillary electrophoresis. Clin. Chem. 44, 1184–1190.
6. Bossuyt, X., Bogaerts, G., Shciettekatte, G., and Blanckaert, N. (1998) Detection and classification of paraproteins by capillary immunofixacion/subtraction. Clin. Chem. 44, 760–769.
7. Clark, R., Katzmann, J.A., Wiegert, E., Namyst-Goldberg, C. S., Oda, R. P., Kyle, R. A., and Landers, J. P. (1996) Rapid capillary electrophoretic analysis of human serum proteins: comparison with high throughput agarose gel electrophoresis. J.Chromarogr. A 744, 205–213.
8. Jenkins, M. A. and Guerin, M. D. (1995) Quantification of serum proteins using capillary electrophoresis. Ann. Clin. Biochem. 32, 493–497.
9. Jenkins, M. A., Kulinskaya, E., Martin, H. D., and Guerin, M. D. (1995) Evaluation of serum protein separation by capillary electrophoresis: prospective analysis of 1000 specimens. J. Chromatogr. B 672, 241–251.
10. Doleman, C. J. A., Siebelder, C. W. M., and Penders, T. J. (1997) Routine serum protein analysis using capillary electrophoresis. Eur. J. Clin. Chem. Clin. Biochem. 35, 393–394.
11. Aguzzi, F. and Poggi, N. (1997) Immunosubtraction electrophoresis. A single method for identifying specific proteins producing the cellulose acetate electropherogram. Ann. Clin. Biochem. 32, 493–497.
12. Klein, G. L. and Jolliff, C. R. (1994) Capillary Electrophoresis for the Routine Clinical Laboratory, Landers, J. P., ed. CRC, Boca Raton FL.
13. Jellum, E., Dollekamp, H., Brunsvig, A., and Gislefoss, R. (1997) Diagnostic applications of chromatography and capillary electrophoresis. J. Chromatogr. B 689, 155–164.
14. Jenkins, M. A., O'Leary, T. D., and Guerin, M. D. (1994) Identification and quantitation of human urine proteins by capillary electrophoresis. J. Chromatogr. B 662, 108–112.
15. Jenkins, M. A. and Guerin, M. D. (1996) Optimization of serum protein separation by capillary electrophoresis (Letter). Clin. Chem. 42, 1886.
16. Blessum, C. R. (1998) Personal communication.

6
Cerebrospinal Fluid Protein Electrophoresis

John R. Petersen and Amin A. Mohammad

1. INTRODUCTION

Cerebrospinal fluid (CSF), a clear colorless fluid with a viscosity similar to water, is produced at a rate of approx 500 mL p/d. The volume averages 135–150 mL in an adult and approx 40 mL in neonates with a turnover rate of 6 h. Approximately two-thirds of the CSF is secreted by the choroid plexuses, whereas the rest comes from leakage of plasma from the capillary bed found in the central nervous system (CNS) and the metabolism of glucose by cells in the CNS.

The normal protein concentration in the CSF is 150–450 mg/L. These proteins are mainly plasma proteins that passively diffuse across the blood-brain barrier *(1)* at a rate that is dependent on the plasma and CSF concentrations, is inversely proportional to the molecular weight, and is dependent on molecular charge. The remainder is locally synthesized within the CNS. Lower molecular weight substances that are uncharged, such as glucose, urea, and creatinine, freely diffuse across the blood–brain barrier, but equilibration can take several hours. Charged small molecules—Na^+, K^+, Ca^{2+}, Mg^{2+}, Cl^-, H^+, and bicarbonate—are actively regulated by specific transport systems.

2. CLINICAL UTILITY OF CSF PROTEIN MEASUREMENT

The analysis of CSF proteins can be useful in the diagnosis and management of a variety of neurological diseases that fall in the following general classifications:

a. Inflammatory conditions that cause a breakdown in the blood–brain barrier;
b. Destructive brain diseases, and
c. Immune response within the CNS.

From: *Clinical and Forensic Applications of Capillary Electrophoresis*
Edited by: J. R. Petersen and A. A. Mohammad © Humana Press Inc., Totowa, NJ

Of these conditions, the most important is detection of an immune response within the CNS. This is because many diseases produce local immune responses leading to an abnormality of the proteins within the CNS. Analysis can be done either directly, by determining the IgG index to determine if interthecal synthesis of immunoglobulins is occurring, or by electrophoretic methods. In order determine the IgG index, it is necessary to measure the immunolglobulin and albumin levels in the serum as well as the CSF. If the ratio (Eq. 1) is greater than a pre-set level that is established by an individual laboratory (usually between 0.64–0.85) then IgG synthesis is occurring within the CNS.

CSF IgG index (CSF IgG/CSF Albumin)/(serum IgG/ serum albumin)　　(1)

Diagnostically, the significance of the IgG index is based on the observation that 70–90% of patients with multiple sclerosis (MS) have an elevated index when first diagnosed *(2)*. Refinement of the index by calculation of specific immunglobulin synthesis has also been developed *(3)*. However, in most instances the original IgG index gives adequate information to the clinician.

The immune process may also produce a polyclonal and, perhaps more importantly, discrete bands (oligoclonal) in the gamma region when CSF is subjected to electrophoresis. The most important application in the fractionation of CSF is in the diagnosis of MS. It has been found that greater than 90% of all patients with MS have oligoclonal bands, whereas only 70–90% have an elevated IgG index *(2)*. However, by combining oligoclonal banding with the IgG index, >95% of MS cases will be abnormal. Oligoclonal band may also be present in 90% patients with subacute sclerosing panencephalitis *(4)*, 60% of patients with neurosyhilis *(5)*, and 40% of patients of patients with viral or bacterial meningitis *(6)*. Discrete bands in the immunoglobulin region may also be seen in patients with infections or other diseases (e.g., multiple myeloma), thus it is advisable to evaluate serum at the same time as the CSF.

3. ELECTROPHORESIS METHODS

3.1. Gel Electrophoresis

Multiple methods such as agarose gel *(4)*, polyacrylamide *(8)*, isoelectric focusing *(8,9)*, and two-dimensional *(10)* electrophoresis have been described to measure the protein profiles associated with the various diseases of the CNS. All of these methods are labor intensive and require an approx 40-fold preconcentration of the CSF in order for the protein bands to be visualized with the stains used (e.g., Coomassie brilliant blue). Because of problems associated with preconcentration, a method using unconcentrated CSF and

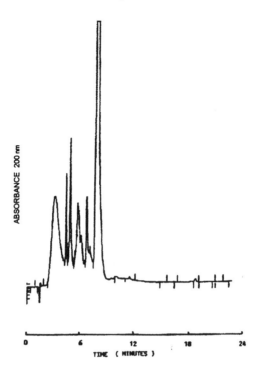

Fig. 1. Typical CSF protein profile using an bare fused silica capillary. Separation buffer was 40 mM borate, pH 10.0, containing 0.4 gL of methyl cellulose. The capillary was 50 μ × 55 cm (35 cm to detection), voltage 25 kV, 30°C, with a 4 s injection of unconcentrated CSF. Reproduced with permission from ref. *(12)*.

silver staining was developed *(11)*. This method has not been used routinely in the clinical laboratory due to the technical difficulties associated with silver staining of the gels. At present of all the methods used for the detection of protein profiles in CSF, agarose gel electrophoresis is probably the most sensitive and routinely used method in the clinical laboratory

3.2. Capillary Electrophoresis (CE)

More recently, capillary electrophoresis (CE) has been used to provide a fast, yet sensitive, method to analyze CSF *(12–14)*. The authors of these articles used a variety of different approaches to analyze CSF.

Crowdrey et al. *(12,13)* analyzed unconcentrated CSF using pH 10.0 borate, buffer, and methylcellulose to minimize electroosmotic flow (EOF). They were able to separate and identify between 20 and 25 peaks (Fig. 1), which included proteins and other components of CSF, under these conditions. Migration of the components of the CSF using these conditions

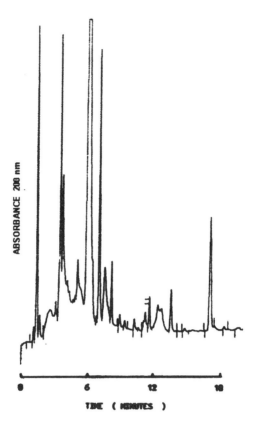

Fig. 2. Typical serum protein profile using a bare fused silica capillary. Separation buffer was 40 m borate, pH 10.0, containing 0.4 gL of methyl cellulose. The capillary was 50 μ × 55 cm (35 cm to detection), voltage 25 kV, 30°C, with a 4 s injection of a 1:5 dilution of serum. Reproduced with permission from ref. *(12)*.

depends on the charge-to-mass ratio, which means that the more acidic components had longer migration times. Using CSF samples from 30 randomly chosen patients, they were able to show differences in the CSF samples. They made no attempt, however, to correlate these differences with disease states. The method was not able to distinguish the fine features in the gamma region when the electropherogram was compared to a serum profile (Fig. 2), making this method unlikely to be used when evaluating a potential MS patient for oligoclonal bands. They were, however, able to detect abnormal proteins in the acidic region (Fig. 3), which may prove to be useful in identifying the underlying pathology of neurologic diseases.

Recently, Sanders et al. *(14)* modified a procedure that had been used to separate serum proteins in order to see if CE could detect oligoclonal bands

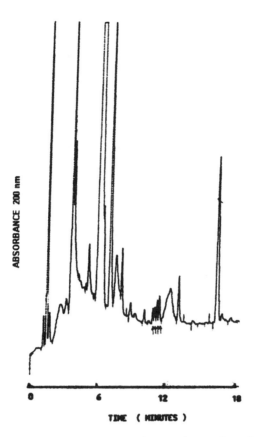

Fig. 3. CSF protein profile that show an abnormal grouping of acidic proteins at approx 11 min using an bare fused silica capillary. Separation buffer was 40 m*M* borate, pH 10.0, containing 0.4 gL of methyl cellulose. The capillary was 50 μ × 55 cm (35 cm to detection), voltage 25 kV, 30°C, with a 4 s injection of unconcentrated CSF. Reproduced with permission from ref. *(12)*.

in CSF from patients with MS. Similar to Crowdrey et al. they also used a high pH (9.25) borate buffer. However, to control EOF they used polyethylene glycol (PEG; MW 8000) and *O*-phosphorylethanolamine (O-PEA) instead of methylcellulose. Using this buffer combination to compare the electropherogram from the CSF (40-fold concnetration) and serum from the same patient they were able to identify oligoclonal bands (Fig. 4). This method gave a concordance of 87% with high-resolution agarose gel electrophoresis (HRAGE) in detection of oligoclonal banding. This is excellent because many times detection of oligoclonal banding between laboratories using the same electrophoresis methods may not compare as well.

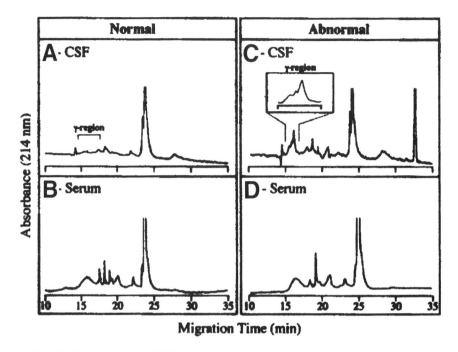

Fig. 4. Separation of CSF (**A** and **C**) that was concentrated as compared to serum (**B** and **D**) that was diluted 1:10. Injection was by pressure (0.5 psi) for 10 s (CSF) or 5 s (serum) in a 75 μ × 87 cm (80 cm to detection) bare fused silica capillary. Separation buffer was 129 m*M* borate, pH 9.25, 0.5% PEG, 75 m O-phosphorylethanolamine. Electrophoresis was at 20 kV with a temperature of 25°C. Reproduced with permission from ref. *(14)*.

Sanders et al. *(14)* also evaluated the ability of CE to identify banding in unconcentrated CSF (Fig. 5). However, because of the lack of sensitivity of their instrumentation, they had to increase the injection volume three- to sixfold over that used for the concentrated CSF. This resulted in a loss of resolution and thus the ability to detect the oligoclonal bands. The authors did speculate that with the newer detection cells (i.e., extended pathlength) that would increase the sensitivity 5–10-fold, a decreased volume of CSF could be injected that may allow detection of the oligoclonal bands.

An interesting feature of the CE method, which uses absorbance at 214 nm to detect the proteins, is the ability to calculate a CSF Ig index. By knowing the total protein concentration of the serum and CSF, the concentration of the albumin and immunoglobulin region can be estimated. Substituting these values into Eq. 1 gives the CSF Ig index. When this result was compared to the result obtained using nephelometry, a good correlation (r = 0.934) was

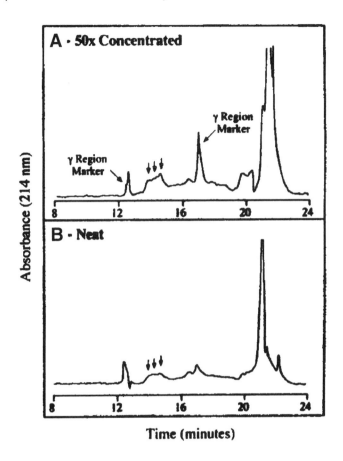

Fig. 5. Comparison of concentrated (50-fold) CSF (**A**) injected for 20 s at 0.5 psi vs unconcentrated CSF injected for 60 s at 0.5 psi. in a 75 μ × 87 cm (80 cm to detection) bare fused silica capillary. Separation buffer was 129 m*M* borate, pH 9.25, 0.5% PEG, 75 m O-phosphorylethanolamine. Electrophoresis was at 20 kV with a temperature of 25°C. Reproduced with permission from ref. *(14)*.

obtained with only 2 discordant results out of 24. This is quite good considering that the immunologic method used unconcentrated CSF, whereas the samples analyzed by CE used CSF concentrated 40- to 60-fold.

4. CONCLUSION

Analysis of proteins and protein profiles in CSF can play an important role in helping the physician identify and sometimes follow the treatment of a disease state. CE may play an important part in speeding up this process by giving additional information that was not previously available, while at the same time reducing the cost of analysis. Although the use of CE to evaluate the protein profiles for abnormalities, such as oligoclonal banding, in CSF appears very promising, it is still in its infancy. Much more work is required, especially in the comparison to current technology (i.e., agarose electrophoresis), in order for CE to be used as a routine method for CSF protein analysis in the clinical laboratory.

REFERENCES

1. Fishman, R. A. (1992) Cerebrospinal Fluid in Diseases of the Nervous System, 2nd ed. W. B. Saunders, Philadelpha, PA.
2. McFarlin, D. E. and McFarlin, H. F. (1982) Multiple sclerosis. N. Engl. J. Med. 307, 1974–1977.
3. Tourtellote, W. W., Haerer, A. F., Fleming, J. O., Murthy, K. N., Levy, J., and Brandes, D. W. (1975) Cerebrospinal fluid (CSF) immunoglobulins-G (IgG) of extravascular orgin in normals and patients with multiple sclerosis (MS): clinical correlation. Trans. Am. Neurol. Assoc. 100, 250–252.
4. Johnson, K. P., Arrigo, S. C., and Nelson, B. J. (1977) Agarose electrophoresis of cerebospinal in multiple sclerosis. Neurology 27, 273–277.
5. Link, H. and Miller, R. (1971) Immunoglobins in muliple sclerosis and infections of the nervous system. Arch. Neurol. 25, 326–344.
6. Olsson, J. E. and Pettersson, B. (1976) A comparsion between agar gel electrophoresis and CSF serum quotients of IgG and albumin in neurological diseases. Acta. Neurol. Scand. 53, 308–322.
7. Epstein, E., Zak, B., Baginski, E. J., and Civin, H. (1976) Interpertation of cerebospinal fluid by gel electrophoresis. Ann. Clin. Lab. Sci. 6, 27–37.
8. Thompson, E. J. (1977) Laboratory diagnosis of multisclerosis: immunological and biochemical aspects. Br. Med. Bull. 33, 28–33.
9. Crowley, G., Gould, B., Rees, J., and Firth, G. (1990) Separation and detection of alkaline oligoclonal IgG band in cerbrospinal fluid using immobilized pH gradients. Electrophoresis 16, 1922–1926.
10. Wiederkehr, F., Ogilivie, A., and Vonderschmitt, D. (1987) Cerbrospinal fluid proteins studied by two-demsional gel electrophoresis and immunoblotting technique. J. Neurochem. 49, 363–372.
11. Mehta, P. D. (1984) Silver staining of unconcentrated cerbrospinal fluid in agarose gel (Panagel) elecctrophoresis. Clin. Chem. 30, 735–736.
12. Cowdrey, G., Firth, M., and Firth, G. (1995) Separation of cerebrospinal fluid proteins using capillary electrophoresis: a potential method for the diagnosis of neurological disorders. Electrophoresis 16, 1922–1926.
13. Cowdrey, G., Firth, M., and Firth, G. (1999) Electrophoresis of cerebrospinal fluid, in Methods in Molecular Medicine, vol. 27: Clinical Applications of Capillary Electrophoresis. Palfrey, S. M., ed., Humana Press, Totowa, NJ.
14. Sanders, E., Katzmann, J. A., Clark, R., Oda, R. P., Shihabi, Z., and Landers, J. P. (1998) Development of capillary electrophoresis as an alternative to high resolution agarose electrophoresis for the diagnosis of multiple sclerosis. Clin. Chem. Lab. Med. 37, 37–45.

7
Lipoprotein Analysis

Rainer Lehmann

1. INTRODUCTION

In the four decades since the first description of the plasma lipoprotein transport system *(1)*, there has been an explosion of knowledge about its component parts, operation, and regulation. Increasingly, the medical community has become aware that defects in lipoprotein metabolism are intimately involved in the pathogenesis of coronary vascular disease (CVD), the major cause of death in most Western countries. Investigations have been made on a broad front, ranging from intensive clinical investigations to fundamental studies on apolipoproteins, the nature and metabolism of lipoprotein, and the action of enzymes and receptors that control the course of lipoprotein metabolism.

The first step in diagnosis of hyper- and hypolipoproteinemias is to define a phenotype (plasma lipoprotein pattern) by chemical analysis of plasma lipids and lipoproteins. Lipoproteins have been separated in at least five different ways, depending on physical, chemical, and immunological properties of the lipid–protein complexes. Lipoproteins are macromolecules with lower hydrated densities than the other plasma proteins, therefore ultracentrifugation (UC), which is also the reference method, has been used to separate various fractions on the basis of differential density *(2–7)*. Lipoproteins can also be separated by gel electrophoresis based on their differing surface charge and molecular size *(8–10)*. They also form insoluble complexes with polyanions and divalent cations and will precipitate by appropriate choice and concentration of polyanions and metal ions *(11–14)*. Lipoproteins may also be separated on the basis of their molecular size by gel or membrane filtration *(15,16)* or isolated by reaction with antibodies to apolipoproteins *(14,17,18)*. Quantification of the various apolipoproteins is predominantly performed by immunoassays *(19,20)*.

From: *Clinical and Forensic Applications of Capillary Electrophoresis*
Edited by: J. R. Petersen and A. A. Mohammad © Humana Press Inc., Totowa, NJ

The aim of this chapter is to provide a short introduction in the topic of lipoprotein metabolism and the clinical relevance of lipoproteins, followed by details of the potential analytical impact of capillary electrophoretic (CE) techniques in this important field. CE methods required for studies on the molecular biology of lipoproteins have not been included (for details on molecular diagnostics, *see* Section 6. or ref. *[21]*).

2. BIOMEDICAL BACKGROUND

2.1. Structure, Classes, and Metabolism of Lipoproteins

Medieval physicians first observed lipoproteins (milky serum) in association with diabetes mellitus, nephrotic syndrome, and overindulgence of alcohol. In the early 1900s studies focused on the metabolism of plasma cholesterol and triglycerides. This approach quickly gave way to the study of the various lipoprotein classes after it was recognized that lipids and cholesterol were merely cargo and that apolipoproteins on the surface of lipoprotein particles were involved in their metabolism.

All of the major lipoprotein particles consist of a shell of amphipathic proteins (apolipoproteins), unesterified cholesterol and phospholipids (hydrophilic on one face and hydrophobic on the other), and a core of triglycerides and cholesterol esters. However, the concentration and characteristics of these particles differ as shown in Table 1. They are classified according to increasing density; chylomicrons (<0.95 g/mL), very low-density lipoproteins (VLDL, 0.95–1.006 g/mL), intermediate-density lipoproteins (IDL, 1.006–1.019), low-density lipoproteins (LDL, 1.019–1.063), and high-density lipoproteins (HDL, 1.063–1.210). Chylomicrons, which are synthesized by and released from the intestinal epithelial cells, consist of more than 80% of triglycerides and are responsible for transporting dietary fat. After release from the epithelial cells, the chylomicrons are metabolized to remnants that are composed mainly of cholesterol. The remnants bind to the hepatic chylomicron-remnant receptor and enter the liver cells, where the proteins are catabolized and cholesterol released. VLDL is a large triglyceride rich particle synthesized by the liver. Normally most of the VLDL is converted to smaller LDL particles through the "VLDL remnants" known as IDL. LDL, a small cholesterol-rich lipoprotein containing only apolipoprotein B-100, has a longer half-life than its precursors, VLDL and IDL. LDL accounts for about 70% of total cholesterol in plasma and is removed from plasma by LDL receptors, which are specific for Apo B-100. The rate of uptake determines plasma LDL concentration and therefore the measured plasma cholesterol concentration. LDL delivers cholesterol to all nucleated cells via endocytosis by the LDL-receptor. HDL, on the other

Table 1
Composition and Properties of Major Lipoprotein Classes

Lipoproteins	Composition (% mass)				Apolipoproteins	Prot./lipid-quotient	Molecular weight (Da) and diameter (nm)	Function	Source
	Chol	PL	TG	Prot					
Chylomicrons	6	4	87	1	A-I, A-IV, B-48, (CI-III, E)[a]	1:100	400,000 kDa >70 nm	Transport	Intestine of dietary fat
VLDL	8–13	6–15	64–80	8–10	A-IV,B-100, C I-III, E	1:11	10,000–80,000 kDa 25–70 nm	Transport of endogenous fat	Liver
LDL	45	25	10	20	B-100, (C, D, E)[a]	1:5	~2300 kDa 19–23 nm	Transport of chol. to peripheral tissues Regulate de novo chol. synthesis	VLDL (via IDL)
HDL	20	30	2–5	48	A-I, A-II, A-IV, C I-III, E	~1:1	~180–1000 kDa 4–10 nm	Transport of cholesterol from peripheral tissues	Liver intestine

Chol, cholesterol; PL, phospholipid; TG, triglyceride; Prot, protein.
[a]The apolipoproteins in brackets are acquired after secretion.

hand, plays an important role in reverse cholesterol transport. A gradient of reverse cholesterol transport is maintained, either by the liver taking up HDL or by transfer via cholesterol ester transferase protein (CETP) of HDL cholesterol ester to Apo B-containing particles, which are also subject to rapid uptake by the liver. Lipoprotein (a) (Lp [a]), whose function is unknown, is also produced by the liver, is similar to LDL, but distinct due to the presence of Apo(a), a glycoprotein with significant homology to plasminogen *(22)*.

Most lipoprotein classes can be separated as discrete subpopulations, e.g. HDL exist in plasma as HDL_1, HDL_2, and HDL_3. These differ in density, size, composition, and physiological function *(4,16,23,24)*. In normal human plasma, the two major subpopulations are HDL_2 and HDL_3. LDL, however, has been separated into at least 12 subfractions *(25–27)* with particle size decreasing with increasing density. The smaller, denser LDL particles seem to be more atherogenic than the larger, lighter particles. Based on the experimental findings, smaller LDL particles have been found to be more susceptible to oxidation in vitro, have a lower binding affinity for the LDL receptors and a lower catabolic rate. They also have a higher concentration of polyunsaturated fatty acids and potentially interact more easily with proteoglycans of the arterial wall *(27)*. For IDL two subpopulations of overlapping density have been isolated *(28)*. Both subpopulations seem to be precursors of two different LDL subclasses. The VLDL subpopulation can be divided into two subspecies, large triglyceride-rich particles and smaller cholesterol ester enriched particles *(28)*. Each of these various classes and subpopulations of lipoproteins play a more or less pivotal role in the pathogenesis of atherosclerosis, some as a risk factor, other as a protective factor. An overview of lipoprotein metabolism is shown in Fig. 1.

2.2. Clinical Relevance and Evaluation of Atherosclerotic Risk

In the 20th century, coronary vascular disease (CVD) has been the major cause of death in the United States. Despite a 26.7% decline in death rates from CVD during the last decade, CVD is still the major cause of death in the Western world *(29)*. In 1995, about one million Americans died of heart and blood vessel diseases (455,152 male deaths and 505,440 female deaths), whereas cancer killed a total of 538,455. The cost of cardiovascular diseases and stroke in 1998 has been estimated at $274.2 billion.

Atherosclerosis is the principal cause of CVD. It is a chronic disease characterized by the focal accumulation of plaque (consisting of cholesterol, lipids, leukocytes, macrophages, smooth muscle cells, and extracellular matrix) in the vessel wall that ultimately leads to obstruction of the lumen through gradual progression, plaque rupture with intraluminal thrombosis, or both *(30)*. If left untreated, atherosclerosis can lead to peripheral vascular dis-

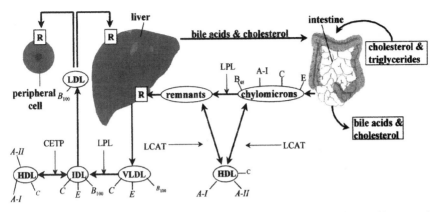

Fig. 1. Pathway of the lipid metabolism (smaller letter size of the apolipoprotein represents lesser quantity). Abbreviations: LPL, lipoprotein lipase; CETP, cholesterol ester transferase protein; LCAT, lecithin:cholesterol acyl transferase; HDL, high-density lipoprotein; VLDL, very low-density lipoprotein; LDL, low-density lipoprotein; B_{100}, apolipoprotein B-100; E, apolipoprotein E; B_{48}, apolipoprotein B-48, A-I, apolipoprotein A-I; A-II, apolipoprotein A-II, C, apolipoprotein C; R, receptor.

ease, heart attack, or stroke. Unfortunately, it is a "silent" disease developing without any symptoms over a long period of time, possibly beginning in childhood. Consequently, early diagnosis to identify individuals at risk is essential.

The importance of serum lipoprotein disturbances as an etiological factor in the development and potentiation of atherosclerosis is now supported by a considerable body of evidence, direct as well as circumstantial, amassed from epidemiological and population studies *(31–35)*. Individuals with atherosclerotic CVD usually have one or more of the four lipoprotein abnormalities: 1) increased LDL, 2) decreased HDL usually associated with increased levels of VLDL, 3) increased level of IDL and chylomicron remnants, and 4) high levels of Lp(a) *(20)*. These abnormalities can be explained by genetic variations in proteins controlling lipid transport: apolipoproteins, processing proteins (lipoprotein and hepatic lipases, cholesterol ester transferase protein, lecithin:cholesterol acyl transferase), and receptors (LDL, chylomicron remnants, and scavenger). LDL oxidation, generated by endothelial cells during LDL transport through arterial walls may also play a proatherogenic role *(22,36,37)*. A new, recently recognized factor associated with a high risk of atherosclerosis is mild hyperhomocysteinemia *(38–41)*. HDL appears to play a protective role by removing cholesterol from peripheral tissues and preventing lipid accumulation in arterial wall. Other main risk factors are hypertension, increasing age, physical inactivity, obesity, smoking, and diabetes mellitus *(42)*.

Lipoprotein metabolism is of particular interest to clinicians involved in diagnosis and treatment of atherosclerosis. Progress resulting in easy-to-handle methods and more detailed informations about the quantitative composition of the various lipoproteins should increase our knowledge and, hopefully, point toward new lines of protection and/or therapy. New analytical methods should facilitate the development of improved screening strategies to help identify individuals that have an increased risk of atherosclerosis.

3. CONVENTIONAL LIPOPROTEIN ANALYSES

In addition to careful history and physical examination, laboratory tests are very important in recognizing and classifying disorders of lipoprotein metabolism by describing lipoprotein profiles and their relation to the risk of CVD. However, measurement of lipids and lipoproteins are among the more difficult and sophisticated clinical laboratory tests and has always presented a challenge to the laboratory.

As a heterogeneous mixture of lipids and proteins, the lipoproteins are not easily defined because significant overlap can exist in the physical properties of the major lipoprotein classes. For example, physical separation, such as chemical precipitation or UC, is the basis for measuring HDL. However, an easy method for the direct measurement of HDL in blood does not exist.

After visual observation of the specimen, the next most useful and reliable tests are determinations of triglyceride and total cholesterol concentrations. These are used as a decision point for the logical progression in the evaluation of a patient suspected of having an abnormality of plasma lipids. However, triglyceride and cholesterol values alone do not address the equally important lipoprotein deficiency states (e.g., decreased HDL levels). It also carries the uncertainty that the atherosclerotic risk will be overestimated in patients with a high cholesterol because of a high HDL cholesterol.

Routine lipoprotein profile consists of measurement of serum cholesterol, triglycerides, LDL-cholesterol (LDL-C), and HDL-cholesterol (HDL-C). This is supplemented in special clinical settings by Lp(a), Apo A-I, and Apo B-100 determination. The routine procedure for lipoprotein quantification is to determine HDL-C in the supernatant after precipitation of apolipoprotein-B-containing lipoproteins (VLDL and LDL), e.g., with dextran sulfate *(11)*. Convenient methods for directly measuring LDL suitable

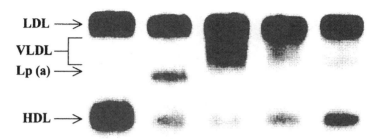

Fig. 2. Agarose gel electrophoresis of sera with different lipoprotein phenotypes (visualization by enzymatic staining of cholesterol). LDL, low-density lipoprotein; VLDL, very low-density lipoprotein; Lp (a), lipoprotein (a); HDL, high-density lipoprotein.

for mass screening are in progress, but not available yet. Currently most routine clinical laboratories estimate LDL-C indirectly using the Friedewald formula: LDL-cholesterol = [total cholesterol] – [total triglycerides/2.2] – [HDL-cholesterol] (mmol/L). This equation holds for triglyceride levels up to, but not above 4.5 mmol/L (400 mg/dl) and becomes inaccurate with increasing IDL levels *(43–46)*. This situation occurs in familial dysbetalipo-proteinemia, diabetes mellitus, chronic renal failure, atherosclerotic vascular disease, and primary biliary cirrhosis. In general, when classifying subjects into categories of CVD risk, LDL cholesterol calculation methods should be used with caution. Perhaps a better, though less used method to quantify HDL-C, Lp(a)-C, VLDL-C, and LDL-C is agarose gel electrophoresis with enzymatic staining for cholesterol *(10)*. All four lipoprotein fractions can be obtained in one run and quantified by a densitometric scan *(see* Fig. 2). This procedure is more time-consuming than precipitation methods, however the method distinguishes between Lp(a)-C and LDL-C and is more accurate than precipitation with respect to LDL-C *(10)*.

Apo A-I and Apo B are usually measured by immunochemical methods. One drawback of immunochemical assays is the influence of the antiserum used, as antibody specificity can lead to appreciable differences in apolipoproteins quantification. Even introduction of an international reference material did not reduce inter-laboratory variability *(47)*.

Epidemiological studies have also suggested that individuals with lower HDL_2-C levels are predisposed to early development of CVD. Thus a significant amount of work has been directed to adapting the polyanion-precipitating reagent technique to HDL subfraction analysis *(12)*. So far, however, no high-throughput method for the analysis of lipoprotein subfractions in clinical routine exists.

In order to understand the complexity of lipoprotein metabolism, methodological advances are required to produce homogeneous lipoproteins in their native forms and to characterize these with respect to both particle size and composition. CE possesses the potential to contribute substantially to a sophisticated diagnosis, prevention, therapy and understanding of atherosclerotic diseases (*see* Section 4.2. and Table 2).

4. LIPOPROTEIN AND APOLIPOPROTEIN ANALYSIS IN RESEARCH AND CLINICAL SETTINGS BY CAPILLARY ELECTROPHORESIS

4.1. Sample Matrix

The matrices of the samples analyzed for lipoprotein and apolipoprotein determination are frequently very complex, e.g., a high total protein concentration, a high content of lipids, a high ionic strength, and so on. Thus, when developing methods it is necessary to focus not only on component separation but also on possible matrix effects. Thus, methods quantifying lipoproteins and apolipoproteins in or isolated from biological specimens have to be sensitive, selective, reproducible, robust, and, for routine clinical use, able to allow a high sample throughput and yield reliable results even in complex matrixes.

A major difficulty in the analysis of highly hydrophobic apolipoproteins is poor solubility or even insolubility in aqueous buffers. This problem can be solved by the use of detergents or organic solvents in the sample buffer (e.g., 20–70% 2-propanol). When using buffers containing organic modifiers, it is crucial to remember that increasing concentrations of organic modifiers decreases the electroendosmotic flow in CE. Thus, at concentrations of 50% of organic solvent, highly hydrophopbic proteins migrate very slowly, resulting in long analysis time and causing peak broadening and reduced mass flow to the detector *(48)*.

The use of detergents to dissolve lipoproteins can also cause problems. This is because the binding of detergent to proteins, including apolipoproteins, alters the Stoke radius and with ionic detergents, the charge of the protein. The number of protein binding sites and the amount of detergent bound in apolipoprotein–detergent complexes are also very important *(49–51)*. When using detergents it is important to realize that the lipids released in the delipidation process can interact with the surfactants in the running buffer. This can produce lipid-loaded micelles generating additional peaks and background in the electropherogram *(52)*. This phenomenon is critical in the CE analysis of the apolipoproteins of VLDL and LDL but can be ignored for HDL *(52,53)*.

4.2. Lipoproteins

4.2.1. Capillary Isotachophoresis

Currently, the major classes of lipoproteins are separated electrophoretically based on their charge, as well as their size, shape, and interaction with supporting medium. The lipoproteins are detected after electrophoresis by nonspecific lipid staining, precipitation with polyanions *(54)*, or enzymatic cholesterol staining *(10,55)*.

In the 1970s and 1980s isotachophoresis in open polytetrafluorethylene-tubes was the dominating "capillary" technique *(56–58)*. As shown in Table 2, it is also the primarily method in the analysis of the various lipoprotein classes by CE *(59–67)*. Capillary isotachophoresis (CITP) is based on the same principle as CZE, except that a discontinuous buffer system is used. This condenses lipoproteins in zones between the leading and terminating constituents. For better separation performance, spacer compounds can be added *(68)*. Quantification is based on the measured zone length, which is proportional to the amount of sample present *(58)*.

Analysis of lipoproteins in "capillaries" was first described in 1981 by Bon et al. *(69)*, demonstrating the preparative isotachophoretic separation of HDL_2 and HDL_3 in a 30-cm long plastic column. In this method the two HDL subclasses were separated into six and ten subfractions. Since then the application of CITP to the analysis of lipoproteins and their subfractions has been intensively evaluated *(59–67)*. A mixture of spacers, such as different mixtures of aminoacids, dipeptides, modified nucleosides, 3-(n-morpholino)-2-hydroxypropanesulfonic acid, and so on, have been tested, enhancing separation *(see* Table 2). Both the composition and concentration of the various spacers define the position of the separated lipoprotein subfractions in CITP. In the first communication on the CITP separation of lipoproteins by Schmitz et al. *(59)*, the resolution of the subfractions was better than the traditional electrophoresis techniques. However, without spacers the separation was not adequate *(59)*. Since then, with a mixture of spacers and different leading and terminating electrolytes, the same group separated 14 distinct lipoprotein subfractions using whole serum or plasma *(60–65)*. Six HDL fractions, chylomicrons, large triglyceride-rich VLDL, small VLDL, IDL, and four LDL fractions were detectable. Visualization of the bands was achieved by pre-incubation (30 min at 4°C) of the serum or ethylenediaminetetraacetic acid (EDTA)-plasma with the nonpolar dye Sudan Black B before injection onto the capillary. The detection was at 570 nm.

CITP-analysis of lipoprotein subclasses isolated by UC from normal, hypercholesterolemic, and hypertriglyceridemic subjects showed that mobility of subclasses does not always correspond to the flotation proper-

Table 2
Survey of Capillary Electrophoretic Applications with Lipoproteins

Detected compounds	Sample	Buffer	Running conditions and capillary	Detection mode	Ref.
Chylomicrons and subfractions of HDL, VLDL, LDL	Serum	Leading electrolyte: 5 mM HCl; 0.2% HPMC, pH 6.5; terminating electrolyte: 10 mM β-alanine, 10 mM histidine, pH 9.0	100 µA for 6 min, then 50 µA for 6 min 500 µm i.d. × 25 cm (PTFE-capillary)	570 nm (prestained with Sudan Black)	(59)
HDL, VLDL, LDL, chylomicrons (all together 14 subpopulations), membrane proteins	Serum, microsome extracts, plasma membranes	Leading electrolyte: 5 mM H_3PO_4; 0.25% HPMC; 20 mM ammediol, pH 9.2 Terminating electrolyte: 100 mM valine; 20 mM ammediol, pH 9.4 Spacer (0.2 mg/mL of each): glycylglycine, alanylglycine, valylglycine, glycylhistidine, histidylleucine, serine, glutamine, methionine, histidine, glycine, 3-methyl-histidine, pseudouridine	Started with 150 µA, than 100 µA, and finally 50 µA 400 µm i.d./15 cm (PTFE-capillary)	570 nm (prestained with Sudan Black)	(60–65)
Lp (a), HDL, LDL, Apo (a)	Commercial standards and UC-isolated lipoproteins	50 mM borate, 3.5 mM SDS, 20% acetonitrile	17.5 kV 75 µm i.d. × 50 cm (uncoated FS-capillary)	214 nm	(71)
HDL, LDL	Commercial standards	Various buffers (sodium-borate, TAPS, and so forth) with different SDS contents	Different voltages 75 µm i.d. × 57 cm. (uncoated FS-capillary)	214 nm	(72)

Lipoprotein	Sample	Electrolyte	Conditions	Detection	Ref
LDL and in vitro oxidized LDL	UC-isolated LDL	40 mM methylglucamine-Tricine, pH 9.0	20 kV 75 µm i.d. × 57 cm (uncoated FS-capillary)	200 nm and 234 nm	(76)
HDL, VLDL, LDL, chylomicrons (all together 14 subpopulations)	Serum	Leading electrolyte: 5 mM HCl; 20 mM ammediol; 0.25% HPMC, pH 6.5 Terminating electrolyte: 20 mM 3-(cyclohexylamino)-1-propane sulfonic acid, pH 10.5 Spacer (final concentration: 56 µg/mL of each): asparatic acid, N,N-bis(2-hydroxyethyl)glycine, N-[2-hydroxyethyl] piperazine-N-9,3-[propane sulfonic acid], glutamine, MOPSO, serine, TAPS, TAPSO, TES, alanylglycine, valylglycine, glycylhistidine	18 kV 180 µm i.d. × 37 cm; (coated FS-capillary)	566 nm (enzymatic cholesterol- or triglyceride-specific staining	(66)
HDL, VLDL, LDL, chylomicrons (all together 9 subpopulations)	Serum	Leading electrolyte: 10 mM HCl, 0.3% HPMC, 17 mM ammediol, pH 8.65 Terminating electrolyte: 20 mM alanine, 17 mM ammediol, pH 10.5 Spacer: ACES, octansulfonic acid, glucuronic acid, N-Tris (hydroxymethyl)methyl-2-aminoethansulfonic acid, N-Tris(hydroxymethyl)methylglycine, N-Tris(hydroxymethyl)methyl-2-aminopropansulfonic acid, serine, glutamine, methionine and glycine	10 kV 180 µm i.d. × 27 cm, (coated FS-capillary)	Ex: 488 nm Em:510nm (LIF), NBD staining	(67)

i.d., inner diameter; PTFE, polytetrafluorethylene; HPMC, hydroxypropylmethyl cellulose; FS, fused silica; MOPSO, 3-(n-morpholino)-2-hydroxypropanesulfonic acid; NBD, 7-nitrobenz-2-oxa-1,3-diazole ceramide in ethylene glycol/DMSO (9:1; v/v; TAPS, N-tris(hydroxymethyl)methyl-3-aminopropane sulfonic acid; TES, n-tris (hydroxymethyl) methyl-2-amino ethane sulfonic acid.

ties of these lipoproteins *(65)*. It was also found that the concentration of the different fractions varied between individuals. Additionally, CITP was able to classify the typical phenotypes of hyperlipoproteinemia *(65)* according to the Frederickson classification *(70)* and World Health Organization (WHO) recommendation. The effects of therapeutic interventions have also been analyzed using CITP *(65)*. It was possible to observe the effects of a 3-hydroxymethylglutaryl (HMG)-CoA reductase inhibitor alone and in combination with bile-acid sequestrants on individual lipoprotein subpopulations. Subpopulations of Apo B-containing lipoproteins in the electropherograms were also shown to be significantly reduced by the HMG-CoA reductase inhibitor. By taking bile-acid sequestrants in addition to the HMG-CoA reductase inhibitor, a further reduction of the Apo B-containing lipoproteins was seen in the CITP separation pattern *(65)*.

Recently, two new approaches of CITP to detect lipoproteins have been described. One, developed by Zorn et al., is to use enzymatic specific staining of the cholesterol or the triglyceride present in the lipoproteins *(66)*. The other method by Schmitz et al., introduced a lipophilic fluorescent dye to stain the lipoproteins *(67)*. Both investigations have been driven by the fact that the lipophilic dye Sudan Black B shows no saturation in lipoprotein staining *(66,67)*.

Following staining of the lipoproteins with cholesterol-specific (cholesterol dehydrogenase and 4-nitrobluetetrazolium) as well as triglyceride-specific staining (glycerol, dihydroxy-acetone, gyceraldehyde, and 4-nitrobluetetrazolium) 14 lipoprotein subfractions were separated by CITP (Fig. 3) with detection at 566 nm. Peaks 1–5 have been identified as HDL subfractions, peaks 8–14 belong to LDL subfractions, and peaks 6–8 include the VLDL fraction and chylomicrons. Peak 8 contains one VLDL and one LDL-fraction. Using triglyceride-specific staining the peaks of the VLDL and chylomicrons dominate (peaks 6–8) whereas cholesterol-specific staining (*see* Fig. 3) causes an increased intensity of the peaks 1–6 (HDL) and 8–14 (LDL).

Following a high lipid diet the electropherograms demonstrate a clear increase in the triglyceride content of peak 6 and 7 (chylomicrons and VLDL) with no significant changes in the HDL and LDL region. After 8 h the triglycerides in subfractions 6 and 7 (VLDL and chylomicrons) shifted to subfractions 8–14 (LDL). In addition, the transition from hypothyroidism to hyperthyroidism also showed a decrease in the cholesterol content of all lipoprotein fractions with the cholesterol-specific staining.

Various fluorescence tagged phospholipid analogs can also be used for specific labeling and quantification of individual lipoprotein classes. The

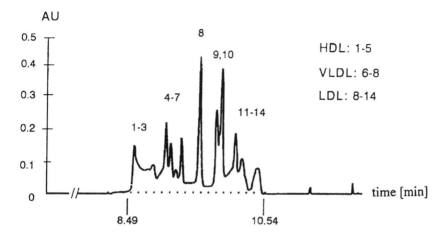

Fig. 3. Capillary isotachophoretic serum lipoprotein profile (enzymatic staining of the cholesterol-content of each lipoprotein subpopulation). Capillary: coated fused silica (37 cm × 180 μm); running conditions: 18 kV; leading electrolyte: 5 mM HCl; 20 mM ammediol; 0.25% HPMC, pH 6.5; terminating electrolyte: 20 mM 3-(cyclohexylamino)-1-propane sulfonic acid, pH 10.5; various spacer have been added to the sample (for details, *see* Table 2); detection: Vis at λ = 566 nm; equipment: Beckman P/ACE 5500. (This figure was kindly provided by Dr. U. Zorn, University of Ulm, Germany.)

compound, 7-nitrobenz-2-oxa-1,3-diazole ceramide (NBD-ceramide), was identified as a good compromise, with respect to saturation and to specific surface area- or particle size-dependent staining. NBD-ceramide, an uncharged, lipophilic dye, labels the phospholipid/cholesterol membrane *(67)*.

The addition of nonfluorescent spacers allows the discrimination of 9 individual lipoprotein subpopulations monitored with laser-induced fluorescence (LIF) detection (ex. 488 nm; em. 510 nm). Four peaks are the result of HDL subpopulations (peak 1–4), one represents chylomicrons (peak 5), and four represent Apo-B containing particles, including VLDL, IDL, and LDL (peak 6–9). An interesting aspect is that analytical CITP is currently the only automatic technique to quantify chylomicrons and IDL particles in human serum. This could be applied to the investigation of the VLDL/IDL subpopulations in patients with CVD *(67)*. The ineffective conversion of VLDL/IDL to LDL by hepatic lipase in CVD patients could also be detected by CITP using LIF detection. Thus CITP allows estimation of highly atherogenic IDL particles simultaneously with HDL and LDL cholesterol levels, improving the estimation of atherosclerotic risk factors *(67)*.

Results of lipoprotein analysis by CITP of 52 patient samples were compared with routine techniques for HDL and LDL quantification *(67)*. Comparison of the results gave correlation's of r = 0.9 and 0.91, respectively, for HDL-C and LDL-C (equations: HDL_{CITP} = 3 + total cholesterol × relative peak area$_{HDL}$/1.53; LDL_{CITP} = –25 + total cholesterol (relative peak area$_{LDL}$/ 0.73). CITP enables the simultaneous quantification of HDL- and LDL-cholesterol within 7 min *(67)* and can be performed on whole serum, plasma, or other biological fluids. Furthermore, CITP analysis of serum lipoprotein patterns may significantly improve the diagnosis of disorders in lipoprotein metabolism (compare Figs. 2 and 3).

In addition to quantification of various lipoprotein subpopulations, CITP allows insight into plasma lipoprotein metabolism. This is done by estimation of the major lipolytic enzyme activities by looking at the appropriate precursor and product. This means the ratio between precursor and product lipoprotein peaks is influenced by a specific lipolytic enzyme thus allowing estimation of lipoprotein conversion rates.

Currently it is difficult to directly quantify HDL by conventional techniques. Most laboratories estimate HDL levels by measuring cholesterol after precipitation of VLDL and LDL with various polyanions (e.g., heparin and manganese chloride). Using CITP prestained (Sudan Black B-, enzymatic-, or fluorescence-stained) serum, lipoproteins can be separated into 9–14 subpopulation and quantified within 7–15 min. The ability of CITP to separate the various lipoproteins is far superior to the results of the current routine procedures. Whether interpretation of this very complex lipoprotein separation pattern adds anything to every day clinical practice has yet to be determined.

CITP has the potential to improve the classification of lipoprotein patterns and to relate it to the risk of CHD. It could permit new insight into pathobiochemistry, etiology, and diagnosis of disorders of lipoprotein metabolism. Furthermore, it has the potential to be used for lipoprotein monitoring during drug therapy, as well as micro-preparation of various lipoprotein subpopulations for further investigations.

4.2.2. Micellar Electrokinetic Capillary Chromatography and Capillary Zone Electrophoresis

Micellar electrokinetic capillary chromatography (MEKC) and capillary zone electrophoresis (CZE) represent other options for the analysis of lipoproteins (*see* Table 2). The addition of a micellar agent, such as sodium dodecyl sulfate (SDS), to the running buffer allows the solubilization of neutral, hydrophobic analytes as well as ion pairs with opposite charge. Two basic principles have to be kept in mind when analyzing lipoproteins by MEKC or CZE: 1) operating at pH values above the *pI* of the lipoprotein particles, leads to negatively charged lipoproteins, keeping them from com-ing in contact with the surface of the fused silica capillary due to repulsion by the negatively charged surface, and 2) the addition of a detergent like SDS to the running buffer at a concentration that will not cause delipidation, enhances the migration of the lipoprotein particles due to incorporation of the detergent.

Cruzado et al. tested various buffers and detergent additives, as well as organic modifiers to achieve an adequate MEKC separation of the various lipoprotein fractions *(52,53,71–73)*. They found that at high pH values HDL and LDL were found to have nearly identical mobilities in different buffers and ionic strengths *(72)*. Addition of SDS or acetonitrile was found to influence significantly the electrophoretic behavior of HDL (high surface polarity) and LDL (low surface polarity). Decreasing the polarity of the running buffer by the addition of acetonitrile resulted in the retaining of an increased amount of SDS by the more hydrophobic LDL particles over the HDL particles. This increases the difference in electrophoretic mobility of both particles. Other lipoproteins like Lp(a) and its reduction products, Lp(a⁻) and Apo(a), can also be separated with sodium borate buffer containing SDS and acetonitrile (for details, *see* Table 2). Under these conditions, LDL and HDL have consistent electrophoretic mobilities that are significantly different from both Lp(a) and Lp(a⁻) *(52,71)*.

Oxidative modifications of LDL appear to be the pathophysiological mechanism implicated in early atherogenesis. Oxidized LDL may also induce several pro-atherogenic mechanisms, such as the regulation of vascular tone by interfering with nitric oxide, in addition to the stimulation of cytokines, chemotactic factors, and transcription factors *(74)*. In view of increasing interest in the role of LDL oxidation in the pathogenesis of atherosclerosis, there is clearly a need for improved methods to evaluate lipoprotein oxidation *(75)*. A recent report by Stocks and Miller *(76)* described a sophisticated CZE procedure using methylglucamine-Tricine buffer to monitor the in vitro oxidation of LDL, which can be initiated by incubation with transition metal catalysts such as Cu^{2+} ions or by exposure to free-radical generating agents. LDL oxidation is characterized by an increase in the electrophoretic mobility as previously shown in agarose gels (77) and an increase in absorbance at 234 nm *(76)*. CZE showed a marked improvement in peak resolution and recovery of LDL relative to earlier MEKC methods *(52,71–73)*. The procedure provides a rapid, sensitive, and precise way of measuring the electrophoretic mobility of LDL (one of the more reliable indicators of LDL modification) with a very high precision (coefficient of variation < 1%). The progressive increase in the electronegativity of LDL particles that occurs during Cu^{2+}-catalyzed auto-oxidation of LDLs, or during reaction with malondialdehyde, can be readily monitored by CZE *(76)*. In addition, the spectral changes, induced by an increase in absorption at 234 nm resulting from the oxidation of fatty acids and cholesterol, can be monitored simultaneously. However, the applicability of the CE technique for the investigation of changes in LDL in vivo has yet to be proved.

Although MEKC is a much easier procedure to run than CITP, the resolving power is not as good. Similar to lipoprotein analysis by agarose gel electrophoresis (Fig. 2), the lipoproteins HDL, VLDL, LDL and Lp(a) can be separated as single peaks, but the subfractions cannot be detected *(52,71–73)*. So far experiments have been performed only with mixtures of UC-isolated lipoproteins. Because the plasma HDL content is usually quantified indirectly as HDL-cholesterol, the MEKC analysis of lipoproteins in serum, prestained plasma, or directly by UV detection, would have a potentially great impact on the routine clinical laboratory diagnosis of dyslipidemias. Contrary to precipitation procedures, the linear relationship of protein concentration to absorption between 195–230 nm guarantees valid quantification. This is because the signal is mainly dependent on the absorption of the peptide bond concentration as long as "Beer-Lambert law" is valid *(78)*.

The conventional way to measure the increase in absorption of oxidized LDL spectrophotometrically can lead to conflicting results, as the compounds added to inhibit or promote oxidation can also contribute significantly to UV absorption. Using electrophoretic separation of the oxidized LDL particles by CZE, these effects can be avoided.

4.3. Apolipoproteins

Apolipoproteins play a pivotal role in lipid homeostasis. Recent publications have suggested that cardiovascular risk profile may be more reliable based on apolipoprotein levels rather than lipid composition of the lipoproteins *(32,79)*. Usually apolipoprotein levels are measured by automated immunoturbidimetric or immunonephelometric assays *(80,81)* For smaller amounts of sample (e.g., in biomedical research) radial immunodiffusion *(82,83)*, rocket electroimmunoassay *(83–86)*, enzyme-linked immunosorbent assay *(87–91)*, or radioimmunoassay *(89,92)* can be used. A general drawback of all immunological determinations of apolipoproteins is caused by the differences in the antibody specificities and epitope recognition *(19,93–95)*. In addition, lipids may mask antigenic sites affecting immunoreactivity *(19,96,97)*. Thus, quantification of apolipoproteins is influenced by the antisera, sample, and methodology used in a particular assay system. This can result in appreciable differences in the amount of each apolipoprotein measured. Examples of completely different, antibody-independent ways to quantify apolipoproteins are: 1) the semi-quantitative densitometric evaluation of stained protein bands on a gel *(98,99)*, and 2) to measure the direct UV signal of the polypeptide bonds at 195–230 nm. In general, the most popular techniques to separate and detect proteins directly nowadays are high-performance liquid chromatography (HPLC) and CE.

Surfactants are the main features of CE analysis of apolipoproteins (*see* Table 3), because the electrophoretic behavior of apolipoproteins is strongly influenced and can be modified by addition of detergent or organic solvents to the running buffer. At concentrations of ≥3.5 mM SDS, lipoproteins are delipidated *(100)*. Knowing this, careful attention should be paid to the fact that lipids released in the delipidation process can associate with the surfactants in the running buffer, producing lipid-loaded micelles. This can generate additional peaks and increased background in the electropherogram *(52)*. This phenomenon is crucial for the apolipoproteins of VLDL and LDL but can be ignored for HDL *(52,53)*.

Tadey and Purdey *(51,101)* performed the fundamental experiments at the beginning of the 1990s. They investigated the influence of various detergents and detergent concentrations, as well as pH on the MEKC separation profile and the migration behavior of apolipoproteins A-I, A-II, B-100, B-48, and C-III from HDL, VLDL and LDL *(51,101)*. The analyses were performed on UC-isolated lipoproteins. Optimal resolution of HDL and LDL apolipoproteins can be achieved by the use of anionic surfactants. Both anionic and cationic detergents (SDS and cetyltrimethylammonium bromide) improve the separation profile of VLDL apolipoproteins. Seven different components of VLDL could be distinguished (not all have yet been identified).

Since then a number of reports using CE to analyze apolipoproteins has followed *(52,53,73,86,102–106)*. The apolipoproteins from HDL (Apo A-I and Apo A-II) gave a very fast and clear-cut separation *(51–53,73,86,101–104,106)*. Using MEKC Apo A-I is separated into two peaks (one major and a small peak) and Apo A-II can be separated into four different fractions (Fig. 4). The heterogeneity in Apo A-II has been previously observed by isoelectric focusing (IEF) showing one major and several minor isoforms *(107)*. Cruzado et al. confirmed this by a detailed characterization of the apolipoproteins from HDL by using a combination of MEKC, reversed-phase HPLC (RP-HPLC), and matrix assisted laser desorption/ionization mass spectrometry (MALDI-MS) *(53)*. They also looked at electropherograms of HDL before and after delipidation and found no differences, meaning that prior delipidation is not required for analysis of these apolipoproteins *(53)*. On the other hand, delipidation of VLDL and LDL

Table 3
Survey of Capillary Electrophoretic Applications with Apolipoproteins

Detected compounds	Sample	Buffer	Running conditions and capillary	Detection mode	Ref.
Apo A-I, Apo A-II, Apo B-100, Apo B-48, Apo C-III	Commercial standard and UC-isolated lipoproteins	Borate buffer with various detergent additives (Triton X-100, SDS, sodium deoxycholate, tetradecyltrimethylammonium bromide, cetyltrimethylammonium bromide)	25 kV 75 and 80 cm in length, (uncoated and PAA-coated FS-capillary)	220 nm	*(51,101)*
Apo A-I, Apo A-II	Standards and UC-isolated HDL	eCAP SDS 14-200 kit (Beckman instruments)	14.1 kV 100 μm i.d. × 47 cm, (PAA-coated FS-capillary)	200 nm	*(102)*
Apo A-I, Apo A-II	UC-isolated HDL and LDL	50 mM sodium borate, 3.5 mM SDS (70% purity), 20% (v/v) acetonitrile, pH 9.7	17.5 kV 75 μm × 56.8 cm (uncoated FS-capillary)	214 nm and MALDI-MS	*(53)*
Apo A-I, Apo A-II, Apo C I-III, Apo B-100, Apo(a), LDL, VLDL, HDL,	Commercial LDL, UC isolated Lp(a)	Apolipoprotein separation: 50 mM sodium borate, 3.5 mM SDS (70% purity), 20% (v/v) acetonitrile, pH 9.1 Lipoprotein separation: 50 mM sodium borate, 0.5 mM SDS (99% purity), pH 9.1	17.5 kV 75 μm i.d. × 56.8 cm, (uncoated FS-capillary)	214 nm and ESI-MS	*(52)*

Apo B-100, LDL	UC-isolated LDL	50 mM sodium borate, various detergents (SDS, sodium myristyl sulfate, sodium cetyl sulfate, sodium decyl sulfate, pH 9.1	17.5 kV 75 μm i.d. × 56.8 cm, (uncoated FS)	214 nm	(73)
Apo B-48, Apo B-100	UC-isolated lipoproteins	DSCE protein analysis kit, SDS content increased to 1% (Bio-Rad laboratories)	15 kV 50 μm × 25 cm, (uncoated FS-capillary)	220 nm	(105)
Apo A-I, Apo A-II, Apo A-IV, Apo E	Commercial standards, UC-isolated HDL	eCAP SDS 14-200 kit (Beckman instruments) or 50 mM Tris, 50 mM Tricine, 6 M urea, pH 8.0	11 or 15 kV 100 μm × 27, 37 or 47 cm, (coated FS-capillary)	214 nm	(86)
Apo A-I, Apo A-II	Commercial standards, UC-isolated HDL, serum	BioRad evaluation buffer (Bio-Rad laboratories)	20 kV 50 μm × 50 cm, (uncoated FS-capillary)	195–220 nm	(103,104)
Apo A-I	Serum	30 mM borate, 0.1% SDS, pH 9.0	12 kV 50 μm × 33 cm, (uncoated FS-capillary)	195 nm	(106)

i.d., inner diameter; FS, fused silica; ESI-MS, electrospray ionization mass spectrometry; MALDI-MS, matrix assisted laser desorption/ionization mass spectrometry; PAA, polyacrylamide; SDS, sodium dodecyl sulfate; UC, ultracentrifugation.

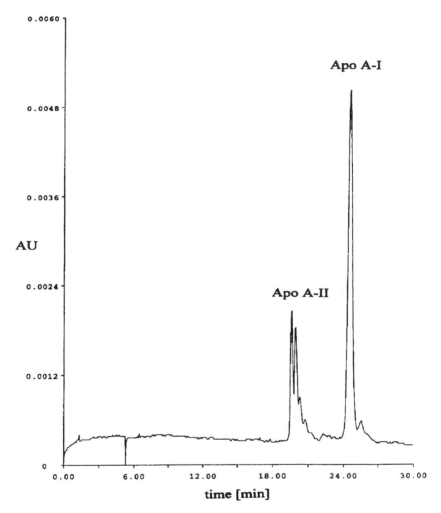

Fig. 4. Capillary electropherogram of a mixture of apolipoprotein A-I and A-II. Capillary: fused silica (50 cm × 50 µm); running conditions: 20 kV; buffer: Bio-Rad LLV evaluation buffer; detection: UV at λ = 220 nm; equipment: Bio-Rad BioFocus 3000 capillary electrophoresis system.

increase the background and generates additional peaks due to the interaction of the released lipids and the surfactant in the buffer *(52)*. This high background prevents the detection of low level apolipoproteins (e.g., Apo E or Apo Cs) *(52)*. To circumvent this problem, they developed a multiple-step procedure in which lipoprotein separated by UC were transferred to a C_{18} reversed-phase liquid-chromatography cartridge. After a series of elu-

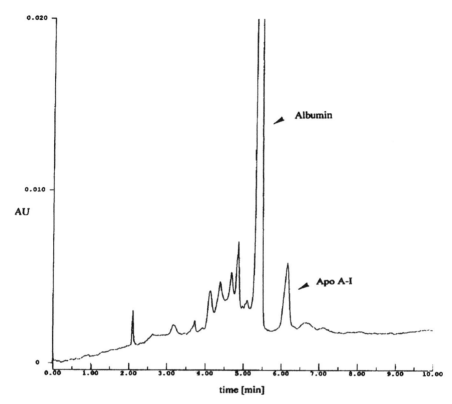

Fig. 5. Serum sample separated by micellar electrokinetic capillary chromatography. Capillary: fused silica (33 cm × 50 μm); running conditions: 12 kV; detection: UV at λ = 195 nm; equipment: Bio-Rad BioFocus 3000 capillary electrophoresis system.

tions, a solution of apolipoprotein in acidified acetonitrile was obtained. During this process, however, Apo B-100 was lost. Goux et al. could demonstrate that in addition to qualitative analyses of HDL apolipoproteins, MEKC could also be used to quantify Apo A-I and A-II *(102)*. Additionally, our group has developed a procedure for the quantification of Apo A-I directly in serum *(103,104,106)* although Apo A-II could not be quantified in serum samples due to the overlap of the albumin and Apo A-II peaks.

Recently we developed a MEKC to analyze routinely Apo A-I levels in human serum. In this study, the MEKC results from 100 samples were compared to the results obtained by a commercial immunonephelometric assay. As shown in Fig. 5, the separation was completed within 8 min, with a reasonable analytical performance *(106)*. Although the detection modes are completely different (CE vs nephelometry) the Apo A-I levels show a linear relationship (slope = 0.93; intercept = + 60; r = 0.59), but the Apo A-I levels for the nephelometric assay are approx 42% higher (mean nephelometry = 160 mg/dL; mean CE = 113 mg/dL). In the area of decreased Apo A-I levels (≤110 mg/dL), associated with a higher atherosclerotic risk, the discrepancy was more obvious. At these levels nephelometry gave values as much as 250% higher than those obtained by CE. At higher levels of Apo A-I both methods gave similar values. Using a certified international Apo A-I reference standard, it was found that the nephelometric results were incorrect. Therefore, it was speculated that individual sample effects, influencing the scattering of light in nephelometry, may be affecting the measurement, especially at low Apo A-I concentrations. The immunonephelometric assay may also be influenced by various polymorphic apolipoprotein forms (over- or underestimation of a specific variant), turbidity of any kind, unspecific binding of the antibody, cross-reactivities, or influences of the sample background *(19,93–97)*. Interference due to hemolysis (free hemoglobin ≤3 g/L) or hyperbilirubinemia (bilirubin ≤714 μmol/L) did not affect the CE results. Also highly lipemic sera (triglyceride ≤27.1 mmol/L), which can not be analyzed by routine immunoassays, gave a well-separated and easy to quantify Apo A-I peak in CE.

Very recently Stocks et al. compared the levels obtained by CZE and MEKC of Apo A-I and Apo A-II isolated by UC from 17 human HDL samples to rocket immunoelectrophoresis *(86)*. Both, the commercial MEKC kit and CZE gave values for Apo A-I and Apo A-II concentrations in human HDL that were in good agreement with those obtained by rocket immuno-electrophoresis. In addition, they showed that the patterns and migration times of rabbit, rat, bovine, and human HDL apolipoproteins (Apo A-I, Apo A-II, Apo A-IV and Apo E) are identical. This is a very important point especially for research projects dealing with animals, because species-specific antibodies that can be difficult to obtain are needed for reliable immunoassay results.

Quantification of Apo B-48 and Apo B-100 may also be useful for metabolic studies, e.g., the potential impact of chylomicron-derived lipids on the hepatic production of lipoproteins *(108)*. The MEKC analysis could be an easy, alternative way to assess chylomicron metabolism in vivo. Currently, the most widely used method (an indirect determination) is to monitor the incorporation and clearance of dietary vitamin A from plasma *(109)*. The peak due to Apo B-100 is not a symmetric peak as demonstrated in other references *(52,73)*, but it is the first time that Apo-B 48 can be directly detected in 1 mL of plasma following an UC-isolation of the lipoprotein fractions.

In 1998 Cruzado et al. described the use of MEKC to study delipidation of LDL by surfactants in conjunction with the development of a method to

Table 4
Test Performance of Capillary Electrophoresis
and Immunoassays for the Quantification of Apolipoproteins

Features	Capillary electrophoresis	Immunoassay
Analysis time	8–30 min	6–180 min
Analytical mode	Sequential	Parallel
Detection mode	Direct (UV-signal)	Indirect (immune reaction)
Interferences and influences on determination	?	Lot variations of antibody specifity epitope characteristic (e.g. polymorphic forms of Apo A-I)
Sample volume (death volume included)	≤10 μL[a]	5–220 μL
Costs per test	~ $0.02[b]	~ $2[c]

[a]Nanoliter injected for analysis.
[b]Consists of a few μL of buffer and a cheap capillary. Calculation based on commercial capillaries (life-time 400 runs) and self-made solutions.
[c]Consists of antibodies, diluent, etc. Estimated commercial price.

quantitate Apo B-100 in VLDL and LDL after isolation by UC. A detergent mixture containing 70% SDS, 25% sodium myristyl sulfate, and 5% sodium cetyl sulfate was found to delipidate the LDL particle more effectively than pure SDS or sodium decyl sulfate. The validity of the results were tested against commercial LDL and plasma standards and gave an accurate determination of Apo B-100 levels within the precision of the standard. In combination with UC-based separation this method bears the potential for the precise determination of Apo B-100 by eliminating systematic error associated with precipitation, resolubilization, losses associated with lipid removal, and variability in chromogenicity and immunoreactivity within the Apo-B-100 protein.

Immunoassay or CE: which method is better? As shown in Table 4 there are a number of pros and cons for both techniques. Currently immunoassays are the generally accepted methods for the routine quantification of apolipoproteins in the clinical and research laboratories. Although reproducible within a particular laboratory, the inter-laboratory comparability is not good. With CE the major drawback is sequential operation that can be overcome by the use of a multi-capillary instrument. Currently a CE instrument with seven capillaries in parallel for routine serum protein analysis is offered on the market *(110–112)*. On the other hand, for laboratories running smaller numbers of samples, a sequential CE instrument is adequate for the overnight analyses of ≥30 apolipoprotein samples. As described earlier, the CE methods should give comparable results between laboratories. However, the apolipoprotein results by CE are not identical to those using nephelometry. In a time with increasing health care costs and lower budgets for research, the price per result also has to be considered. Since the costs of an analysis using CE are extremely low, when compared to immunoassay, apolipoprotein determination using CE should be considered as an economical alternative (*see* Table 4).

5. CONCLUSION AND FUTURE PERSPECTIVES

Lipoproteins, in addition to apolipoprotein identification and quantification, will continue to play an important role in the understanding of the pathogenesis of atherosclerosis for many years. Further development efforts will be directed towards the development of increasingly affordable, rapid, reliable, and automated technologies. CE with its various modes has several advantages when compared to the current procedures for lipoprotein and apolipoprotein analyses. These advantages are extreme analytical flexibility, using small quantities of low cost separation buffer, ability to use of a variety of detection modes, small sample size (nanoliter), high speed, efficiency, and reproducibility. It is also possible to install fully automated procedures. Furthermore, CE allows a rapid change from one buffer system to another: in other words, change from one analytical procedure to another.

In this chapter it becomes obvious that use of CE for lipoprotein analysis is still in its infancy. LDL, which is routinely only detected as one fraction, can be subdivided in up to six fractions by CITP that may yield new insights in the pathophysiology of the LDL-subfractions. It is possible that new areas in the study of atherogenesis may be achieved by the analysis of HDL subfractions. Since CE first separates then detects the lipoproteins, immunoassay problems caused by antibodies are eliminated. In addition, since multiple apolipoproteins can be determined in one run, CE is a good alternative to procedures like gel electrophoresis or UC. In the future, with a multicapillary instrument and with on-line sample pretreatment, it could well be competitive to automated special analyses. For broader acceptance of lipoprotein and apolipoprotein analysis by CE, three things are needed: 1) The development of chemical reagent kits, instruments, and software suitable for daily clinical laboratory use; 2) an increase of sensitivity and sample throughput; and 3) comparison and evaluation of various applications with current laboratory methods under daily laboratory conditions. In addition special attention needs to be paid to accuracy, reproducibility, speed, and susceptibility to disturbances (methods, capillaries, CE instruments). Other important criteria are ease of use in routine work situations, possibly automation, low cost per test, inexpensive and long-lasting reagents, widely accessible methodology, and clinically relevant reference ranges. Until now the number of reports evaluating these applications in comparison to the traditional procedures is low, however, this is likely to change in the near future.

Taken together, high-efficiency separations based on charge-to-mass ratio have been achieved through a combination of buffer modifiers and uncoated or permanently coated capillaries. Use of dynamically coated capillaries and separations based on the molecular weight have not yet been tested, but may further improve separation of the lipoproteins. CE offers more than simple improvement in quantitative and qualitative analyses of lipoprotein and apolipoproteins. It also offers the possibility of monitoring the reaction rates of apolipoproteins with different surfactants, lipoprotein degradation, lipoprotein metabolism, as well as therapeutic effects on lipoprotein classes. The use of CITP in the analysis of lipoproteins may facilitate the development of new clinical screening methods, possibly leading to new diagnostic markers or patterns, better prognostic evaluation, and new therapeutic modalities. Of course, as with all new developments, it is likely that some things may not turn out to be as important as expected. But I am also confident that many as yet unanticipated discoveries will be made as a result of the increased performance of this analytical technique. Nevertheless, the impact that these additional CE applications will have on diagnosis and treatment of atherosclerosis greatly depends on the success of transferring them from the academic research laboratories to the commercial marketplace.

REFERENCES

1. Gofman, J. W., DeLalla, O., and Glazier, F. (1954) The serum lipoprotein transport system in health, metabolic disorders, atherosclerosis and coronary heart disease. Plasma 2, 413–484.
2. Patsch, J. R., Sailer, S., Kostner, G., Sandhofer, F., Holasek, A., and Braunsteiner, H. (1974) Separation of the main lipoprotein density classes from human plasma by rate-zonal ultracentrifugation. J. Lipid. Res. 15, 356–365.
3. Chung, B. H., Wilkinson, T., Geer, J. C., and Segrest, J. P. (1980) Preparative and quantitative isolation of plasma lipoproteins: rapid, single discontinuous density gradient ultracentrifugation in a vertical rotor. J. Lipid Res. 21, 284–291.
4. Groot, P. H., Scheek, L. M., Havekes, L., van Noort, W. L., and van't Hooft, F. M. (1982) A one-step separation of human serum high density lipoproteins 2 and 3 by rate-zonal density gradient ultracentrifugation in a swinging bucket rotor. J. Lipid Res. 23, 1342–1353.
5. Skinner, E. R. (1992) The separation and analysis of high-density lipoprotein (HDL) and low-density lipoprotein (LDL) subfractions, in Lipoprotein Analysis (Skinner, E.R. and Converse, J. L. eds.), IRL Press, Oxford, pp. 85–118.

6. Nauck, M., Winkler, K., Wittmann, C., Mayer, H., Luley, C., Marz, W., and Wieland, H. (1995) Direct determination of lipoprotein(a) cholesterol by ultracentrifugation and agarose gel electrophoresis with enzymatic staining for cholesterol. Clin. Chem. 41, 731–738.

7. Jialal, I., Hirany, S. V., Devaraj, S., and Sherwood, T. A. (1995) Comparison of an immunoprecipation method for direct measurement of LDL-cholesterol with beta-quantification (ultracentrifugation). Am. J. Clin. Pathol. 104, 76–81.

8. Raymond, S., Miles, J. L., and Lee, J. C. (1966) Lipoprotein patterns in acrylamide gel electrophoresis. Science 151, 346, 347.

9. Campos, E., Fievet, P., Caces, E., Fruchart, J. C., and Fievet, C. (1994) A screening method for abnormally high lipoprotein(a) concentrations by agarose lipoprotein electrophoresis. Clin. Chim. Acta. 230, 43–50.

10. Nauck, M., Winkler, K., Marz, W., and Wieland, H. (1995) Quantitative determination of high-, low-, and very-low-density lipoproteins and lipoprotein(a) by agarose gel electrophoresis and enzymatic cholesterol staining. Clin. Chem. 41, 1761–1767.

11. Bachorik, P. S. and Albers, J. J. (1986) Precipitation methods for quantification of lipoproteins, in Methods in Enzymology (Segrest, J. P. and Albers, J. J., eds.), Academic, New York, NY, pp. 78–100.

12. Gidez, L. I., Miller, G. J., Burstein, M., Slagle, S., and Eder, H. A. (1982) Separation and quantitation of subclasses of human plasma high density lipoproteins by a simple precipitation procedure. J. Lipid Res. 23, 1206–1023.

13. Vogel, S., Contois, J. H., Couch, S. C., and Lammi Keefe, C. J. (1996) A rapid method for separation of plasma low and high density lipoproteins for tocopherol and carotenoid analyses. Lipids 31, 421–426.

14. Nauck, M., März, W., and Wieland, H. (1998) New immunoseparation-based homogeneous assay for HDL-cholesterol compared with three homogeneous and two heterogeneous methods for HDL-cholesterol. Clin. Chem. 44, 1443–1451.

15. Rudel, L. L., Marzetta, C. A., and Johnson, F. L. (1986) Separation and analysis of lipoproteins by gel filtration, in Methods in Enzymology (Segrest, J. P. and Albers, J. J., eds.), Academic, New York, NY, pp. 45–57.

16. Weisgraber, K. H. and Mahley, R. W. (1980) Subfractionation of human high density lipoproteins by heparin-Sepharose affinity chromatography. J. Lipid Res. 21, 316–325.

17. Cheung, M. C. and Albers, J. J. (1984) Characterization of lipoprotein particles isolated by immunoaffinity chromatography. Particles containing A-I and A-II and particles containing A-I but no A-II. J. Biol. Chem. 259, 12,201–12,209.

18. Nauck, M., Marz, W., Haas, B., and Wieland, H. (1996) Homogeneous assay for direct determination of high-density lipoprotein cholesterol evaluated. Clin. Chem. 42, 424–429.

19. Labeur, C., Shepherd, J., and Rosseneu, M. (1990) Immunological assays of apolipoproteins in plasma: methods and instrumentation. Clin. Chem. 36, 591–597.

20. Jialal, I. (1996) A practical approach to the laboratory diagnosis of dyslipidemia. Am. J. Clin. Pathol. 106, 128–138.

21. Lehmann, R., Voelter, W., and Liebich, H. M. (1997) Capillary electrophoresis in clinical chemistry. J. Chromatogr. B 697, 3–35.

22. Jialal, I. (1998) Evolving lipoprotein risk factors: lipoprotein (a) and oxidized low-density lipoproteins. Clin. Chem. 44, 1827–1832.
23. Blanche, P. J., Gong, E. L., Forte, T. M., and Nichols, A. V. (1981) Characterization of human high-density lipoproteins by gradient gel electrophoresis, Biochim. Biophys. Acta 665, 408–419.
24. Li, Z., McNamara, J. R., Ordovas, J. M., and Schaefer, E. J. (1994) Analysis of high density lipoproteins by a modified gradient gel electrophoresis method. J. Lipid Res. 35, 1698–1711.
25. Campos, H., Blijlevens, E., McNamara, J. R., Ordovas, J. M., Posner, B. M., Wilson, P. W. F., Castelli, W. P., Schaefer, E. J. (1992) LDL particle size distribution: results from the Framingham Offspring Study. Arterioscler. Thromb. 12, 1410–1419.
26. Nichols, A. V., Krauss, R. M., and Musliner, T. A. (1995) Nondenaturing Polyacrylamide Gradient Gel Electrophoresis, in Methods in Enzymology (Segrest, J. P. and Albers, J. J., eds.), Academic, New York, NY, pp. 417–431.
27. Halle, M., Berg, A., Baumstark, M. W., and Keul, J. (1998) LDL subfraction profile and coronary heart disease: a review. Z. Kardiol. 87, 317–330.
28. Musliner, T. A., McVicker, K. M., Iosefa, J. F., and Krauss, R. M. (1987) Metabolism of human intermediate and very low density lipoprotein subfractions from normal and dysbetalipoproteinemic plasma. In vivo studies in rat. Arteriosclerosis 7, 408–420.
29. National Center for Health Statistics (1997) Final 1995 State Mortality. US Census Bureau, Hyattsville, MD.
30. McGorisk, G. M. and Treasure, C. B. (1996) Endothelial dysfunction in coronary heart disease, Curr. Opin. Cardiol. 11, 341–350.
31. Prati, P., Vanuzzo, D., Casaroli, M., Di Chiara, A., De Biasi, F., Feruglio, G. A., and Touboul, P. J. (1992) Prevalence and determinants of carotid atherosclerosis in a general population. Stroke 23, 1705–1011.
32. Luc, G., Fievet, C., Arveiler, D., Evans, A. E., Bard, J. M., Cambien, F., Fruchart, J. C., et al. (1996) Apolipoproteins C-III and E in apoB- and non-apoB-containing lipoproteins in two populations at contrasting risk for myocardial infarction: the ECTIM study. Etude Cas Temoins sur 'Infarctus du Myocarde. J. Lipid Res. 37, 508–517.
33. Criqui, M. H., Denenberg, J. O., Langer, R. D., and Fronek, A. (1997) The epidemiology of peripheral arterial disease: importance of identifying the population at risk. Vasc. Med. 2, 221–226.
34. Avins, A. L. and Browner, W. S. (1998) Improving the prediction of coronary heart disease to aid in the management of high cholesterol levels: what a difference a decade makes. JAMA 279, 445–449.
35. McNamara, J. R., Shah, P. K., Nakajima, K., Cupples, L. A., Wilson, P. W., Ordovas, J. M., and Schaefer, E. J. (1998) Remnant lipoprotein cholesterol and triglyceride reference ranges from the Framingham Heart Study. Clin. Chem. 44, 1224–1232.
36. Guretzki, H. J., Gerbitz, K. D., Olgemoller, B., and Schleicher, E. (1994) Atherogenic levels of low density lipoprotein alter the permeability and composition of the endothelial barrier. Atherosclerosis 107, 15–24.

37. Vogel, R. A. (1997) Coronary risk factors, endothelial function, and athero-sclerosis: a review. Clin. Cardiol. 20, 426–432.
38. McCully, K. S. (1998) Homocysteine, folate, vitamin B6, and cardiovascular disease. JAMA 279, 392, 393.
39. Welch, G. N. and Loscalzo, J. (1998) Homocysteine and atherothrombosis. N. Engl. J. Med. 338, 1042–1050.
40. Duell, P. B. and Malinow, M. R. (1998) Lipid and metabolism—homocyst(e)inemia and risk of atherosclerosis: a clinical approach to evalua-tion and management. Endocrinologist 8, 170–177.
41. Hoogeveen, E. K., Kostense, P. J., Beks, P. J., MacKaay, A. J. C., Jakobs, C., Bouter, L. M., et al. (1998) Hyperhomocysteinemia is associated with an increased risk of cardiovascular disease, especially in non–insulin-dependent diabetes mellitus: a population-based. Arterioscler. Thromb. Vasc. Biol. 18, 133–138.
42. Grundy, S. M., Balady, G. J., Criqui, M. H., Fletcher, G., Greenland, P., Hiratzka, L. F., et al. (1998) Primary prevention of coronary heart disease: Guidance from Framingham: a statement for healthcare professionals from the AHA task force on risk reduction. Circulation 97, 1876–1887.
43. Senti, M., Pedro Botet, J., Nogues, X., and Rubies Prat, J. (1991) Influence of intermediate-density lipoproteins on the accuracy of the Friedewald formula. Clin. Chem. 37, 1394–1397.
44. Matas, C., Cabre, M., La Ville, A., Prats, E., Joven, J., Turner, P. R., et al. (1994) Limitations of the Friedewald formula for estimating low-density lipo-protein cholesterol in alcoholics with liver disease. Clin. Chem. 40, 404–406.
45. Marniemi, J., Maki, J., Maatela, J., Jarvisalo, J., and Impivaara, O. (1995) Poor applicability of the Friedewald formula in the assessment of serum LDL cho-lesterol for clinical purposes. Clin. Biochem. 28, 285–289.
46. Senti, M., Pedro Botet, J., Rubies Prat, J., and Vidal Barraquer, F. (1996) Sec-ondary prevention of coronary heart disease in patients with extracoronary ath-erosclerosis: a need for accuracy of low density lipoprotein determination, Angiology. 47, 241–246.
47. Boerma, G. J. M., Bruijn, A. M., and van Teunenbroek, A. (1994) Reference values for apolipoprotein A-I and apolipoprotein B in serum still depend on choice of assay techniques, Eur. J. Clin. Chem. Clin. Biochem. 32, 923–927.
48. Weinmann, W., Maier, C., Baumeister, K., Przybylski, M., Parker, C. E., and Tomer, K. B. (1994) Isolation of hydrophobic lipoproteins in organic solvents by pressure-assisted capillary electrophoresis for subsequent mass spectromet-ric characterization. J. Chromatogr. A 664, 271–275.
49. Helenius, A. and Simons, K. (1972) The binding of detergents to lipophilic and hydrophilic proteins. J. Biol. Chem. 247, 3656–3661.
50. Makino, S., Tanford, C., Reynolds, J. A. (1974) The interaction of polypeptide components of human high density serum lipoprotein with detergents. J. Biol. Chem. 249, 7379–7382.
51. Tadey, T. and Purdy, W.C. (1993) Effect of detergents on the electrophoretic behaviour of plasma apolipoproteins in capillary electrophoresis. J. Chromatogr. A 652, 131–138.

52. Macfarlane, R. D., Bondarenko, P. V., Cockrill, S. L., Cruzado, I. D., Koss, W., McNeal, C. J., et al. (1997) Development of a lipoprotein profile using capillary electrophoresis and mass spectrometry. Electrophoresis 18, 1796–1806.

53. Cruzado, I. D., Song, S., Crouse, S. F., O'Brien, B., Macfarlane, R. D., and O'Brien, B.C. (1996) Characterization and quantitation of the apoproteins of high-density lipoprotein by capillary electrophoresis. Anal. Biochem. 243, 100–109.

54. Bartholome, M., Wieland, H., and Seidel, D. (1980) Quantification of plasma lipoprotein cholesterol: a simple procedure for enzymatic determination of cholesterol in electrophoretically separated lipoproteins. Clin. Chim. Acta 104, 101–105.

55. Neubeck, W., Wieland, H., Habenicht, A., Muller, P., Baggio, G., and Seidel, D. (1977) Improved assessment of plasma lipoprotein patterns. III. Direct measurement of lipoproteins after gel-electrophoresis. Clin. Chem. 23, 1296–1300.

56. Everaerts, F. M., Beckers, J. L., and Verheggen, T. P. E. M. (1976) Isotachophoresis: Theory, Instrumentation and Applications, Amsterdam, The Netherlands, Elsevier, pp. 1–384.

57. Bocek, P., Gebauer, P., Dolnik, V., and Foret, F. (1985) Recent developments in isotachophoresis. J. Chromatogr. 334, 157–195.

58. Krivankova, L., Gebauer, P., and Bocek, P. (1996) Isotachophoresis, in Methods in Enzymology (Karger, B. L. and Hancock, W. S., eds.), Academic, New York, NY, pp. 375–401.

59. Schmitz, G., Borgmann, U., and Assmann, G. (1985) Analytical capillary isotachophoresis: a routine technique for the analysis of lipoproteins and lipoprotein subfractions in whole serum. J. Chromatogr. 320, 253–262.

60. Josic, O., Zeilinger, K., Reutter, W., Böttcher, A., and Schmitz, G. (1990) High-performance capillary electrophoresis of hydrophobic membrane proteins. J. Chromatogr. 516, 89–98.

61. Nowicka, G. and Schmitz, G. (1990) Characterization of subpopulations of Apo B containing lipoproteins separated by analytical capillary isotachophoresis. Klin. Wochenschr. 68, 119,120.

62. Nowicka, G., Brüning, T., Grothaus, B., Kahl, G., and Schmitz, G. (1990) Characterization of apolipoprotein B-containing lipoproteins separated by preparative free flow isotachophoresis. J. Lipid. Res. 31, 1173–1186.

63. Nowicka, G., Brüning, T., Böttcher, A., Kahl, G., and Schmitz, G. (1990) Macrophage interaction of HDL subclasses separated by free flow isotachophoresis, J. Lipid. Res. 31, 1947–1963.

64. Josic, O., Böttcher, A., and Schmitz, G. (1990) High-performance capillary isotachophoresis of serum lipoproteins and membrane proteins. Chromatographia 30, 703–706.

65. Schmitz, G. and Möllers, C. (1994) Analysis of lipoproteins with analytical capillary isotachophoresis. Electrophoresis 15, 31–39.

66. Zorn, U., Wolf, C.-F., Wennauer, R., Bachem, M. G., and Grünert, A. (1997) Kapillarelektrophoretische Differenzierung von Lipoproteinen. Diagnostik Digest 7, 22–26.

67. Schmitz, G., Mollers, C., and Richter, V. (1997) Analytical capillary isotachophoresis of human serum lipoproteins. Electrophoresis 18, 1807–1813.

68. Stover, F. S. (1989) Spacer performance in the cationic isotachophoresis of proteins. J. Chromatogr. 470, 201–208.

69. Bon, G. B., Cazzolato, G., and Avogaro, P. (1981) Preparative isotachophoresis of human plasma high density lipoproteins HDL 2 and HDL 3. J. Lipid. Res. 22, 998–1002.

70. Fredrickson, D. S. (1971) An international classification of hyperlipidemias and hyperlipoproteinemias. Ann. Intern. Med. 75, 471–472.

71. Hu, A. Z., Cruzado, I. D., Hill, J. W., McNeal, C. J., and Macfarlane, R. D. (1995) Characterization of lipoprotein (a) by capillary zone electrophoresis. J. Chromatogr. A 717, 33–39.

72. Cruzado, I. D., Hu, A. Z., and Macfarlane, R. D. (1996) Influence of dodecyl sulfate ions on the electrophoretic mobilities of lipoprotein particles measured by HPCE. J. Cap. Elec. 3, 25–29.

73. Cruzado, I. D., Cockrill, S. L., McNeal, C. J., and Macfarlane, R. D. (1998) Characterization and quantitation of apolipoprotein B-100 by capillary electrophoresis. J. Lipid Res. 39, 205–217.

74. Westhuyzen, J. (1997) The oxidation hypothesis of atherosclerosis: an update. Ann. Clin. Lab. Sci. 27, 1–10.

75. Jialal, I. and Devaraj, S. (1996) Low-density lipoprotein oxidation, antioxidants, and atherosclerosis: a clinical biochemistry perspective. Clin. Chem. 42, 498–506.

76. Stocks, J. and Miller, N. E. (1998) Capillary electrophoresis to monitor the oxidative modification of low density lipoproteins. J. Lipid Res. 39, 1305–9.

77. Rice Evans, C., Leake, D., Bruckdorfer, K. R., and Diplock, A. T. (1996) Practical approaches to low density lipoprotein oxidation: whys, wherefores and pitfalls. Free Radic. Res. 25, 285–311.

78. Tietz, N. W. (1987) Fundamentals of Clinical Chemistry, 3rd ed. (Tietz, N. W., ed.), W.B. Saunders, Philadelphia, PA, pp. 53–84.

79. Marques Vidal, P., Ruidavets, J. B., Cambou, J. P., Cambien, F., Chap, H., and Perret, B. (1995) Distribution, fatty acid composition and apolipoprotein A-I immunoreactivity of high density lipoprotein subfractions in myocardial infarction. Atherosclerosis 112, 29–38.

80. Marcovina, S. M., Albers, J. J., Henderson, L. O., and Hannon, W. H. (1993) International federation of clinical chemistry standardization project for measurements of apolipoprotein A-I and B. III. Comparability of apolipoprotein A-I values by use of international reference material. Clin. Chem. 39, 773–781.

81. Contois, J. H., McNamara, J. R., Lammi-Keefe, C. J., Wilson, P. W. F., Massov, T., and Schaefer, E. J. (1996) Reference intervals for plasma apolipoprotein A-I determined with a standardized commercial immunoturbidimetric assay: results from the Framingham Offspring Study. Clin. Chem. 42, 507-514.

82. Reman, F. C. and Vermond, A. (1978) The quantitative determination of apolipoprotein A-I (apo-lp-Gln I) in human serum by radial immunodiffusion assay (RID). Clin. Chim. Acta 87, 387–394.

83. Havekes, L., Hemmink, J., and de Wit, E. (1981) Low-density-lipoprotein apoprotein B in plasma as measured by radial immunodiffusion and rocket immunoelectrophoresis. Clin. Chem. 27, 1829–1833.
84. Micic, S., Arends, J., Norgaard Pedersen, B., Christoffersen, K., and Andersen, G. E. (1988) Simultaneous quantification by double rocket immunoelectrophoresis of apolipoproteins A-I and B in blood spotted on filter paper. Clin. Chem. 34, 2452–2455.
85. Holmquist, L. and Vesterberg, O. (1986) Quantification of human serum apolipoprotein A-I by zone immunoelectrophoresis assay and a procedure for the preparation of an A-I standard. Clin. Chim. Acta 156, 131–143.
86. Stocks, J., Nanzeem Nanjee, M., and Miller, N. E. (1998) Analysis of high density lipoprotein apolipoproteins by capillary zone and capillary SDS gel electrophoresis. J. Lipid Res. 39, 218–227.
87. Bojanovski, M., Gregg, R. E., Wilson, D. M., and Brewer, H. B., Jr. (1987) Semi-automated enzyme-linked immunosorbent assay (ELISA) for the quantification of apolipoprotein B using monoclonal antibodies. Clin. Chim. Acta 170, 271–280.
88. Leroy, A., Olivier, P., Vu Dac, N., and Fruchart, J. C. (1989) Characterization of two monoclonal antibodies to human apolipoprotein A-I that also bind to rabbit apolipoprotein A-I. Application to ELISA evaluation of rabbit serum apo A-I. Clin. Chim. Acta 179, 85–95.
89. Wang, X. L., Wilcken, D. E., and Dudman, N. P. (1990) Neonatal apo A-I, apo B, and apo(a) levels in dried blood spots in an Australian population. Pediatr. Res. 28, 496–501.
90. Sorell, L., Rojas, G., Rodriguez, M., Ramos, C., Torres, L., and Torres, M. B. (1995) A sandwich ELISA based on anti-apo(a) and anti-apo B monoclonal antibodies for lipoprotein(a) measurement. Clin. Chim. Acta 236, 59–70.
91. Kee, P., Bais, R., Sobecki, S. K., Branford, S., Rye, K. A., and Barter, P. J. (1996) Indirect sandwich enzyme-linked immunosorbent assay (ELISA) for plasma apolipoprotein E. Ann. Clin. Biochem. 33, 119–126.
92. Mei, J. V., Powell, M. K., Henderson, L. O., Smith, S. J., Cooper, G. R., Marcovina, S. M., and Hannon, W. H. (1994) Method-dependent variations in the stability of apolipoprotein B in a stabilized liquid reference material. Clin. Chem. 40, 716–722.
93. Pruvot, I., Fievet, C., Durieux, C., Dac, N. V., and Fruchart, J.C. (1988) Electroimmuno- and immunonephelometric assays of apolipoprotein A-I by using a mixture of monoclonal antibodies. Clin. Chem. 34, 2048–2052.
94. Adolphson, J. L. and Albers, J. J. (1989) Comparison of two commercial nephelometric methods for apoprotein A-I and apoprotein B with standardized apoprotein A-I and B radioimmunoassays. J. Lipid. Res. 30, 597–606.
95. Riesen, W. F., Sturzenegger, E., Imhof, C., and Mordasini, R. (1986) Quantitation of apolipoprotein B by polyclonal and monoclonal antibodies. Clin. Chim. Acta 154, 29–40.
96. Mao, S. J. T., Miller, J. P., and Gotto, A. M., Sparrow, J. T. (1980) The antigenic structure of apolipoprotein A-I in human high density lipoproteins. J. Biol. Chem. 255, 3448–3453.

97. Schonfeld, G., Chen, J.-S., and Roy, R. G. (1977) Use of antibody specificity to study the surface disposition of apoprotein A-I on human high density lipoproteins. J. Biol. Chem. 252, 6655–6659.

98. Sigalov, A. B. (1993) Comparison of apolipoprotein A-I values assayed in lyophilized and frozen pooled human sera by a non-immunochemical electrophoretic method and by immunoassay. Eur. J. Clin. Chem. Clin. Biochem. 31, 579–583.

99. Maguire, G. F., Lee, M., and Connelly, P. W. (1989) Sodium dodecyl sulfate-glycerol polyacrylamide slab gel electrophoresis for the resolution of apolipoproteins. J. Lipid. Res. 30, 757–761.

100. Tanford, C., Nozaki, Y., Reynolds, J. A., and Makino, S. (1974) Molecular characterization of proteins in detergent solutions. Biochemistry 13, 2369–2376.

101. Tadey, T. and Purdy, W. C. (1992) Characterization of plasma apolipoproteins by capillary electrophoresis. J. Chromatogr. 583, 111–115.

102. Goux, A., Athias, A., Persegol, L., Lagrost, L., Gambert, P., and Lallemant, C. (1994) Capillary gel electrophoresis analysis of apolipoproteins A-I and A-II in human high-density lipoproteins. Anal. Biochem. 218, 320–324.

103. Lehmann, R., Liebich, H., Grübler, G., and Voelter, W. (1995) Capillary electrophoresis of human serum proteins and apolipoproteins. Electrophoresis 16, 998–1001.

104. Liebich, H. M., Lehmann, R., Weiler, A. E., Grübler, G., and Voelter, W. (1995) Capillary electrophoresis, a rapid and sensitive method for routine analysis of apolipoprotein A-I in clinical samples. J. Chromatogr. A 717, 25–31.

105. Proctor, S. D. and Mamo, J. C. (1997) Separation and quantification of apolipoprotein B-48 and other apolipoproteins by dynamic sieving capillary electrophoresis. J. Lipid Res. 38, 410–414.

106. Lehmann, R., Beck, A., Häring, H. U., and Voelter, W. (2000) Determination of apolipoprotein A-I serum levels—Capillary electrophoresis versus clinical routine immunonephelometric assay, Electrophoresis (submitted).

107. Lackner, K. J., Edge, S. B., Gregg, R. E., Hoeg, J. M., and Brewer, H. B. (1985) Isoforms of apolipoprotein A-II in human plasma and thoracic duct lymph. J. Biol. Chem. 260, 703–706.

108. Azrolan, N., Odaka, H., Breslow, J. L., and Fisher, E. A. (1995) Dietary fat elevates hepatic apoA-I production by increasing the fraction of apolipoprotein A-I mRNA in the translating pool. J. Biol. Chem. 270, 19,833–19,838.

109. Karpe, F., Bell, M., Bjorkegren, J., and Hamsten, A. (1995) Quantification of postprandial triglyceride-rich lipoproteins in healthy men by retinyl ester labeling and simultaneous measurement of apolipoproteins B-48 and B-100. Arterioscler. Thromb. Vasc. Biol. 15, 199–207.

110. Bienvenu, J., Graziani, M. S., Arpin, F., Bernon, H., Blessum, C., Marchetti, C., Righetti, G., et al. (1998) Multicenter evaluation of the Paragon CZE 2000 capillary zone electrophoresis system for serum protein electrophoresis and monoclonal component typing. Clin. Chem. 44, 599–605.

111. Bossuyt, X., Schiettekatte, G., Bogaerts, A., and Blanckaert, N. (1998) Serum protein electrophoresis by CZE 2000 clinical capillary electrophoresis system. Clin. Chem. 44, 749–759.

112. Bossuyt, X., Bogaerts, A., and Schiettekatte, G., and Blanckaert, N. (1998) Detection and classification of paraproteins by capillary immunofixation/subtraction. Clin. Chem. 44, 760–764.

8

Clinical Analysis of Structural Hemoglobin Variants and Hb A$_{1c}$ by Capillary Isoelectric Focusing

James M. Hempe, Alfonso Vargas, and Randall D. Craver

1. INTRODUCTION

Capillary isoelectric focusing (cIEF) for analysis of hemoglobin (Hb) variants has two major clinical applications: 1) diagnosis and management of congenital hemoglobinopathies, and 2) assessment of glycemic control in subjects with diabetes. For congenital Hb disorders, like sickle-cell disease or beta thalassemia, the specific identification and precise quantification of both normal and abnormal structural Hb variants is required. Assessment of glycemic control for diabetes management, on the other hand, requires separation and quantification of a post-translational variant, Hb A$_{1c}$, that is a chemically modified (glycated) form of normal adult Hb A.

A major benefit of the cIEF format for the clinical laboratory is that both of these applications can be fulfilled using the same analytical instrument, cIEF procedure, and set of simple and inexpensive reagents. Operated by a single medical technologist or other trained laboratorian, cIEF in this format can meet the routine diagnostic needs of many hospital laboratories for analysis of both structural Hb variants and Hb A$_{1c}$. With newer CE instruments, advanced software, and higher capacity autosamplers, high-through-put applications are possible. Despite clear diagnostic and economic advantages, dedicated commercial CE systems have not been developed for these clinical applications. The purpose of this chapter is to describe the use of cIEF for the analysis of both structural and post-translational Hb variants, and to describe the advantages of using a single instrument and analytical procedure for both Hb variant and Hb A$_{1c}$ analyses in a clinical laboratory environment.

From: *Clinical and Forensic Applications of Capillary Electrophoresis*
Edited by: J. R. Petersen and A. A. Mohammad © Humana Press Inc., Totowa, NJ

2. cIEF OF HEMOGLOBINS

Human hemoglobins are tetrameric peptides consisting of two α globins, and either two β, γ, or δ globins that make up normal Hb variants, Hbs A, F, and A_2, respectively *(1,2)*. During electrophoresis, the tetramers migrate as $\alpha\beta$, $\alpha\gamma$, or $\alpha\delta$ dimers that are separated by cIEF due to differences in molecular surface charge *(1)*. Amino acid substitutions or deletions, or the post-translational modification of the dimers by complexation with other compounds can alter the charge and thus the migration of the Hb variant.

A detailed description of our method has been presented elsewhere *(3)*. Briefly, a coated capillary is filled with carrier ampholytes (mixture of pH 6–8 and 3–10) in a liquid polymer (methylcellulose) solution. A small volume of hemolyzed blood is pressure-injected (10 s) into the capillary inlet. The inlet is immersed in dilute phosphoric acid solution at the anode while the capillary outlet is immersed in dilute sodium hydroxide solution at the cathode. Constant voltage (30 kV) is applied across the electrodes generating an electric field of 1111 V/cm. A linear pH gradient is established within 2–3 min, and each Hb variant becomes concentrated (focused) in a narrow band at its isoelectric point (pI). Pressure is then used to mobilize the focused protein zones (with the voltage still applied) past the detector window where absorbance at 415 nm (specific for heme moieties) is measured. Detector output is collected by a computer and displayed on-screen as a series of absorbance peaks. Data analysis software is used to integrate the absorbance output to determine the area under the curve above the baseline for each Hb variant peak. The amount of each variant present is then expressed as a proportion (%) of total Hb, i.e., the area of each peak is divided by the total area of all peaks. Because most Hb variants have different pIs, they can be identified by where they focus in the capillary. Peak identification is based on the calculation of the pI of the unknown peaks from a by linear regression equation of pI vs elution time of known Hb variants in a standard sample. The entire process takes about 18 min per sample, with analytical sensitivity to 0.5% of total Hb, and specificity based on pI ± 0.01 pH units.

3. DIAGNOSIS OF CONGENITAL HEMOGLOBIN DISORDERS BY cIEF

3.1. Overview of the Application

Structural hemoglobinopathies and thalassemias are congenital hemoglobin disorders that cause anemia, morbidity, and mortality resulting from abnormal Hb function *(1,2)*. These diseases arise from genetic mutations that alter the amino-acid composition, structure, and function of the α, β, γ, and/or δ globins that make up hemoglobin tetramers. The presence of abnormal structural hemoglobin variants, like Hb S (sickle hemoglobin), is commonly used to determine Hb phenotype and diagnose structural hemoglobinopathies like sickle cell disease. In contrast, thalassemia syndromes are caused by mutations or gene deletions that alter the production or processing of normal globin. Only normal structural globins are produced, but in abnormal proportions such that quantification of normal Hb variants in the blood, especially Hbs A_2 and F, can be diagnostic of thalassemia syndromes.

The need for analytical methods to identify and quantify structural Hb variants is primarily confined to hospital laboratories, commercial reference laboratories, and state-supported neonatal screening laboratories. Although there are over 600 known mutations in the genes that regulate hemoglobin structure *(4)*, most of the demand for analysis of structural Hb variants is for diagnosis and management of a limited number of hemoglobinopathies. For example, mutations in the β globin gene produce Hbs S, E, and C, the three most common abnormal hemoglobin variants in the world. In the homozygous state, these mutations cause sickle-cell disease, Hb E disease, and Hb C disease, respectively. Most routine assays performed by clinical laboratories in the United States are related to the diagnosis and management of these diseases, which may occur in heterozygous combinations or with β thalassemia.

3.2. Comparison of cIEF to Conventional Methods

To meet the diverse needs of a clinical laboratory, tests used to evaluate patients with suspected congenital hemoglobin disorders must be able to 1) identify many normal and abnormal structural Hb variants and 2) precisely measure the proportions of these variants in the blood. In this regard, the information provided by cIEF for the diagnosis of hemoglobinopathies and thalassemias is vastly superior to that provided by conventional clinical assays *(5–8)*. Conventional methods include alkaline electrophoresis, acid electrophoresis, or gel IEF for the identification of major Hb variants, minicolumn ion exchange chromatography for analysis of Hb A_2, and alkali denaturation for quantification of Hb F. The information provided by all of these assays is provided by a single cIEF assay. Autosampling and computer-assisted data collection give cIEF automation features comparable to HPLC, but with the added advantages of lower sample and reagent requirements, low-cost consumables, and protocol simplicity.

3.3. Clinical Application of cIEF Laboratory Results

A detailed description of the method we use and its diagnostic advantages and limitations for routine Hb variant analysis has been published *(3)*.

We have also demonstrated elsewhere the practical use of cIEF in the hematological evaluation of patients with common congenital Hb disorders that make up the bulk of the analytical workload for most laboratories, i.e., sickle cell disease, Hb C disease, and β thalassemia *(5–8)*. Hb E, commonly found in patients of Asian ancestry, cannot be separated from Hbs O-Arab and C-Harlem by cIEF, but a probable identification can be made on the basis of the pI of the unknown variant, the results of a sickle solubility test for Hb C-Harlem, and family history. Minor variants like Hb Constant Spring and Hb A_2' are easily detected and measured by cIEF *(8)*. As a result, cIEF is the only analytical procedure needed for the primary laboratory examination of patients with suspected hemoglobinopathies. The need for follow-up testing is minimal so that use of a specialized reference laboratory is an economically viable way to identify rare unknown Hb variants or to confirm a preliminary identification made by cIEF.

3.3.1. Monitoring Patients with Known Hemoglobinopathies

Over the last 5 years, 31% of the samples sent to our laboratory were for longitudinal monitoring of the efficacy of hypertransfusion, chemotherapy, or bone-marrow transplantation in patients with known Hb disorders, especially sickle-cell disease. The goal in each treatment for sickle cell disease is to decrease the proportion of Hb S in the blood and increase the proportions of functional Hbs, especially Hbs A and F, to limit sickling. Rapid turnaround of test results can be important for patients where more than one transfusion may be needed before a surgical procedure. Easy analytical run setup and the ability to insert a sample into a priority position after the beginning of a run is one of the benefits of cIEF.

The use of cIEF for 1) diagnosis of sickle-cell disease; 2) assessing the effects of transfusion of normal blood into a patient with sickle-cell disease; and 3) evaluation of a subject with sickle-cell disease treated with hydroxyurea, a chemotherapeutic agent used to upregulate the expression of γ globin genes and the production of Hb F is shown in Fig. 1. The levels of Hbs S, A, and F are also monitored in subjects with sickle-cell disease following bone-marrow transplantation to replace erythrocyte progenitor stem cells. Similarly, assessment of Hb F level can help in the diagnosis of chronic myelogenous leukemia.

3.3.2. Assessment of Patients with Suspected Hemoglobinopathies

In addition to common Hb variants, cIEF can also detect many uncommon abnormal structural Hb variants, even if the exact identity of the variant cannot be immediately determined. A good example of the diagnostic power of cIEF is demonstrated in Fig. 2, which shows an electropherogram of the

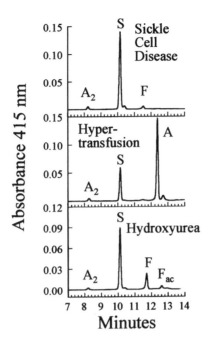

Fig. 1. Monitoring patients with known hemoglobinopathies. These electrophero-grams show the structural Hb variants present in blood from three patients with sickle cell disease that were either untreated (**A**), undergoing hypertransfusion with blood from a donor with normal Hb phenotype (**B**), or treated with hydroxyurea to induce Hb F synthesis (**C**). The goal of both transfusion therapy and hydroxyurea chemo-therapy is to reduce the proportion of Hb S and increase the proportions of Hbs A or F, respectively. Acetylated fetal Hb F_{ac}, a normal post-translational modification of Hb F, is also apparent in the patient treated with hydroxyurea.

Hb variants present in the blood from a patient with an unusual Hb disorder. In this case, the electropherogram showed three large peaks migrating in positions similar to that expected for Hbs C (~7.9 min), S, and A. The pattern was similar to what might be observed in a subject with Hb S/C disease undergoing hypertransfusion, except that the proportions of Hbs C and S would be expected to be more similar. Unlike less sensitive conventional assays, however, cIEF provided additional information that facilitated a more comprehensive determination of the Hb phenotype. Two other abnormal peaks were also seen, including a very small peak eluting at around 6 min, and a larger peak partially separated from Hb S and appearing as a shoulder anodal to the Hb S peak. Except for Hbs A_2, S, and A, none of the other peaks in this sample could be identified based on pI by comparison to Hb variants previously encountered in our laboratory. Although the Hb pheno-

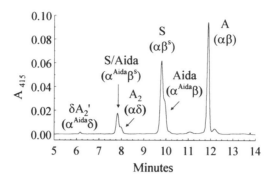

Fig. 2. Identification of uncommon Hb variants. Hb S trait/Aida trait is a rare compound heterozygous condition with a clinical presentation similar to that of Hb S trait. cIEF analysis of the patient's blood indicated a phenotype including one normal β globin allele (Hb A), one abnormal β globin allele (Hb S), 6 β Glu^-(Val), three normal α globin alleles, and one abnormal α globin allele (Hb Aida, 64 α Asp^-(Asn). This combination of normal and abnormal alleles produced four major αβ Hb variants, including Hbs A, S, Aida (pI = 7.188, apparent as a large shoulder anodal to Hb S), and S/Aida hybrid (pI = 7.430, apparent as a small peak anodal to Hb A_2). Two minor αδ Hb variants are also apparent, including normal Hb A_2 and an α variant of Hb A_2 (Hb $αA_2'$, pI = 7.617).

type of this patient could not specifically identified, we could inform the physician that the patient exhibited the sickle-cell mutation in one β globin gene, and an unknown mutation in one α globin gene. Identification of a α globin mutation was based on the following evidence. First, unusual minor cIEF peaks present at less than 1% of total Hb are usually either α or δ variants of Hb A_2. Second, a mutation in a single α globin gene results in the production of an abnormal αβ variant that represents about 25% of the normal variant. With Hbs A_2, S, and A identified based on pI, the proportions and migration positions of the three unknown peaks could only be interpreted to be evidence of three α variants, one α variant for each of the three common Hb variants present. The sample was sent to a reference laboratory (Mayo Laboratories, Rochester, MN) where the unusual major Hb variants were identified as Hb Aida and Hb S/Aida hybrid. The Hb phenotype was thus that of Hb S trait/Hb Aida trait, a rare double heterozygous condition with a clinical presentation similar to that of Hb S trait.

This example shows the power of cIEF by providing the information needed to identify both routine and unusual Hb phenotypes. One can expect to at least detect, if not tentatively identify, most unusual variants due to the high-resolution and peak detection sensitivity of cIEF. The calculated pI of Hb variants in an unknown sample is a very reproducible and specific indi-

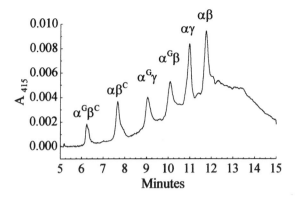

Fig. 3. Neonatal screening by cIEF. Blood collected on filter paper for neonatal screening was extracted in hemolyzing reagent and analyzed by cIEF. The sample was observed to contain Hb A ($\alpha\beta$), Hb C ($\alpha\beta^C$, a β variant of Hb A), Hb G-Philadelphia ($\alpha^G\beta$, an α variant of Hb A), Hb F ($\alpha\gamma$), an α variant of Hb F ($\alpha^G\gamma$), and an α variant of Hb C ($\alpha^G\beta^C$). With further development, cIEF has potential for both high-throughput screening and for follow-up confirmation of abnormal variants identified by a screening method.

cator of the identity of all of the more common Hb variants. Because cIEF for Hb variant analysis is relatively new, however, there is limited information about the pI of many unusual Hb variants. Nevertheless, a probable identity can often be inferred by comparing relative focusing positions on cIEF to that reported by gel IEF *(9–11)* or alkaline electrophoresis *(2,4)*. We have reported the pI of a number of common and uncommon Hb variants analyzed by cIEF in our laboratory *(8)* using commercially available control samples, samples verified by a reference laboratory, and proficiency testing samples.

3.3.3. Neonatal Screening

Neonatal screening to identify individuals with congenital Hb disorders is well-established in many countries because of the prevalence of these diseases, and because early diagnosis and intervention can markedly improve the outcome of sickle-cell disease and other hemoglobinopathies. We have previously shown that cIEF can be used to perform rapid assays (<4 min) to identify Hbs S and A in blood dried on filter paper *(5)*. The use of high-resolution cIEF for identification of an unusual Hb phenotype in a neonatal screening application is shown in Fig. 3. In this electropherogram, six Hb variants are shown in blood from a single subject dried on filter paper and sent to our laboratory for analysis. The thought process to identify the underlying Hb phenotype was as follows. Only two structural Hb variants are normally expressed in neonates, Hbs F and A (evident as αγ and αβ dimers). Homozygous abnormal alleles of both maternal and paternal β globin genes, like the mutations that give rise to sickle-cell disease, would also give rise to only two structural variants, e.g. Hbs F and S. Three structural Hb variants would be expected in neonates with one normal and one abnormal allele of the β globin gene because both normal and abnormal αβ globin variants would be present along with Hb F. In contrast, four structural Hb variants would be expected in subjects with one mutation in the four α globin genes because both normal and abnormal α variants of both Hbs F and A would be present. In the present case (Fig. 3), the six variant peaks separated by cIEF are attributable to the combination of two mutations in two different globin genes. Four peaks (Hbs A, F, C, and G-Philadelphia) were identified by comparing the calculated pI to pIs previously determined for known Hb variants. The identities of the remaining two variant peaks were then deduced based on what would be expected in a neonate with the double heterozygous phenotype of Hb C trait/Hb G-Philadelphia trait.

Although high-resolution cIEF is analytically suitable for neonatal screening, its role in very high-throughput analysis (e.g., 500 samples/d in many neonatal screening laboratories) has not yet been shown to be technically or economically feasible. The main reason is that autosampler capacity on early generation cIEF instruments was unsuitable for high-throughput applications. In addition, there has been little interest in pursuing this market by manufacturers of capillary electrophoresis (CE) instrumentation. This is regrettable because cIEF could clearly be run on newer generation instruments with higher capacity autosamplers (e.g., 96-well plate format) serving as a low-cost and precise method for high-throughput screening of Hb variants from blood dried on filter paper.

A secondary role for cIEF in current neonatal screening programs as a confirmatory analytical method may be indicated, however. Most high-throughput screening programs presently use high-performance liquid chromatography (HPLC), gel electrophoresis, or gel IEF. The trend has been toward increasing use of automated HPLC, however, the higher cost per test compared to conventional gel systems has proven prohibitive to full-scale conversion to HPLC. High-efficiency separations are not as important as cost for neonatal screening because most laboratories only report specific identification for a limited number of abnormal Hb variants, e.g., Hbs S, E, C, and Bart's. A designation as "other" is sufficient for all other uncommon Hb variants because once identified as abnormal by the primary screening method the samples are usually re-analyzed by a secondary method to confirm and/or identify the Hb phenotype. The cIEF method described here would work well as a secondary identification assay for neonatal screening.

4. MONITORING GLYCEMIC CONTROL
IN DIABETIC PATIENTS

Our research with Hb variants clearly indicated that the same cIEF methodology used for the analysis of structural Hb variants could also be used for the analysis of posttranslational or chemically modified Hb variants. Posttranslational hemoglobins include oxidation products *(8)* like methemoglobins and Hb A_3 (glutathione adduct), and glycation products like Hb A_{1c}. Adding additional tests to an existing platform and reagent system is attractive because of the potential for decreasing the instrument cost per test. Oxidation products, however, are only measured in a small number of specialized laboratories to help diagnose congenital methemoglobinemias, a class of disorders resulting in the oxidation of heme iron and decreased heme oxygen binding *(2,4)*. However, many laboratories, including ours, measure Hb A_{1c} as an indicator of the long-term glucose control in diabetic patients. The following is an initial report of our research and development of cIEF for the analysis of Hb A_{1c} and its clinical use in the evaluation of diabetic patients.

4.1. Overview of the Application

Diabetes causes chronic high blood glucose leading to 1) hyperglycosylation of proteins and cellular structures, and 2) accumulation of toxic metabolites because of abnormal glucose metabolism *(12)*. These metabolic disruptions lead to retinopathy, neuropathy, nephropathy, and other complications of the disease such that diabetes is the leading cause of blindness, end-stage renal disease, and lower-extremity amputations. Treatment of these disorders in the 16 million people in the United States with diabetes costs at least $100 billion annually, accounting for approx 15% of the national health care budget and 25% of Medicare costs *(13)*. The Diabetes Control and Complications Trial (DCCT) *(14)* showed conclusively that intensive management of blood glucose, through frequent administration of insulin, markedly decreases the long-term complications of diabetes. The DCCT also concluded that glycohemoglobin is a good long-term indicator of average blood glucose and is therefore a good laboratory test of glucose status *(15)*. It is now widely accepted that optimal diabetes management should include frequent assessment of glycohemoglobin to evaluate the efficacy of each patient's individual glycemic management program.

Significant controversy remains, however, regarding the best way to measure glycohemoglobin. Part of the problem relates to analyte heterogeneity since glycohemoglobins are a diverse group of compounds with a variety of different sugar moieties bound to hemoglobin at a number of different molecular sites *(12)*. Glycohemoglobin fractions that have been measured clinically to assess glycemia include total glycohemoglobin (e.g., by affinity chromatography) and various subcomponents like Hb A_{1c}, a posttranslational modification of adult Hb A where glucose is nonenzymatically bound to the N-terminal valine of β globin in a stable ketoamine arrangement. It is the most abundant glycohemoglobin, representing around 5–7% of total hemoglobin in nondiabetic individuals, and over 25% in poorly controlled diabetic subjects. Hb A_{1c} is easily separated by most charge-based assay systems, and was the specific analyte used to monitor glycemia in the DCCT. Thus, largely because of the DCCT and despite continued controversy, Hb A_{1c} has become the de facto gold standard laboratory test for assessing glycemic control in diabetic individuals.

4.2. Comparison of cIEF to Conventional Methods

Even if one accepts Hb A_{1c} as the best indicator of long-term glucose status, the selection of a specific method to measure Hb A_{1c} remains problematic. The choice is confounded by the wide variety of commercial analyzers that measure Hb A_{1c} based on different structural or charge-based separation protocols. This includes chromatography (both ion-exchange and affinity), electrophoresis, and immunoassay, each of which is subject to characteristic interferences and problems *(12)*. For example, immunoassays provide no information about the Hb phenotype of a patient. This represents a particular problem for the management of patients with sickle-cell trait or other abnormal Hb phenotypes because these individuals have inherently lower proportions of Hb A_{1c} as a result of the presence of other Hb variants.

Most of the commercially available tests for Hb A_{1c} are HPLC-based systems in hospital and reference laboratories and immunoassays in physician's offices. Because test results are widely variable with different analytical methods, national and international programs have been developed to standardize glycohemoglobin results *(16–18)*. Standardization is considered important because of the importance of longitudinal assessment of diabetic patients and standardization of management practices. The apparent need for standardization, however, also reflects the instability of the analytical market for Hb A_{1c} testing.

To our knowledge, cIEF is the only method that, in addition to analyzing for Hb A_{1c}, can also identify and quantify structural Hb variants using the same reagents. Some commercial HPLC systems can be used for both Hb A_{1c} and Hb variant analysis, however, different columns and/or buffers are needed. Currently CE kits, which include all necessary reagents, are now commercially available for analysis of both Hb variants and Hb A_{1c} by capillary zone electrophoresis (CZE) *(19–21)*. These assays are both rapid (<6 min) and relatively precise (CV < 6%), but separate proprietary buffer systems are used to analyze Hb variants and Hb A_{1c}.

4.3. Method Development of cIEF for Hb A_{1c} Analysis

The analytical properties of the cIEF method we have used to assess structural Hb variants appeared suitable for the analysis of Hb A_{1c}, including separation and quantification. However, prior to clinical application of the method it was necessary to select a method for eliminating interference from labile Hb A_{1c}, an unstable aldimine intermediate that is the precursor in the formation of the stable ketoamine. A more detailed report of the analytical properties of the cIEF method described here, including normal ranges, precision, linearity, and so on, will be published.

4.3.1. Removal of Labile Hb A_{1c}

Stable Hb A_{1c}, not the labile fraction, reflects long-term average blood glucose and thus glycemic control. Because labile and stable Hb A_{1c} are similarly charged, they coelute or comigrate in most charge-based separation systems. Detailed accounts of the analytical implications of this interference have been reported *(22–24)* and have led to the development of a number of protocols for eliminating the labile fraction based on dissociation of the unstable complex, like erythrocyte (RBC) hemolysis and incubation at low pH or RBC incubation in saline.

4.3.1.1. Effects of Low pH

We determined that low pH incubation was unsuitable for removal of labile Hb A_{1c} because of the formation of oxidation products that affect the quantification of Hb variants. Although incubating RBC hemolysates at low pH, rapidly (<30 min) and efficiently removed labile Hb A_{1c}, low pH also promoted the oxidation of heme iron ($Fe^{2+} \rightarrow Fe^{3+}$) and the post-translational formation of methemoglobin. We examined the formation of these oxidation products in a series of buffers over the wide pH range of 4.0–7.5, including buffers prepared in our laboratory and the commercially available hemolyzing reagent used with the Bio-Rad Diamat HPLC. Our results indicate that the same pH conditions that promoted the rapid dissociation of labile Hb A_{1c} also promoted heme iron oxidation.

The effect of low pH on Hb oxidation is clearly demonstrated in Fig. 4. In this experiment, RBCs were hemolyzed in Bio-Rad Diamat hemolyzing reagent at 37°C for 30 min, then repeatedly analyzed 25 times in succession over a period of over 10 h. The electropherograms shown in the figure were obtained at 0 and 3 h, and clearly show the increase in methemoglobin intermediate fractions with time. These results highlight the instability of the Hb at low pH and the adverse effects of low pH on analytical reproducibility. It is important to note that increasing oxidation over time would prohibit automation of the sampling process since a variable time between hemolysis and analysis would affect reproducibility.

There are two main reasons for questioning low pH as a method for eliminating interference by labile Hb A_{1c}. First, the effects of low pH on heme iron oxidation and the optical properties and quantification of Hb are well-documented *(25–28)*. In this case Hb with iron in the oxidized state has a lower extinction coefficient than Hb with iron in the reduced state. This means that a solution containing oxidized Hb will have lower absorbance at 415 nm than a solution containing the same concentration of Hb in the reduced state. Thus, the presence of low pH-induced methemoglobin in a sample will lead to underestimation of total Hb as measured by any method using absorbance at 415 nm. If the estimate of total Hb is inaccurate, then the measurement of Hb A_{1c} expressed as a percent of total Hb will also be inaccurate.

A second reason to question the use of low pH incubation for removal of labile Hb A_{1c} is that increased production of posttranslationally modified Hb variants leads to analytical speciation. This is a problem because conversion of native Hb variants into distinct subcomponents, i.e., methemoglobin fractions, is concentration dependent and can markedly affect analytical results. For example, Hb A is sufficiently abundant such that oxidation leads to the production of enough stable methemoglobin fractions of Hb A to become detectable above baseline in the absorbance plot *(see* Fig. 4). Although Hb A_{1c} is also oxidized under similar conditions, methemoglobin A_{1c} fractions either coelute with other species (e.g., Hb A) or are not detectable above baseline.

The analytical problems presented by Hb oxidation at low pH are not unique to cIEF. Any assay using absorbance detection can be expected to be susceptible to similar interference. It should be noted that this problem would go unnoticed, however, in assays that cannot separate oxidized and reduced Hb subcomponents. The effect of methemoglobin on measurement of Hb A_{1c} when using low pH to remove interference by labile Hb A_{1c} needs more attention and further study. It seems obvious, however, that low pH incubation simply replaces the interference of labile Hb A_{1c} with the equally problematic interference caused by methemoglobin formation.

4.3.1.2. SALINE INCUBATION

Because rapid removal of the labile component by hemolysis of RBC at low pH appeared analytically unsuitable due to the presence of treatment-induced oxidation products, we evaluated saline incubation as an alternative

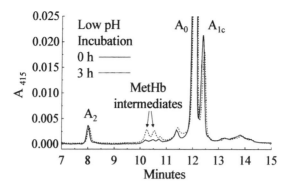

Fig. 4. Removal of labile Hb A_{1c} by low pH: formation of Hb oxidation products. Labile Hb A_{1c} must be removed from blood prior to the measurement of stable Hb A_{1c} for assessment of long-term glucose control. A common method used to eliminate interference by labile Hb A_{1c} is incubation of erythrocytes at low pH (~ pH 5.0) to dissociate glucose from labile Hb A_{1c}. These electropherograms show the time-dependent effect of low pH on Hb in erythrocytes incubated in Bio-Rad Diamat hemolyzing reagent for 30 min then analyzed by cIEF. Small amounts of methemoglobin (MetHb) intermediates were observed even when the sample was analyzed immediately (0 h). Markedly more MetHb was observed when the same sample was analyzed 3 h later. Repeated analysis of the sample over 10 h showed that the measured amount of Hb A_{1c} progressively decreased from 12.3–9.7% while MetHb progressively increased from 1.0 to 10.0% as the sample simply sat at low pH in the autosampler. This indicates that low pH is not a suitable method for the removal of labile Hb A_{1c}.

method for removing the labile Hb A_{1c} fraction. Initially we used a modification of the commonly used method of adding 100 μL of RBC to 1 mL of saline (1:10) and incubating the cells in a water bath overnight (18 h) at 37°C. However, overnight incubation resulted in the production of detectable amounts of oxidation products, including some methemoglobin but more importantly Hb A_3, the glutathione adduct of Hb A *(8)*. In a series of experiments, we evaluated the production of oxidation products and the disappearance of labile Hb A_{1c} over time and at different temperatures. We observed that 1) labile Hb A_{1c} was not efficiently removed at room temperature (~25°C), 2) oxidation products were not usually detected in samples hemolyzed in a solution containing 10 mmol/L KCN and 5 mmol/L EDTA until after more than 8 h of incubation at 37°C, and 3) removal of labile Hb A_{1c} was relatively complete within 5–6 h of incubation at 37°C. Based on these results, we adopted a 6–8 h incubation of RBC in saline (1:10 v/v) at 37°C as our protocol for removing labile Hb A_{1c}. Although somewhat cumbersome in an 8 h work day, we have used this method for over two years

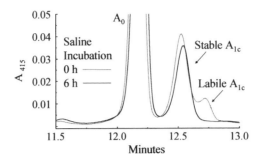

Fig. 5. Removal of labile Hb A_{1c} by saline incubation. Hb A_{1c} in blood from a diabetic subject was analyzed by cIEF before and after the erythrocytes were incubated in isotonic saline for 6 h at 37°C. Labile Hb A_{1c} migrated slightly anodal to stable Hb A_{1c} and was efficiently removed by incubation in saline for 6 h.

with good clinical results to analyze the relatively small number of samples routinely received by our laboratory (usually <40/wk).

The efficient removal of labile Hb A_{1c} by this saline incubation protocol is demonstrated in Fig. 5. In this case, blood was collected from a diabetic subject in poor control and analyzed by cIEF both before and after saline incubation for 6 h. Prior to incubation, two small, partially resolved peaks were observed anodal to Hb A. These peaks were attributed to stable and labile Hb A_{1c}, respectively, by comparing relative focusing positions to that previously reported with gel IEF *(29)*. Moreover, the more anodal peak was not present following saline incubation, as would be expected by the dissociation of labile Hb A_{1c}. It should be noted that this sample contained an unusually high proportion of labile Hb A_{1c}, and that in most samples the labile fraction appears merely as a shoulder on the stable Hb A_{1c} peak. It is also possible that an intensive effort to improve cIEF separation for on-line resolution of stable and labile Hb A_{1c} could abolish the need for sample pretreatment to eliminate the labile fraction.

4.3.2. Correlation with Hb A_{1c} Analysis by HPLC

After selecting a 6-h saline incubation for the removal of labile Hb A_{1c}, we next compared cIEF quantitative results with those obtained by ion-exchange HPLC on the same samples. This was made possible thanks to the cooperation of Dr. Randie Little (Department of Child Health, University of Missouri School of Medicine, Columbia, MO). Samples analyzed by the HPLC method *(30)* were shipped as whole blood on ice to our laboratory and immediately analyzed by cIEF. In one comparison, erythrocytes from 40 different samples were incubated in saline overnight (~15–18 h) at 37°C prior to analysis by both HPLC and cIEF. In the second comparison, the

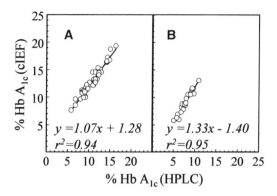

Fig. 6. Correlation of cIEF and HPLC results. Hb A_{1c} results were compared in two sets of samples analyzed by cIEF and ion exchange HPLC. Samples in both (**A**) and (**B**) were prepared from erythrocytes incubated in saline overnight prior to analysis by HPLC. Samples analyzed by cIEF were prepared from erythrocytes incubated in saline for 18 h (**A**) or 6 h (**B**) prior to analysis. Good correlation was observed in both comparisons, though both proportional (slope) and fixed (intercept) bias were affected by the duration of saline incubation prior to analysis by cIEF.

same incubation protocol was used for 21 samples analyzed by HPLC, but using a shorter 6-h incubation for samples analyzed by cIEF.

Figure 6 shows the correlation of the HPLC and cIEF results in these two experiments. Excellent correlation ($R^2 \geq 0.94$) was observed between the HPLC and cIEF methods in both experiments, regardless of the duration of saline incubation. A positive proportional bias (1.07 vs 1.33) was observed for the cIEF assay in both experiments, whereas a more variable fixed bias (+1.28 vs –1.40) was found in samples incubated in saline for 18 and 6 h, respectively. It seems likely that the lower proportional bias compared to the HPLC reference method observed in the 18 h incubation experiment was attributable to the similar incubation protocol used by both laboratories. Because of the problems with oxidation products described above, however, we chose to use the shorter 6 h incubation in our laboratory.

4.3.3. Longitudinal Assessment of Individual Patients with Diabetes

The use of cIEF to monitor Hb A_{1c} in children with Type I diabetes at scheduled quarterly clinic visits over a 2-yr period is shown in Fig. 7. Patients in "good control" actively monitor their glycemic status and adjust their diet, exercise, and insulin as needed to keep blood glucose at or near-normal levels. Consequently, these patients tend to have consistently near normal Hb A_{1c} values over time. In contrast, patients in "poor control" are usually noncompliant, do not monitor blood glucose, skip clinic visits, and

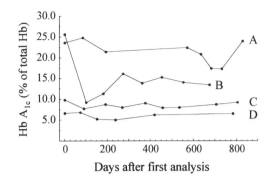

Fig. 7. Using cIEF to monitor long-term glucose status in diabetic subjects. Hb A$_{1c}$ measured by cIEF was used to evaluate diabetic children over a 2-yr period. Examples of the clinical application of the results include patients: (**A**) in poor control with chronic elevated Hb A$_{1c}$; (**B**) with newly diagnosed diabetes where the first observation was from blood collected prior to the advent of insulin therapy; (**C**) in good control with near normal Hb A$_{1c}$ levels; and (**D**) in a subject with both diabetes and sickle-cell trait Hb phenotype.

take little or no action to control their chronic hyperglycemia. As a result, these patients tend to have high and often variable Hb A$_{1c}$ values at each clinic visit. Individuals recently diagnosed with Type I diabetes initially have a very high Hb A$_{1c}$ at their first clinic visit due to poor control of glycemic status prior to diagnosis. This is frequently followed by a "honeymoon period" of low Hb A$_{1c}$ values for about a year after glycemia management is implemented, then an increase in Hb A$_{1c}$ as the body adjusts to a state of controlled chronic hyperglycemia. Diabetic subjects with sickle-cell trait have inherently less Hb A$_{1c}$ than those with normal Hb phenotype when expressed as a percentage of total Hb. These results clearly indicate the clinical relevance of cIEF for measuring Hb A$_{1c}$ to monitor glycemic control over time.

5. CONCLUSION

Our institution is a 200-bed pediatric hospital. We offer both Hb variant and Hb A$_{1c}$ analyses three days a week throughout the year. With our present procedure, sample to sample run time is approx 18 min including all rinses and injections, or about 3 samples/h. With a P/ACE 2200 (Beckman Instruments, Fullerton, CA) samples can run unattended during the day or overnight, with a maximum of 20 samples (~7 h) loaded on the autosampler at one time. This means about 40 samples can be analyzed in one working day. This number of samples would require 2–3 technologist hours per day for instrument setup, data reduction and reporting, and routine administrative responsibilities.

Annually, we perform approx 400 tests to diagnose or monitor congenital hemoglobinopathies, especially sickle-cell disease, and over 1000 tests for Hb A_{1c} to manage diabetic patients. Reagents and consumables, including capillaries, cost only a few cents per test. Controls are inexpensively prepared in our laboratory from RBC and can be stored at $-70°C$ (not at $-20°C$) in hemolyzing reagent for at least 2 yr. Between-run imprecision (% CV) for a normal control containing 2.7% Hb A_2 and 97.3% Hb A was 3.5 and 0.1%, respectively, based on 50 replicate analyses performed on different days over a 5-mo period with multiple capillaries *(8)*. Between run imprecision for controls containing 8.3 and 15.6% Hb A_{1c} was 2.3 and 2.0% CV, respectively, in 40 replicate analyses performed on different days over a 5-mo period.

Given the advantages of capillary electrophoresis for the analysis of hemoglobin variants, including both structural and posttranslational variants, it is surprising that a major manufacturer of analytical instrumentation has not yet had the foresight to develop a commercially available system for these applications.

REFERENCES

1. Bunn, H. F. and Forget, B. G. (1986) Hemoglobin: molecular, genetic and clinical aspects. W. B. Saunders Company, Philadelphia, PA.
2. Fairbanks, V. F. (1980). Hemoglobinopathies and thalassemias. Brian C. Decker, New York.
3. Hempe, J. M. and Craver, R. D. (1999) Laboratory diagnosis of structural hemoglobinopathies and thalassemias by capillary isoelectric focusing, in Methods in Molecular Medicine, vol. 27: Clinical Applications of Capillary Electrophoresis (Palfrey, S. M., ed.), Humana, Totowa, NJ, pp. 81–98.
4. Schmidt, R. M. (1993) Laboratory diagnosis of hemoglobinopathies, in Hematology: Clinical and Laboratory Practice (Bick, R. L., ed.), Mosby, St. Louis, MO, pp. 327–390.
5. Hempe, J. M., Granger, J. G., Warrier, R. P., and Craver, R. D. (1997) Analysis of hemoglobin variants by capillary isoelectric focusing. J. Cap. Elec. 4, 131–35.
6. Hempe, J. M. and Craver, R. D. (1994) Quantification of hemoglobin variants by capillary isoelectric focusing. Clin. Chem. 40, 2288–2295.
7. Craver, R. D., Abermanis, J. G., Warrier, R. P., Ode, D. L., and Hempe, J. M. (1997) Hemoglobin A_2 levels in healthy persons, sickle cell disease, sickle cell trait, and β-thalassemia by capillary isoelectric focusing. Am. J. Clin. Pathol 107, 88–91.
8. Hempe, J. M., Granger, J. G., and Craver, R. D. (1997) Capillary isoelectric focusing of hemoglobin variants in the pediatric clinical laboratory. Electrophoresis 18, 1785–1795.
9. Basset, P., Beuzard, .Y, Garel, M. C., and Rosa, J. (1978). Isoelectric focusing of human hemoglobin: Its application to screening, to the characterization of 70 variants, and to the study of modified fractions of normal hemoglobins. Blood 51, 971–982.

10. Koepke, J. A., Thoma, J. F., and Schmidt, R. M. (1975) Identification of human hemoglobins by use of isoelectric focusing in gel. Clin. Chem. 21, 1953–1955.
11. Black, J. (1984) Isoelectric focusing in agarose gel for detection and identification of hemoglobin variants. Hemoglobin 8, 117–127.
12. Goldstein, D. E., Little, R. R., Lorenz, R. A., Malone, J. I., Nathan, D., and Peterson, C. M. (1995) Tests of glycemia in diabetes. Diabetes Care 18, 896–909.
13. Harris, M. I. and Eastman, R. C. (1996) Early detection of undiagnosed non-insulin-dependent diabetes mellitus. JAMA 276, 1261,1262.
14. The Diabetes Control and Complications Trial Research Group. (1993) The effect of intensive treatment of diabetes on the development and progression of long-term complications in insulin-dependent diabetes mellitus. The Diabetes Control and Complications Trial Research Group. New Engl. J. Med. 329, 977–986.
15. The Diabetes Control and Complications Trial Research Group. (1987) Diabetes Control and Complications Trial (DCCT): results of feasibility study. The DCCT Research Group. Diabetes Care 10, 1–19.
16. Weykamp, C. W., Penders, T. J., Miedema, K., Muskiet, F. A., and van der, Slik, W. (1995) Standardization of glycohemoglobin results and reference values in whole blood studied in 103 laboratories using 20 methods. Clin. Chem. 41, 82–86.
17. Bodor, G. S., Little, R. R., Garrett, N., Brown, W., Goldstein, D. E., and Nahm, M. H. (1992) Standardization of glycohemoglobin determinations in the clinical laboratory: three years of experience. Clin. Chem. 38, 2414–2418.
18. Little, R. R., Wiedmeyer, H. M., England, J. D., Wilke, A. L., Rohlfing, C. L., Wians, F. H., Jr., et al. (1992) Interlaboratory standardization of measurements of glycohemoglobins. Clin Chem 38, 2472–2478.
19. Doelman, C. J., Siebelder, C. W., Nijhof, W. A., Weykamp, C. W., Janssens, J., and Penders, T. J. (1997) Capillary electrophoresis system for hemoglobin A1c determinations evaluated [see comments]. Clin. Chem. 43, 644–648.
20. Mario, N., Baudin, B., Bruneel, A., Janssens, J., Vaubourdolle, and M. (1999) Capillary zone electrophoresis for the diagnosis of congenital hemoglobinopathies. Clin. Chem. 45, 285–288.
21. Cotton, F., Lin, C., Fontaine, B., Gulbis, B., Janssens, J., and Vertongen, F. (1999) Evaluation of a capillary electrophoresis method for routine determination of hemoglobins A2 and F. Clin. Chem. 45, 237–243.
22. Mullins, R. E. and Austin, G. E. (1986) Sensitivity of isoelectric focusing, ion exchange, and affinity chromatography to labile glycated hemoglobin. Clin. Chem. 32, 1460–1463.
23. Bisse, E., Berger, W., and Fluckiger, R. (1982) Quantitation of glycosylated hemoglobin. Elimination of labile glycohemoglobin during sample hemolysis at pH 5. Diabetes 31, 630–633.
24. Mortensen, H. B. and Christophersen, C. (1982) Glycosylation of human hemoglobin A. Kinetics and mechanisms studied by isoelectric focusing. Biochim. Biophys. Acta 707, 154–163.
25. Bunn, H. F. and Drysdale, J. W. (1971) The separation of partially oxidized hemoglobins. Biochim. Et Biophys. Acta 229, 51–57.

26. Tomoda, A., Takeshita, M., and Yoneyama, Y. (1978) Analysis of met-form hemoglobin in glucose-deleted human red cells. FEBS Lett 88, 247–250.
27. Zijlstra, W. G., Buursma, A., and Meeuwsen-van der Roest, W. P. (1991) Absorption spectra of human fetal and adult oxyhemoglobin, de-oxyhemoglobin, carboxyhemoglobin, and methemoglobin. Clin. Chem. 37, 1633–1638.
28. Tomoda, A., Yoneyama, Y., and Tsuji, A. (1981) Changes in intermediate haemoglobins during autoxidation of haemoglobin. Biochem. J. 195, 485–492.
29. Stickland, M. H., Perkins, C. M., and Wales, J. K. (1982) The measurement of haemoglobin A1c by isoelectric focussing in diabetic patients. Diabetologia 22, 315–317.
30. Goldstein, D. E., Little, R. R., England, J. D., Wiedmeyer, H. M., and McKenzie, E. M. (1986) Methods for quantitating glycosylated hemoglobins: high performance liquid chromatography and thiobarbituric acid colorimetry, in Methods in Diabetes Research (Larner, J., Pohl, S. L., and Clarke, W. L., eds.), Wiley, New York, pp. 475–504.

III
Metabolic Diseases

9

Amino Acid Analysis

Mary Kathryn Linde

1. INTRODUCTION

Sequencing of biological or synthetic peptides has sparked interest in the separation and quantitation of amino acids by capillary electrophoresis (CE). Because amino acids comprise a group of negatively charged, positively charged and neutral molecules, it has been difficult to separate and quantitate all amino acids using a single procedure. Today many proteins and peptides that require sequencing are frequently available in only microgram (µg) quantities necessitating quantitation of the amino acids at extremely low concentrations. Although a few amino acids contain aromatic groups that strongly absorb in the ultraviolet (UV) range, the majority lacks strongly absorbing chromophore groups. This lack of sensitivity further complicates the ability to separate amino acids.

CE does offer advantages in solving some of these problems. Specifically, CE requires only a small sample size, although nanomolar (n*M*) are still required, and the separation can be finished quickly, sometimes within minutes.

Jorgenson and Lukacs *(1,2)* first used CE to separate and detect amino acids in 1981. They demonstrated rapid separation and fluorescent detection of both peptides and amino acid derivatives. After derivatization with 5-dimethylaminonaphthalene-1-sulfonyl chloride (dansyl) they were able to separate a mixture of dansylated amino with a separation efficiency of approx 250,000 theoretical plates *(2)*. They also demonstrated that the separation was proportional to voltage applied and that by increasing the voltage up to 30 kV, efficiencies exceeding 400,000 theoretical plates can be achieved within 10–30 min *(1)*. This pioneering work demonstrated that the simple, rapid separations found with CE can be an alternative to high-performance liquid chromatography (HPLC).

From: *Clinical and Forensic Applications of Capillary Electrophoresis*
Edited by: J. R. Petersen and A. A. Mohammad © Humana Press Inc., Totowa, NJ

Amino acid identification and quantification is of prime importance for medical diagnosis *(3,4)* as well as biomedical and industrial research. Thus, as methods and instrumentation have become available throughout the 1980s, the use of CE for amino acid separation and identification has expanded.

2. DETECTION

Derivatization to produce either a strongly UV absorbing or fluorescent chromophore prior to injection onto the capillary have been investigated to enhance the detection of amino acids.

2.1. Ultraviolet

In early studies, UV absorption was the most common method to detection amino acids or amino-acid derivatives separated by CE. There were, however, several drawbacks. The short pathlength of the capillary and the low molar absorptivities of the amino acids or derivatives limited the detection limits. Even so, the strong UV absorbance of the coenzyme pyrroloquinoline quinone was shown to provide sensitive detection of derivatized amino acids *(5)*. Additionally, cyclic 3-phenyl-2-thiohydantoin derivatives that absorb strongly at 254 nm are produced by the reaction of phenylisothiocyanate and amino acids *(6)*. However, the formation of the thiohydantoin derivatives from the amino and carboxylic acid groups of the amino acid eliminates one of the properties (the zwitterionic charge) that helps in the separation of many of the amino acids.

2.2. Fluorescence

Fluorescence, both lamp based and laser induced, has been found to be more useful for the highly sensitive detection required for amino acids separated by CE *(7)*. During the 1980s, most investigators used lamp based fluorescence *(1,8–10)*. Albin et al. *(11)* described a lamp-based fluorescence detector to measure amino acid derivatives of 9-fluorenylmethyl chloroformate at concentrations as low as 10 ng/mL. Lui and coworkers *(12)* synthesized 3-(4-carboxybenzoyl)-2-quinolinecarboxyaldehyde to produce fluorescent isoindole products and were able to effectively detect 17 amino acids with lamp-based fluorescence.

Laser-induced fluorescence (LIF) dramatically improved sensitivity but because of the limited number of commercially available lasers the number of derivatizing agents were limited to those with excitation spectra that match those of commonly used lasers. The argon ion laser has been the most popular in LIF because of its output at 488 nm that matches the excitation maxima of fluorescein isothiocyanate *(7)*. Lui et al. *(13)* used a chiral reagent, 4-(3-isothiocyanatopyrrolidin-1-yl)-7-nitro-2,1,3-benzoxadiazole to produce fluorescent diastereomeric derivatives with a 488 nm excitation maximum. A helium-cadmium laser with emission lines at 325 or 442 nm has been used *(14)* in some applications. Tetramethylrhodamine isothiocyanate amino-acid derivatives have been sucessfully detected using a helium-neon laser *(15)*. In additon, laser modifications have resulted in a semiconductor laser *(15)* and diode laser *(16)*, both of which are reported to improve efficiency. Timperman et al. *(17)* have also reported a highly sensitive LIF wavelength-resolved detection system

A sheath flow cell was used as a post-column reactor for fluorescence derivatization by Cobel and Timperman *(18)*. They described a simple laser-induced fluorescence detection method for proteins and amino acids in which fast-reacting o-phthaldialdehyde-2-mercaptoethanol was added to the sheath fluid for derivatization. Fluorescent excitation using a helium-cadmium laser (325 nm excitation) allowed emissions to be collected with a microscope objective and focused through a slit to a photon-counting photomultiplier tube. Lowest limits of detection were for glycine which showed detection limits at 2.3×10^{-8} *M*. A UV (krypton fluoride) laser (244 nm excitation) was used by Chan and associates *(19)* for measurement of native tryptophan fluorescence after separation by micellar electrokinetic chromatography (MEKC).

2.3. Indirect Fluorescence

Some investigators reported measurement of native amino acids by indirect fluorescence detection *(9,10)*. The principle of this method of detection is dependent on the presence of a strongly fluorescing background electrolyte to produce a high background signal. The nonflorescent analyte passing through the detector displaces some of the fluorescing-background electrolyte, resulting in a decrease in background signal. Indirect detection was described by Bruin et al. *(20)* using salicylate at pH 11.0 as the background electrolyte to detect underivatized amino acids. The method was reported to be more sensitive for low electrolyte concentrations. Ma and coworkers *(21)* also studied the use of quinine sulfate as the background electrolyte for detection of cationic amino acids. In addition, Lee and Lin *(22)* studied nine different background electrolytes for detection of underivatized amino acids. They found π-amino salicylic acid and 4-(*N,N*-dimethyl)aminobenzoic acid in a basic solution to be the most useful. They also found that adding cationic surfactants reduced the electroosmotic flow. In a later study *(23)*, they added cyclodextrins in reduce electroosmosis and enhance selectivity.

2.4. NMR

Sweedler et al. *(24)* found proton nuclear magnetic resonance (NMR) a useful detection system. They circumvented the inherently low sensitivity of NMR, which requires the use of large diameter flow cells, by wrapping a microcoil directly around the capillary to construct a 5.0 nL cell. Even though the sensitivity was less than that of UV detection systems, NMR detectors can provide an alternative for on-column detection.

2.5. MS

Electrospray ionization to create gas phase ions from the nonvolatile components separated by CE allowed structural analysis through mass spectroscopy (MS). This combination of CE and MS was reported by Garcia and Henion *(25)*. They attempted to overcome the incompatibilities between the two systems by the use of gel-filled capillaries to decouple the electrophoresis buffer from the ionization source. They provided much structural information on separated dansylated-amino acids.

2.6. Electrochemical

Although most underivatized amino acids are not electroactive, some reports of electrochemical detection methods do appear promising. Underivatized amino acids were detected by electrochemical detection using a copper electrode above pH 12.0 *(26)*. Dinitrophenyl-derivatized amino acids have also been detected using a reductive electrochemical system *(27)*. O'Shea et al. *(28)* described the use of carbon-fiber electrodes with an electrical isolation circuit. Using this system, they were successful in detection of glutamic acid and aspartic acids, which are easily oxidized following reaction with naphthalene-2,3-dicarboxaldehyde.

2.7. Other

Waldron and Dovichi *(29)* reported a thermooptical detector system that used a krypton fluoride laser as the energy source. The method was found to be sensitive at the 1 μM level for 3-phenyl-2-thiohydantoin-amino acids. Other workers investigated chemoluminescence *(30,31)* and nucleation light-scattering *(32)* detection.

3. DERIVATIZATION

Although derivatization alters the electrophoretic properties of amino acids, it has been the only method to detect amino acids at the concentrations required (p*M*). This has led to a plethora of derivatizing agents (*see* Table 1).

Table 1
Common Agents for Amino Acid Derivatization

Derivatizing agent	Reference
5-dimethylaminonaphthalene-1-sulfonyl chloride (dansyl)	*(1,2,25,47,49, 55,56,58, 62,64–66,68, 73–77,114)*
Fluorescein isothiocynate	*(11)*
Fluorescamine	*(11)*
Pyrroloquinoline quinone	*(5)*
3-phenyl-2-thiohydantoin	*(6,52)*
o-phthaldialdehyde	*(11,40,42–44, 92)*
Naphthalene-2,3-dicarboxaldehyde	*(16,44)*
9-fluorenylmethyl chloroformate	*(35,70,77,110)*
(+)- and (-)-1-(-fluroenyl) ethyl chloroformate	*(36)*
3-(4-carboxybenzoyl)-2-quinolinecarboxaldehyde	*(12)*
4-(3-isothiocyanatophrrolidin-l-yl)-7-nitro-2,1,3-benzoxadiazole	*(13)*
6-aminoquinoyl-*N*-hydroxysuccinimidyl carbamate	*(37,71,77)*
Tetramethylrhodamine isothiocyanate	*(15)*
Pyronin succinimidyl ester	*(38)*
Dicarbocyanine succinimidyl ester	*(39)*
o-phthaldialdehyde in tandem with dicarbocyanine succinimidyl ester	*(40)*
1-methoxycarbonylindolizine-3,5-dicarbaldehyde	*(41)*
2-(9-anthry)ethyl chloroformate	*(36)*
Tetramethylrhodamine thiocarbamyl	*(57)*
(S)-1-(1-naphthyl)ethyl isothiocyanate	*(67)*
(S)-1-phenylethyl isothiocyanate	*(67)*
N-tert-butoxycarbonyl	*(69)*
N-acetylcysteine and *o*-phthaldialdehyde	*(86)*
2,3,4,6-tetra-*O*-acetyl-1-thio-β-D-glucopyranose to *o*-phthaldialdehyde	*(87)*
(+)-*OO*-dibenzoyl-L-tartaric anhydride	*(88)*
o-phthaldialdehyde-2-mercaptoethanol	*(18)*
Phenylthiocarbamyl	*(32,98)*
Monobromobimane	*(104)*
4-aminosulfonyl-7-fluoro-2,1,3-benzoxadiazole	*(112)*

3.1. Pre-Column

The dansyl amino acids derivatives, as described by Jorgenson and Lukacs *(1,2)*, have been the most frequently reported, especially in early studies. The dansyl derivatives are still used as the standard to assess the utility and efficiency of new techniques or modifications of previous methods. The fluorescence is easily detected and, although quantum yields are reduced in the aqueous environment of CE *(8)*, results are reproducible.

Fluorescein, another popular fluorescent label for biochemical molecules in early CE studies, has both excitation and emission spectra in the visible wavelength range *(11)* allowing for easy detection. However, undesirable side reactions of fluorescein isothiocynate (FITC) used in the derivatization process have prevented its widespread use when the molecule of interest is at low concentration. Another fluorogenic molecule, fluorescamine, which has similar properties to FITC has also been used *(33)*. The problem with this label was that the sensitivity was insufficient for many applications.

A substituted isoindole ring, formed through the reaction between anime group on an amino acid and o-phthaldialdehyde, results in derivatives that show both a strong absorbance at 260 and 340 nm *(11)* and also fluoresce at 475 nm. Unlike FITC, o-phthaldialdehyde does not produce florescent side products, making it a more usable reagent. However, when compared to another popular fluorogenic derivatizing agent, naphthalene-2,3-dicarboxaldehyde, the derivatives formed with o-phthaldialdehyde are much less stable. Naphthalene-2,3-dicarboxaldehyde derivatives, like fluorescein, have excitation and emission spectra in the visible range, 462 nm and 490 nm, respectively. They became popular in chiral separations (*see* Section 4.2.) *(34)* even though the narrow Stokes shift presented a potential source of error on some instruments.

The fluorogenic label, 9-fluorenylmethyl chloroformate, forms amino derivatives that strongly absorb at 265 nm and fluoresce at 315 nm. Both primary and secondary amines can be derivatized with this reagent *(35)*. Wan and associates *(36)* used a related agent, (+)- and (-)-1-(-fluroenyl) ethyl chloroformate, in the analysis of amino-acid enantiomerics (*see* Section 4.2.). Liu and others *(12)* reported a highly sensitive method for separation of primary amines derivatized with 3-(4-carboxybenzoyl)-2-quinolinecarboxaldehyde. They used LIF as the method of detection (*see* Section 2.). In another study *(13)* these same investigators separated amino-acid residues labeled with the reagent, 4-(3-isothiocyanatopyrrolidin-l-yl)-7-nitro-2,1,3-benzoxadiazole, which has an excitation maximum of 480 nm.

Many of these amino-acid derivatives are unstable, which prevented long-term storage of the compounds, thus limiting the ability to have purified standards for unknown identification. Improved stability was achieved using 6-aminoquinoyl-*N*-hydroxysuccinimidyl carbamate *(37)* as the derivatizing agent. Amino-acid derivatives were prepared with this reagent using protein or peptide hydrolysates were much more stable in both HPLC and CE applications.

LIF (*see* Section 2.) because of its sensitivity, sparked investigations with many fluorophores was used to produce amino-acid derivatives. The 540 nm optimal excitation wavelength of Tetramethylrhodamine isothiocyanate *[15]*), produced by a helium–neon laser, allowed a low-cost detection method. A synthesized label, pyronin succinimidyl ester, was excited with a semiconductor laser *(38)*. Mank and Yeung *(39)* labeled amino acids with the dicarbocyanine using dicarbocyanine succinimidyl ester. A diode laser (667 nm emission) was used in this study to produce the excitation wavelength along with a low-cost detection method.

3.2. On-Column

Although most derivatizations have been developed using pre-column techniques, on-column and post-column derivatizations have also been investigated. On-column derivatization has been achieved at the inlet of the capillary column where derivatizing reagent and sample were allow to react for a period of time before the electrophoresis was begun. Two variations have been described *(8)*. In one method, the tandem mode, a plug of the derivatizing reagent was injected into the capillary inlet preceding a plug of the sample solution. In the sandwich mode, a plug of derivatizing reagent was injected at the capillary inlet, followed by a plug of the sample solution and then by another plug of the derivatizing reagent. Taga and Honda *[40]*) used o-phthaldialdehyde in a tandem mode with dicarbocyanine succinimidyl ester that capitalized on the mobility differences in of the two reactants. Although derivatization was enhanced, there was a loss in resolution. Another fluorescent-derivitizing reagent, 1-methoxycarbonylindolizine-3,5-dicarbaldehyde (excitation at 409 nm and emission at 482 nm), has been used in a sandwich mode to produce a highly sensitive method *(41)*.

Gilman and Ewing *(16)* demonstrated amino-acid, on-column derivatization and detection of separated amino acids from injected intact cells. Single cells were injected into the column inlet. Once in the capillary, the cells were lysed and the released amino acids derivatized with naphthalene-2,3-dicarboxaldehyde. The amino acids within the cells were able to be detected and quantitated at attomole concentrations.

3.3. Post-Column

Pre-column and on-column derivatization allows for several potential errors. For example, the derivatizing agent may react more efficiently with one amino acid than another, thus quantitative errors may occur. At the same time derivatized standards may not directly relate to the same level of amino acid in an unknown mixture *(8)* because of matrix differences and/or differences in affinity of the derivatizing agent. Derivatized amino acids may show different migration rates relative to each other as compared to their underivatized form, allowing possible qualitative problems. By using post-column derivatization, many of the potentially erroneous results of pre-column and on-column derivatization can be eliminated.

As with other derivatizing modes, the most extensively studied post-column agents have been fluorogenic. Albin and workers *(11)* introduced o-phthaldialdehyde by differential electroosmotic flow at a gap junction reactor, which was further modified by Gilman and Ewing *(42)* to allow introduction of the derivatizing agent by diffusion. Both o-phthaldialdehyde and naphthalene-2,3-dicarboxyaldehyde, along with LIF, were used to develop a highly sensitive analytical method for glycine. Zhu and Kok *(43)* introduced o-phthaldialdehyde through a porous tube connecting the capillary and the reactor tube. Using a lamp rather than LIF, they were able to detect amino acids at concentrations of 2 µm. Using a coaxial design, Zhang and Yeung *(44)* constructed a reactor that used a power source separate from that used by the CE instrument. Using o-phthaldialdehyde as the post-column derivatizing agent and LIF, they were able to detect concentrations of 2.2×10^{-8} *M* for six amino acids. These and other post-column derivatization methods for fluorescence and chemiluminescence detection was reviewed by Zhu and Kok *(45)*.

4. METHODS OF SEPARATION

4.1. Micellar Electrokinetic Capillary Chromatography (MEKC)

Pure mixtures have been used in the great majority of the studies involving separation of amino acids. However, low-peak capacity of the methods used limited the use of CE in separating more complex mixtures. Using micellar electrokinetic capillary chromatography (MEKC), separation of neutral along with charged components was possible based on their partitioning between the aqueous phase and a pseudo-stationary phase *(46)*. MEKC was shown very effective in separation of complex mixtures of amino acids. Ong and coworkers *(47)* successfully separated 15 dansylated amino acids in less than 30 min using 40 m*M* sodium docecyl sulfate (SDS) in a phosphate-borate buffer. The first separation of all 20 natural amino acids was reported by Skocir and coworkers *(48)* using 102 m*M* SDS in 20 m*M* borax buffer, pH 9.2, and a column temperature of 10°C. Matsubara and Terabe *(49)* subsequently resolved 24 dansylated amino acids in 70 min at pH 2.4 using a neutral surfactant and a Tween 20-phosphate buffer (Fig. 1).

Terabe and his coworkers *(50)* also showed that addition of urea to SDS buffers enhanced separation of amino acids derivatized by 3-phenyl-2-thiohydantin. Using this derivatizing agent, Castagnola and associates *(51)*

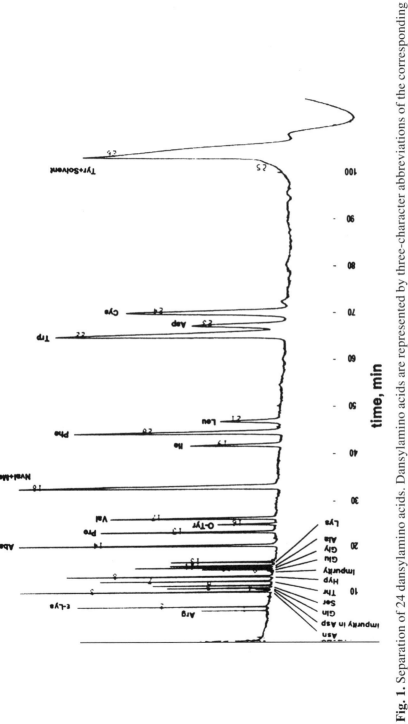

Fig. 1. Separation of 24 dansylamino acids. Dansylamino acids are represented by three-character abbreviations of the corresponding amino acids (_-Lys is _-dansyllysine, O-Tyr is O-dansyltyrosine, Cys is didansylcystine, and Lys and Tyr are didansyl derivatives). A fused silica capillary, 25 µm × 34 cm (19 cm to detector) was used for the separation. Electrophoretic buffer is 100 mM Tween-20, 25 mM sodium phosphate, pH 2.4; applied voltage was 16 kV; detection was at 200 nm.

studied the effect of various buffer conditions, SDS concentrations, and amount of derivatizing agent added. By optimizing the conditions, they were able to resolve 18 amino acids simultaneously in 15 min. Furthering this work, Kim and coworkers *(52)* compared the surfactants, SDS and dodecyltrimethyl ammonium bromide, and indicated that SDS gave the best separation for analysis of Edman degradation products using 3-phenyl-2-thiohydantin as the derivatizing agent. Using a 50 m*M* SDS in 25 m*M* phosphate buffer, they could resolve all natural amino acids except leucine and isoleucine. Still another study demonstrated the use of mixed cationic-anionic micelles for separation of these derivatized amino acids *(53)*.

MEKC separation and resolution of other derivatized amino acids were also investigated. Ueda and coworkers *(34)* found that using naphthalene-2,3-dicarboxaldehyde they were able to separate the derivatized amino acids in about 25 min using SDS buffer to which β-cyclodextrin was added. DeSilva and Kuwana *(54)* subsequently used cyclodextrin-modified MEKC to separate several amino acids using naphthalene-2,3-dicarboxaldehyde. They assessed the importance of SDS for the separation in addition to the effect of neutral hydroxypropyl beta-cyclodextrin and charged carboxy-methyl beta-cyclodextrin on the resolution. Chan and associates *(35)* separated 18 amino acids derivatized with 9-fluorenylmethyl chloroformate using a SDS-borate surfactant at pH 9.2. Wan et al. *(36)* used a SDS-phosphate-borax-urea system to separate 2-(9-anthry)ethyl chloroformate derivatized amino acids. Mank and Yeung *(39)* separated 18 amino acids derivatized with dicarbocyanine using SDS-borate-MeOH at 30 kV.

Although fused silica capillaries work well and are easier to use, coated capillaries have the potential to improve the separation of derivatized amino acids. In this regard Sun et al. *(55)* synthesized and evaluated anionic-polymer-coated capillaries with a pH-independent electroosmotic flow to separate dansylated amino acids. In addition, Janini et al. *(56)* developed a technique called reversed-flow MEKC in which polyacrylamide coated capillaries were used to suppress the electroosmotic flow (EOF). Reversing the polarity of the instrument was necessary because the SDS micelle migration was anodic and the EOF was negligible under these conditions. Using this system with SDS-acetate, pH 4.2, was used to separate 15 dansylated amino acids. They also studied the effect of cetyltrimethyl ammonium bromide.

Other modifications have been reported to improve separation and resolution of amino acids that were difficult to analyze. Culbertson and Jorgenson *(57)* used flow-counterbalanced CE to control the analyte migration to separate components with closely related mobilities, such as leucine and isoleucine derivatized with tetramethylrhodamine thiocarbamyl. Simultaneous pH and ionic-strength effects and buffer selection were investigated by Camillari and Okafo *(58)*, who reported improved separation of dansylated amino acids when using D_2O to increase the viscosity.

4.2. Chiral Separations

Amino acids have at least one chiral carbon and, with few exceptions, exist in two optically active enantiomeric forms, dextrorotatory (D) and levarotatory (L). These optical isomers behave differently in biological systems. For example, enzyme activity is often specific for a particular optical isomer and different enantiomeric forms of a drug may produce different therapeutic effects. In living organisms, proteins contain the D-enantiomeric form of amino acids, whereas nucleic acids contain the L form. The fact that the enantiomeric amino acids have different properties and functions of enantiomers make their separation critically important (*see* Table 2 for a listing of the chiral separation of amino acids). Separation and quantitation of these forms has been achieved by a variety of methods, such as anionic-polymer-coated capillaries *(55)*, addition of an optically active molecule to the migration buffer, which acts as a chiral selector, and by chiral derivatization prior to analysis creating a diastereomer.

Studies by Wan and associates *(36)* using (+)- and (-)-1-(-fluroenyl) ethyl chloroformate, showed that after converting enantiomers of amino acids into diastereomers, separation, identification, and quantitation of the optical isomers was possible at 3×10^{-8} *M*. In another set of experiments Liu and others *(13)* used CE to separate D- and L-amino acid residues using the fluorescent chiral reagent 4-(3-isothiocyanatopyrrolidin-l-yl)-7-nitro-2,3-benzoxadiazole. Using 25 m*M* acetate buffer, pH 4.0, 10 m*M* Triton X-100 they were able to separate derivatized D,L-proline and D,L-valine. Without the addition of Triton X-100, no separation was seen; thus, they suggested that the partitioning coefficients for the various diasteromers between the micelles and the solution was of prime importance in their separation. They applied this method to the determination of D- and L-amino acids using the peptide, gramicidin D, as the test case. This study demonstrated that CE showed higher efficiencies than HPLC under the same conditions.

Gassmann and associates *(59)* separated dansylated D- and L-amino acids by the interaction between the respective amino acid and a Copper (II) complex of L-histidine present in the support electrolyte. They reported separation and detection of femtomole amounts of racemic mixtures of dansylated amino acids within 10 min. In a later study *(60)*, Copper II-L-aspartamine in the run buffer was also shown to be an effective chiral selector. Direct chiral resolution of underivatized amino acids by ligand-exchange capillary zone electrophoresis (CZE) was described by Vegvari and coworkers *(61)*. Using

Table 2
Common Chiral Selectors Used for Separation of Enantiomers of Amino Acids

Chiral selector	Reference
L-histidine/Cu II complex	*(59)*
L-asparatamine/Cu II complex	*(60)*
Didecyl-L-alanine	*(62)*
α-cyclodextrin	*(63)*
β-cyclodextrin	*(36,63,67,76)*
γ-cyclodextrin	*(36,63,70,71)*
Heptakis-(2,6-di-o-methyl)-β-cyclodextrin	*(63)*
γ-cyclodextrin and sodium deoxycholate	*(64)*
β-cyclodextrin and urea	*(66)*
Heptakis-2,3,4-tri-*O*-methyl-β-cyclodextrin	*(67)*
Hydroxypropyl-β-cyclodextrin	*(69)*
Hydroxypropyl-γ-cyclodextrin	*(69)*
n-alkyl-β-D-glucopyranosides	*(72)*
Sulfobutyl ether-β-cyclodextrin	*(73,74)*
Bovine albumin and dextrins	*(75)*
Restocetin	*(77)*
Vancomycin	*(78)*
Sodium-*N*-dodecanoyl-L-valinate	*(79)*
Sodium-*N*-dodecanoyl-L-serine	*(80)*
β-escin	*(83)*
Digitonin	*(83)*
Sodium-*N*-dodecanoyl-L-glutamate	*(81,82)*
Digitonin and sodium taurodexycholate	*(82)*
Digitonin and sodium docecyl sulfate	*(83)*
Seriodal-glycoside surfactant-borate complex	*(84)*
L-phenylalanine anilide and methacrylic acid	*(85)*
L-phenylalanine anilide and 2-vinylpyridine	*(85)*
Triethanolamine-phosphoric acid with α-cyclodextrin	*(89)*
Teicoplanin	*(90)*

N-(2-hydroxy-octyl)-L-4-hydroxyproline/Cu (II) as a selector, amino acids containing aromatic residues and histidine were resolved. In all the cases, *in situ* diasteromers were formed enhancing separation. Cohen et al. *(62)* was also able to separate dansylated D- and L-amino acids using the chiral detergent, didecyl-L-alanine, dissolved in a solution of SDS, forming mixed micelles. The chiral detergent incorporated in the SDS micelles with the hydrophilic chiral L-alanine regions orientated to the surface where an interaction with chiral amino acids could occur.

Early studies of Snopek et al. *(63)* showed the simple and robust utility of cyclodextrin as stereospecific selectors or electrolyte modifiers. They showed that α-, β- and γ-cyclodextrin as well as heptakis-(2,6-di-o-methyl)-β-cyclodextrin were effective in chiral separation for both CZE and isotachophoresis. They used a poly(tetrafluoroethylene) capillary and a conductivity detector to resolve model isomeric compounds. Terabe et al. *(64)* advanced this work by a modification of the MEKC technique for enantiomeric separation by adding a mixture of β-cyclodextrins and γ-cyclodextrins. They then applied this technique for the separation of 10 pairs of dansylated-amino acids. The best separations, however, were achieved using a mixture of both cyclodextrins in SDS. Good separations were also achieved with addition of β-cyclodextrins, γ-cyclodextrins, and with mixtures of γ-cyclodextrin and sodium taurodeoxycholate. Penn and coworkers *(65)* also studied the mechanisms involved in micelle-assisted separations using β-cyclodextrins in SDS to separate dansylated amino acids.

The use of urea was also found to enhance the separation of dansylated amino acids with β-cyclodextrins *(66)*. In addition, Bonfichi et al. *(67)* achieved efficient chiral separations using heptakis-2,3,6-tri-*O*-methyl-β-cyclodextrin and β-cyclodextrin. These workers used (*S*)-1-(1-naphthyl)-ethyl isothiocyanate and (S)-1-phenylethyl isothiocyanate for derivatization prior to separations.

Chiral separations of dansylated amino acids have also been accomplished by adding high molecular weight anionic and cationic surfactants to cyclodextrins *(68)*. The modified cyclodextrins, hydroxypropyl-β-cyclodextrin and hydroxypropyl-γ-cyclodextrin, were also shown to improve the chiral separations of *N*-tert-butoxycarbonyl amino acids *(69)*. In addition, Wan and associates *(16)* studied various combinations of SDS, 2-propanol, β-cyclodextrins, and γ-cyclodextrins in the enantiomeric separation of 2-(9-anthry)ethyl chloroformate derivatized amino acids. They were able to resolve 12 and 13 amino acids with various surfactant combinations. Riester et al. *(70)* reported on the chiral separation of 9-fluorenylmethyl chloroformate derivatives of amino acids using γ-cyclodextrins along with SDS. Swartz et al. *(71)* described the simultaneous MEKC separation of a mixture of six amino-acid enantiomers derivatized with 6-aminoquinoyl-*N*-hydroxysuccinimidyl carbamate. The use of n-alkyl-β-D-glucopyranosides to separate enantiomers has described by Desbene and Fulchic *(72)*.

Many variations of MEKC have been used to separate enantiomers of dansyl-amino acids. For example, negatively charged sulfobutyl ether-β-cyclodextrin was found to be useful by Desiderio and Fanali *(73)* to separate the enantiomers of dansylated amino acids. Similarly, Janini et al. *(74)* used sulfobutyl ether-β-cyclodextrin to separate enantiomers of 12 dansylated amino acids. In addition, Sun and coworkers *(75)* explored the use of affinity interactions between macromolecules and amino acids using bovine albumin and dextrins to separate dansylated amino acids. Dansylated amino acids have also been separated with *N*-methylformamide and β-cyclodextrin *(76)*.

Armstrong et al. *(77)* introduced the use of the macrocyclic antibiotic, ristocetin, as a chiral selector. Using this antibiotic the chiral separation of a large groups of amino acids derivatized with 5-dimethylaminoaphthalene-1-sulfonyl chloride, 6-aminoquinoyl-*N*-hydroxy succinimidyl carbamate, or 9-fluorenylmethylchloroformate was possible. Resolutions equal to or greater than those of cyclodextrin were achieved. Another macrocyclic antibiotic, vancomycin, was also found to be an effective chiral selector *(78)*.

Amino acids derivatized with 3-phenyl-2-thiohydantoin have also been separated in MEKC using chiral surfactants, such as sodium-*N*-dodecanoyl-L-valinate *(79)*, sodium-*N*-dodecanoyl-L-serine *(80)*, and sodium-*N*-dodecanoyl-L-glutamate *(81)*. The formation of mixed micelles using sodium-*N*-dedecanoyl-L-glutamate along with a mixture of digitonin and sodium taurodexycholate *(82)* or digitonin with SDS effectively separated phenylthiohydantoin-amino acids *(83)*. Others showed that chiral micelles consisting of steriodal-glycosides borate complexes could also be used *(84)*. Additionally, Lin and coworkers *(85)* reported on the highly specific separation of amino-acid enantiomers using an on-column prepared molecular imprinted polymer. L-Phenylalanine anilide was used as the print molecule and methacrylic acid and/or 2-vinylpyridine as the functional monomers to prepare the on-column polymer.

Investigators have also designed procedures that produce derivatized amino acids that were diastereomers *(39,59)*, thus separation did not need to be chiral selective. Houben et al. *(86)* used N-acetylcysteine and o-phthaldialdehyde to derivatize D,L-valine forming diastereomers prior to separation. Tivesten and Folestad *(87)* produced diastereomers by adding 2,3,4,6-tetra-*O*-acetyl-1-thio-β-D-glucopyranose to the o-phthaldialdehyde for precolumn-labeling of D- and L-amino acids. They added polymer modifiers to achieve optimal conditions for the separation of 17 labeled amino acids. Scheutzner et al. *(88)* optimized conditions by adjusting pH and solvent composition to separate diastereomer derivatives of (+)-*OO'*-dibenzoyl-L-tartaric anhydride in CZE.

The critical need to determine optical purity of raw materials as well as final products prompted the chiral separation and quantitation of tryptophan, a frequent starting material in pharmaceutical synthesis. In this regard Altria et al. *(89)* not only detected but quantitated 0.1% L-tryptophan in the presence of the D-enantiomer using a triethanolamine-phosphoric acid containing α-cyclodextrin. A good example of this type of separation is shown in

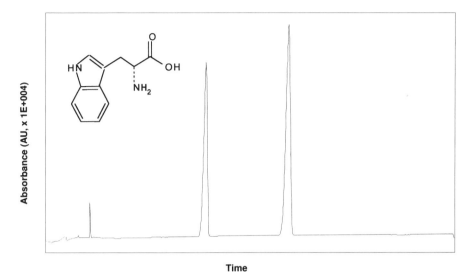

Fig. 2. Separation of tryptophan in the presence of highly sulfated α-cyclo-dextrin. The instrument was a MDQ system from Beckman Coulter Inc. A fused silica capillary, 50 μm × 31.5 cm, was used for the separation. Buffer was 25 m*M* TEA phosphate, pH 2.5, to which was added 5% highly α-cyclodextrin; voltage was 15 KV (reversed polarity). The sample was pressure injected at 0.3 psi for 4 s with UV detection at 200 nm.

Fig. 2. Tesarova et al. *(90)* also compared separation of *N*-tert-butyloxy-carbonyl (t-Boc) amino acids, important precursors in peptide synthesis, and their nonblocked analogs on a teicoplanin-based chiral stationary phase. The mobile-phase composition was optimized using various ratios of acetoni-trile and 1% triethylamine/acetate buffer to achieve separation in 8–12 min. The retention and enantioresolutions were compared and the investigators concluded that native unblocked amino acids have better interaction with the teicoplanin stationary phasse, were better enantioresolved than blocked amino acids, and finally that the amino group plays an important role in the steroselective stationary phase-analyte interaction.

Direct chiral resolution of underivatized amino acids by ligand-exchange CZE was described by Vegvari and coworkers *(61)*. Using *N*-(2-hydroxy-octyl)-L-4-hydroxyproline/Cu (II) as a selector, amino acids containing aro-matic residues and histidine were resolved.

5. MICROCHIP TECHNOLOGY

The challenges of microchip technology have also been applied to CE analysis of amino acids. By fusing a cover glass over glass or quartz plates into which small channels were micromachined, tiny capillary channels are formed. Such channels function as open-tubular capillaries on the microchip and was used by Seiler et al. *(91)* to rapidly separate phenylthiocarbamyl amino acids in <2 min. Amino acids, derivatized with o-phthaldialdehyde have been separated within a few seconds using either a chip-based precolumn *(92)* or a chip-based postcolumn *(93)* derivatization reaction. The micromachining of CE injectors and separation on glass chips has also been studied by Fan and Harridan *(94)* by studying the flow at the capillary junction under various defined conditions. Von Heeren and associates *(95)* have used MEKC on microchips. They were able to separate six FITC-labeled amino acids in a few seconds. On-column sample gating was described by Monning and Jorgenson *(96)*. In their system most of the sample, which was continuously introduced into the capillary, was destroyed by photolysis, but that which survived became the sample plug. FITC-labeled amino acids were separated in about 1.5 s. In a later study, 5-FITC-labeled amino acids were separated in 120 ms *(97)*.

6. CLINICAL AND BIOMEDICAL APPLICATIONS

The most useful application for CE in amino-acid analysis is elucidating the structure of both natural and laboratory-synthesized proteins and polypeptides. In 1991, Bergman and associates *(98)* demonstrated the utility of CE for preparative purposes because of its reproducibility. These workers also demonstrated that amino-acid composition and sequence analysis of proteins could be achieved using phenylthiocarbamyl derivatized amino. Rapid, reliable results on extremely small sample accelerated industrial adaptations. For example, the aromatic amino acids in citrus juice were measured by Cancalon and Byran *(99)* and in cheddar cheese by Strickland et al. *(100)* using CE.

Although the utility of amino-acid identification and quantitation in biological samples is more limited than for industrial uses, their measurement in specific cases can give crucial information about the disease state. Separation of amino acids in biological fluids is also much more difficult than when using pure substances. There is the potential for matrix interference, such as the reaction of the derivatizing agent with other components, and in addition, difficulty in comparing solvent-based standards to amino acids in the samples. Thus amino-acid separation and quantitation in biological samples is more problematic than analysis of model laboratory mixtures. Methods developed using model mixtures frequently do not work when applied to biological samples, making assay modifications necessary. Dankava and Kaniansky *(101)* assessed limitations of various modes of CZE in the separation of enantiomers in model and urine matrices. Tryptophan was used as the model analyte and a 90-component mixture of UV light-absorbing organic anions served as the model matrix. Using on-line coupled isotacophoretic sample pretreatment for high sample-load capacity, they were able to separate samples corresponding to 3–6 μL of undiluted urine.

Cerebrospinal fluid analysis to monitor amino-acid levels using MEKC was reported by Berquist et al. *(102)* using an on-line derivatization and microdialysis sampling technique. Continuous in vivo monitoring of glutamate and aspartate in neurotransmitters of rats using CZE has been reported by Zhou and coworkers *(103)*. An automated procedure for in vivo monitoring cysteine and glutathione in rat caudate nucleus was also reported by Lada and Kennedy *(104)*. In this study, microdialysis was coupled on-line with CZE. The dialysates were derivatized on-line with monobromo-bimane and transferred to the capillary by a flow-gated interface. Separated thiols were measured on-line by a helium-cadmium LIF. Glutamate in microdialysates of striated muscle were measured with CE in an off-line procedure *(105)*. Additionally, phenylthiohydantoin derivatives of 3- and 4-hydroxyproline were separated using MEKC in bovine skeletal muscle collagen *(106)*.

Diagnostic applications of CE for amino-acid analysis have also expanded. Glutamine measured by CZE and LIF detection in cerebrospinal fluid of children with meningitis was reported by Tucci and coworkers *(107)*. They found glutamine concentration was lower in children with viral and bacterial meningitis and proposed that the lower concentrations might be caused by glutamine use by the bacteria. They confirmed the diagnostic utility of this analytical method in the critical differentiation of meningitis. Shihabi and Friedberg *(108)* and Lehmann et al. *(109)* reviewed amino-acid analysis in serum, urine, other body fluids and tissues.

Jellum and coworkers *(110)* described a multi-component analytical system to determined diagnostic metabolites, such as cysteine and homocysteine, in urine of patients with various aminoacidopathies and other metabolic disorders. They used a diode-ray detector for fluorescence detection of metabolites derivatized with 9-fluorenylmethyl chloroformate and separated by CZE. They modified and expanded this study using gas chromatography-mass spectroscopy (GC-MS) in a study on sera of patients collected prior to disease symptoms and held in the Janus-bank *(111)*. Kang et al. *(112)* determined 4-aminosulfonyl-7-fluoro-2,1,3-benzoxadiazole-derivatized homocysteine, glutathione, and cysteine in plasma. Causse et al. *(3)* separated and determined homocysteine in plasma using FITC as the derivatizing agent and an argon ion laser for detection. The detection of this intermediary metabolite in the methionine pathway is useful to detect not only genetic metabolic disorders, but also the potential risk for atherosclerosis and some thromboembolic diseases.

Tagliaro et al. *(4)* used CZE in the determination of serum phenylalanine in a rapid, inexpensive method for diagnosis of phenylketonuria. Also, cysteine in human blood, plasma and urine has been separated and quantitated at the attomole level using an end-column amperometric detection with a gold/mercury amalgam electrode *(113)*. In addition, enantiomeric forms of amino acids derived from novel depsipeptide antitumor antibiotics were analyzed by a metal chelate MEKC method using a cyclodextrin *(114)*. The amino acids were hydrolyzed and derivatized with either dansyl chloride for UV-absorbance detection or with FITC for LIF detection. Enantiomeric identities of serine, beta-hydroxyl-*N*-methy-valine were confirmed and a nonchiral aminoacid, sarcosine, was found.

7. CONCLUSION

CE is used for separation and analysis of amino acids, however, its use has mainly been outside the clinical arena. CE has been shown to be extremely useful in the food, wine, and biotechnology areas. Although CE provides faster separation and turn-around time, the driving force in clinical laboratories, HPLC and GC, are still the mainstays. Perhaps as more diagnostic applications using CE are developed, it will replace HPLC as the method of choice for rapid amino-acid analysis.

REFERENCES

1. Jorgenson, J. W. and Lukacs, K. D. (1981) High-resolution separations based on electrophoresis and electroosmosis. J. Chromatogr. 218, 209–216.
2. Jorgenson, J. W. and Lukacs. K. D. (1981) Zone electrophoresis in open-tubular glass capillaries. Clin. Chem. 27, 1551–1553.
3. Causse, E., Terrier, R., Champagne, S., Nertz, M., Valdiguie, P., Salvayre, R., and Couderc, R. (1998) Quantitation of homocysteine in human plasma by capillary electrophoresis and laser-induced fluorescence detection. J. Chromatogr. A 817, 181–185.
4. Tagliaro, F., Moretto, S., Valentini, R., Ganibaro, G., Antonioli, C., Moffa, M., and Tato, L. (1994) Capillary zone electrophoresis determination of phenylalanine in serum: a rapid inexpensive and simple method for diagnosis of phenylketonuria, Electrophoresis 15, 94–97.
5. Esaka, Y., Yamaguchi, Y., Kano, K., and Goto, M. (1993) Separation of amino acid-oxazole derivatives of the redox coenzyme pyrroloquinoline quinone by capillary zone electrophoresis. J. Chromatogr. 652, 225–232.
6. Otsuka, K., Terabe, S., and Ando T. (1985) Electrokinetic chromatography with micellar solutions: separation of phenylthiohydantoin-amino acids. J. Chromatogr. 332, 219–226.

7. Wu, S. and Dovichi, N. J. (1989) High-sensitivity fluorescence detector for fluorescein isothiocyanate derivatives of amino acids separated by capillary zone electrophoresis. J. Chromatogr. 480, 141–155.
8. Smith, J. T. (1997) Developments in amino acid analysis using electrophoresis. Electrophoresis 18, 2377–2392.
9. Kuhr, W. G. and Young, E. S. (1988) Indirect fluorescence detection of native amino acids in capillary zone electrophoresis. Anal. Chem. 60, 1832–1834.
10. Kuhr, W. G. and Young, E. S. (1988) Optimization of sensitivity and separation in capillary zone electrophoresis with indirect fluorescence detection. Anal. Chem. 60, 2642–2646.
11. Albin, M., Weinberger, R., Sapp, E., and Moring, S. (1991) Fluorescence detection in capillary electrophoresis: evaluation of derivatizing reagents and techniques. Anal. Chem. 63, 417–422.
12. Liu, J., Hsieh, Y., Wiesler, D., and Novotny, M. (1991) Design of 3-(4-carboxybenzoyl)-2-quinolinnecarboxaldehyde as a reagent for ultra sensitive determination of primary amines by capillary electrophoresis using laser fluorescence detection. Anal. Chem. 63, 408–412.
13. Liu, Y., Schneider, M., Sticha, C. M., Toyooka, T., and Sweedler, J. V. (1998) Separation of amino acid and peptide steroisomers by nonionic micelle-mediated capillary electrophoresis after chiral derivatization. J. Chromatogr. A 800, 345–354.
14. Ueda, T., Michell, R., Kitamura, F., and Metcalf, T. (1992) Separation of naphthalene-2,3-dicarboxaldehyde-labeled amino acids by high-performance capillary electrophoresis with laser-induced fluorescence detection. J. Chromatogr. 593, 265–274.
15. Zhao, J. Y., Chen, D. Y., and Dovichi, N. J. (1992) Low-cost laser-induced fluorescence detection for micellar capillary zone electrophoresis. Detection to the zeptomol level of tetramethylrhodamine thiocarbamyl amino acid derivatives. Anal. Chim. Acta 608, 117–120.
16. Gilman, S. D. and Ewing, A. G. (1996) Analysis of single cells by capillary electrophoresis with on-column derivation and laser-induced fluorescence detection. Anal. Chem. 67, 58–64.
17. Timperman, A. T., Khatib, K., and Sweedler, J. V. (1995) Wavelength resolved fluorescence detection in capillary electrophoresis. Anal. Chem. 67, 139–144.
18. Coble, P. G. and Timperman, A. T. (1998) Fluorescence detection of proteins and amino acids in capillary electrophoresis using a post-column sheath flow reactor. J. Chromatogr. A. 829, 309–315.
19. Chan, K. C., Muschik, G. M., and Issaq, H. J. (1995) Separation of tryptophan and related indoles by micellar electrokinetic chromatography with KrF laser-induced fluorescence detection. J. Chromatogr. A 718, 203–210.
20. Bruin, G. J., van Asten, A. C., Xu, X., and Poppe, H. (1992) Theoretical and experimantal aspects of indirect detection in capillary electrophoresis. J. Chromatogr. 608, 97–107.

21. Ma, Y., Zhang, R., and Cooper, C. L. (1992) Indirect photometric detection of polyamines in biological samples separated by high performance capillary electrophoresis. J. Chromatogr. 608, 93–96.

22. Lee, Y. H. and Lin, T. I. (1994) Capillary electrophoretic determination of amino acids with indirect absorbance detection. J. Chromatogr. A 680, 287–297.

23. Lee, Y. H. and Lin, T. I. (1995) Capillary electrophoretic determination of amino acids. Improvement by cyclodextrin additives. J. Chromatogr. A 716, 335–346.

24. Wu, N., Peck, T. L., Webb, A. G., Magin, R. L., and Sweedler, J. V. (1994) H-NMR spectroscopy on nanoliter scale for static on line measurements. Anal. Chem. 66, 3849–3857.

25. Garcia, F. and Henion, J. D. (1992) Gel-filled capillary electrophoresis/mass spectrometry using liquid junction ion spray interface. Anal. Chem. 649, 985–990.

26. Ye, J. and Baldwin, R. P. (1994) Determination of amino acids and peptides by capillary electrochemical detection at a copper electrode. Anal. Chem. 66, 2669–2674.

27. Malone, M. A., Weber, P. L., Smyth, M. R., and Lunte, S. M. (1994) Reductive electrochemical detection for capillary electrophoresis. Anal. Chem. 66, 3782–3787.

28. O'Shea, T. J., Greenhagen, R. D., Lunte, S. M., Lunte, C. E., Smyth, M. R., Radzik, D. M., and Watanabe, N. (1992) Capillary electrophoresis with electrochemical detection employing on-column nafion joint. J. Chromatogr. 593, 305–312.

29. Waldron, K. C. and Dovichi, N. J. (1992) Sub-femtomole determination of pheylthiohydantoin-amino acids: capillary electrophoresis and thermooptical detection. Anal. Chem. 64, 1396–1399.

30. Wu, N. A. and Huie, C. W. (1993) Peroxyoxalate chemiluminescence detection in capillary electrophoresis. J. Chromatogr. 634, 309–315.

31. Liao, S.-Y. and Whang, C.-W. (1996) Indirect chemiluminescence detection of amino acids separated by capillary electrophoresis. J. Chromatogr. A 736, 247–254.

32. Szostek, B. and Koropchak, J. A. (1996) Condensation nucleation light scattering detection for capillary electrophoresis. Anal. Chem. 68, 2744–2752.

33. Shippy, S. A., Jankowski, J. S., and Sweedler, J.V. (1995) Analysis of trace level peptides using capillary electrophoresis with UV laser-induced fluorescence. Anal. Chim. Acta 307, 163–171.

34. Ueda, T., Mitchell, R., Kitamura, F., Metcalf, T., Kuwana, T., and Nakamoto, A., (1991) Chiral separation of naphthalene-2,3-dicarboxaldehyde-labeled amino acid enantiomers by cyclodextrin-modified micellar electrokinetic chromatograhy with laser induced fluorescence detection. Anal. Chem. 63, 2971–2981.

35. Chan, K. C., Janini, G. D., Muschik, G. M., and Issaq, J. J. (1993) Laser-induced fluorescence detection of 9-fluorenylmethyl chloroformate derivatized amino acids in capillary electrophoresis. J. Chromatogr. 653, 93–97.

36. Wan, H., Andersson, P. E., Engstroem, A., and Blomberg, L. G. (1995) Direct and indirect chiral separation of amino acids by capillary electrophoresis. J. Chromatogr. A 704, 3018–3022.

37. Cohen, S. A. and Michaud, D. P. (1993) Synthesis of a fluorescent derivatizing agent 6-aminoquinolyl-N-hydroxysuccinimidyl carbamate and its application for analysis of hydrolysate amino acids via high-performance liquid chromatography. Anal. Biochem. 211, 279–284.

38. Fuchigami, T., Imasak, T., and Shiga, M. (1993) Subatomole detection of amino-acids by capillary electrophoresis based on semi-conductor fluorescence detection. Anal. Chim. Acta 282, 209–213.

39. Mank, A. J. G. and Yeung, E. S. (1995) Diode laser-induced fluorescence detection in capillary electrophoresis after pre-column derivatization of amino acids and small peptides. J Chromatogr. A 708, 309–321.

40. Taga, A. and Honda, S. (1996) Derivatization at capillary inlet in high performance capillary electrophoresis: its reliability in quantitation. J. Chromatogr. A 742, 243–250.

41. Oguri, S., Uchida, C., Miyake, Y., and Miki, Y. (1995) 1-methoxy-carbonylindolizine-3,5-decarbaldehyde as a derivatization reagent for amine compounds in high performance capillary electrophoresis. Analyst, 120, 63–68.

42. Gilman, S. D. and Ewing, A. G. (1995) Post-column derivatization for capillary electrophoresis using naphthalene-2,3-dicarboxyaldehyde and 2 mercaptoethanol. Anal. Methods Instrum. 2, 133–141.

43. Zhu, R. and Kok, W. T. (1995) Post column reaction system for fluorescence detection in capillary electrophoresis. J Chromotogr. A 716, 113–133.

44. Zhang, I. and Yeung, E. S. (1996) Postcolumn reactor in capillary electrophoresis for laser-induced fluorescence detection. J. Chromatogr. A 734, 331–337.

45. Zhu, R. and Kok, W. T. (1998) Post-column derivatization for fluorescence and chemiluminescence detection in capillary electrophoresis. J. Pharm. Biomed. Anal. 17, 985–999.

46. Terabe, S., Otsuka, K., and Ando, T. (1984) Electrokinetic chromatography with micellar solution and open tubular capillary. Anal. Chem. 56, 111–113.

47. Ong, C. P., Ng, C. L., Lee, H. K., and Li, S. F. Y. (1991) Separation of dns-amino acids and vitamins by micellar electrokinetic chromatography. J Chromatogr. 559, 537–545.

48. Skocir, E., Vindevogel, J., and Sandra, P. (1994) Separation of 23 dansylated amino acids by micellar electrokinetic chromatography at low-temperatures. Chromatographia 39, 7–10.

49. Matsubara, N. and Terabe, S. (1994) Separation of 24 dansylamino acids by capillary electrophoresis with a non-ionic surfactant. J. Chromatogr. A 680, 311–315.

50. Terabe, S., Ishihama, Y., Nishi, H., Fukuyama, T., and Otsuka K, (1991) Effect of urea addition in micellar electrokinetic chromatography. J. Chromatogr. 545, 359–368.

51. Castagnola, M., Rossetti, D. V., Cassiano, L., Rabino, R., Nocca, G., and Giardina, B. J. (1993) Optimization of phenylthiohydantoinamino acid sepa-

ration by micellar electrokinetic capillary electrophoresis. J. Chromatogr. 638, 327–334.

52. Kim, N. J., Kim, J. H., and Lee, K.-J. (1995) Application of capillary electrophoresis to amino acid sequencing of peptides. Electrophoresis 16, 510–515.

53. Ong, C. P., Ng, D. L., Lee, H. K., and Li, S. F. Y. (1994) The use of mixed surfactants in micellar electrokinetic chromatography. Electrophoresis 15, 1273–1275.

54. DeSilva, K. and Kuwana, T. (1997) Separation of chiral amino acids by micellular electrokinetic chromatography with derivatized cyclodextrins. Biomed. Chromatogr. 11, 230–235.

55. Sun, P., Landman, A., Barker, G. E., and Hartwick, R. A. (1994) Synthesis and evaluation of anionic-polymer-coated capillaries with pH dependent electroosmotic flows for capillary electrophoresis. J. Chromatogr. A 685, 303–312.

56. Janini, G. M., Muschik, G. M., and Issaq, H. J. (1996) Separation of pyridine carboxylic acid isomers and related compounds by capillary zone electrophoresis. Effect of cetyltrimethylammonium bromide on electroosmotic flow and resolution. J. Chromatogr. B 683, 29–35.

57. Culbertson, C. T. and Jorgenson, J. W. (1994) Flow counterbalanced capillary electrophoresis. Anal. Chem. 66, 955–962.

58. Camilleri, P. and Okafo, G. (1991) Simultaneous pH and ionic strength effects and buffer selection in capillary electrophoretic techniques. J. Chromatogr. 541, 489–495.

59. Gassmann, E., Luo, J. W., and Zare, R. N. (1985) Electrokinetic separation of chiral compounds. Science 230, 813, 814.

60. Gozel, P., Gassmann, E., Michelson, H., and Zare, R. N. (1987) Electrokinetic resolution of amino acid enantiomers with copper (II)-aspartame. Anal. Chem. 59, 44–49.

61. Vegvari, A., Schmid, M. G., Kilar, F., and Gubitz, G. (1998) Chiral separation of alpha-amino acids by ligand-exchange capillary electrophoresis using N-(2-hydroxy-octyl)-L-4-hydroxyproline as a selector. Electrophoresis 19, 2109–2012.

62. Cohen, A. S., Terabe, S., Smith, J. A., and Karger, B. L. (1987) High performance capillary electrophoresis separation of bases, nucleosides, and oligonucleotides: retention manipulation via micellar solutions and metal additives. Anal. Chem. 59, 1021–1027.

63. Snopek, J., Soini, H., Novotny, M., Smalkova-Keulemansova, E., and Jelinek, I. (1991) Selected applications of cyclodextrin selectors in capillary electrophoresis. J. Chromatogr. 559, 215–222.

64. Terabe, S., Miyashita, Y., Ishihama, Y., and Shibata, O. (1993) Cyclodextrin-modified micellar electrokinetic chromatography separations of hydrophobic and enantiomeric compounds. J. Chromatogr. 636, 47–55.

65. Penn, S. G., Lui, G., Bergstroem, E. T., Goodall, D. M., and Loran, J. S. (1994) Systematic approach to treatment of enantiomeric separations in capillary electrophoresis and liquid chromatography. I. Initial evaluation using propranolol and dansylated amino acids. J. Chromatogr. A 680, 147–155.

66. Yoshinaga, M. and Tanaka, M. (1995) Effect of urea addition on chiral separation of dansylamino acids by capillary zone electrophoresis with cyclodextrins. J. Chromatogr. A 710, 331–337.

67. Bonfichi, R., Dallanoce, C., Lociuro, S., and Spada, A. (1995) Free-solution capillary resolution of chiral amino acids via derivatization with monochiral isothiocyanates. Part I. J. Chromatogr. A 707, 355–365.

68. Ozaki, H., Ichihara, A., and Terabe, S. (1995) Micellar electrokinetic chromatography using high-molecular mass surfactants: comparison between anionic and cationic surfactants and effects of modifiers. J. Chromatogr. 709, 3–10.

69. Yowell, G. G., Fazio, S. D., and Vivilecchia, R. (1996) Direct chiral separation of amino acids derivatized with 2-(9-anthryl) ethyl chloroformate by capillary electrophoresis using cyclodextrins as chiral selectors. Effect of organic modifiers on resolution and enantiomeric elution order. J. Chromatogr. A 745, 73–79.

70. Riester, D., Wiesmueller, K.-H., Stoll, D., and Kuhn, R. (1996) Racemization of amino in solid phase peptide synthesis investigated by capillary electrophoresis. Anal. Chem. 68, 2361–2365.

71. Swartz, M. E., Mazzeo, J. R., Grover, E. R., and Brown, P. R. (1995) Separation of amino acid enantiomers by micellar electrokinetic capillary chromatography using synthetic chiral surfactants. Anal. Biochem. 231, 65–71.

72. Desbene, P. L. and Fulchic, C. E. (1996) Utilization of n-alkyl-β-D-glucopyranosides in enantiomeric separation by micellar electrokinetic chromatography. J. Chromatogr. A 749, 257–269.

73. Desiderio, C. and Fanali, S. (1995) Use of negatively charged sulfobutyl ether-β-cyclodextrin for enantiomeric separation by capillary electrophoresis. J. Chromatogr. A 716, 183–196.

74. Janini, G. M., Muschik, G. M., and Issaq, H. J. (1996) Electrokinetic chromatography in suppressed electroosmotic flow environment: use of a charged cyclodextrin for the separation of enantiomers and geometric isomers. Electrophoresis 17, 1575–1583.

75. Sun, P., Wu, N., Barker, G. and Hartwick, R. S. (1993) Chiral separations using dextran and bovine serum albumin as run buffer additives in affinity capillary electrophoresis. J. Chromatogr. 648, 475–480.

76. Valko, I. E., Siren, H., and Riekkola, M.-L. (1996) Chiral separation of dansyl-amino acids in nonaqueous medium by capillary electrophoresis. J. Chromatogr. A 737, 263–272.

77. Armstrong, D. W., Gasper, M. P., and Rundlett, K. L. (1995) Highly enantioselective capillary electrophoresis: separations with dilute solutions of the macrocyclic antibiotic ristocetin. J. Chromatogr. A 689, 285–304.

78. Vespalec, R., Corstjens, H., Billiet, H. A. H., Frank, J., and Luyden, K. C. A. M. (1995) Enantiomeric separation of sulfur-and selenium-containing amino acids by capillary electrophoresis using Vancomycin as a chiral selector. Anal. Chem. 67, 2501–2514.

79. Otsuka, K., Kawahara, J., Tatekawa, K., and Terabe, S. (1991) Chiral separations by micellar electrokinetic chromatography with sodium N-dodecanoyl-L-valinate. J. Chromotogr. 559, 209–214.

80. Otsuka, K., Karuhaka, K., Higashimori, M., and Terabe, S. (1994) Optical resolution of amino acid derivatives by micellar electrokinetic chromatography with sodium N-dodecanoyl-L-serine. J. Chromotogr. A 680, 317–320.

81. Otsuka, K., Kawakami, H., Tamaki, W., Terabe, S., Otsuka, K., Kawahara, J., Tatekawa, K., and Terabe, S. (1995) Chiral separations by micellar electrokinetic chromatography with sodium N-dodecanoyl-L-glutamate. J. Chromatogr. A, 716, 319–322.

82. Otsuka, K., Kawahara, J., Kawaguchi, Y., Koike, R., Hisamitsu, T., and Terabe, S. (1993) Optical resolution by high-performance capillary electrophoresis and micellar electrokinetic chromatography with sodium N-dodecanoyl-L-glutamine and digitonin. J. Chromotogr. 652, 253–257.

83. Kurosu, Y., Murayama, K., Shindo, N., Shisa, Y., and Shioka, N. (1996) Optical resolution of phenylthiohydantoin-amino acids by capillary electrophoresis and identification of the phenylthiohydantoin-D-amino acid residue of [D-ala^2]-methionine enkephalin. J. Chromatogr. A 752, 279–286.

84. Mechref, Y. and El Rassi, Z. (1996) Micellar electrokinetic capillary chromatography with in-situ charged micelles: VI. Evaluation of novel chiral micelles consisting of steroidal-glycoside surfactant-borate complexes. J. Chromatogr. A 724, 285–296.

85. Lin, J. M., Nakagama, T., Uchiyama, K., and Hobo, T. (1997) Capillary electrochromatographic separation of amino acid enantiomers using on-column prepared molecularly imprinted polymer. J. Pharm. Biomed. Anal. 15, 1351–1358.

86. Houben, R. J. H., Gielen, H., and Vanderwa, S. (1993) Automated preseparation derivatization on a capillary electrophoresis instrument. J. Chromatogr. A. 634, 317–322.

87. Tivesten, A. and Folestad, S. (1995) Separation of precolumn-labeled D-and L- amino acids by micellar electrokinetic chromatography with UV fluorescence detection. J. Chromatogr. A 708, 323–337.

88. Schuetzner, W., Caponecchi, G., Fanali, S., Rizzi, A., and Kenndler, E. (1996) Separation of diastereomers by capillary zone electrophoresis in free solution with polymer additive and organic solvent component. Effect of pH and solvent composition. J. Chromatogr. A 719, 411–420.

89. Altria, K. D., Harkin, P., and Hindson, M. G. (1996) Quantitative determination of tryptophan enantiomers of capillary electrophoresis. J. Chromatogr. B 686, 103–110.

90. Tesarova, E., Bosakova, Z., and Pacakova, V. (1999) Comparison of enantioselective separation of N-tert-butyloxycarbonyl amino acids and their non-blocked analogues on teicoplanin-based chiral stationary phase. J. Chromatogr. A 838, 121–129.

91. Seiler, K., Harrison, D. J., and Manz, A. (1993) Planar glass chips for capillary electrophoresis: repetitive sample injection, quantitation and separation efficiency. Anal Chem. 65, 1481–1488.

92. Jacobson, S. C., Hergenroeder, R., Moore, A. W., Jr., and Ramsey, J. M. (1994) Precolumn reactions with electrophoretic analysis integrated on a microchip. Anal. Chem. 66, 4127–4132.

93. Jacobson, S. C., Koutny, L. B., Hergenroeder, R., Moore Jr., A. W., and Ramsey, J. M. (1994) Microchip capillary electrophoresis with an integrated postcolumn reactor. Anal. Chem. 66, 3472–3476.
94. Fan, Z. H. and Harrison, D. J. (1994) Micromachining of capillary electrophoresis injectors and separation on glass chips and evaluation of flow at capillary intersections. Anal Chem. 66, 177–184.
95. von Heeren, F., Verpoorte, E., Manz, A., and Thormann, W. (1996) Micellar electrokinetic chromatography separations and analyses of biological samples on a cyclic planar microstructure. Anal. Chem. 68, 2044–2053.
96. Monnig, C. A. and Jorgenson, J. W. (1991) On column sample gating for high-speed capillary zone electrophoresis. Anal. Chem. 63, 802–807.
97. Moore, A. W., Jr. and Jorgenson, J. W. (1993) Study of zone broadening in optically gated high-speed capillary electrophoresis. Anal. Chem. 65, 3550–3560.
98. Bergman, T., Agerberth, B., and Jornvall, H. (1991) Direct analysis of peptides and amino acids from capillary electrophoresis, FEBS Lett. 283, 100–103.
99. Cancalon, P. F. and Bryan, C. R. (1993) Use of capillary electrophoresis monitoring citrus juice composition. J. Chromatogr. 652, 555–561.
100. Strickland, M., Weimer, B. C., and Broadbent, J. R. (1996) Capillary electrophoresis of cheddar cheese. J. Chromatogr. A 731, 305–313.
101. Dankava, M. and Kaniansky, D. (1999) Capillary zone electrophoresis separation of enantiomers present in complex ionic matrices with on-line isotachophoretic sample pretreatment. J. Chromatogr. A 838, 31–38.
102. Bergquist, J., Gilman, S. D., Ewing, A. G., and Ekmann, R. (1994) Analysis of human cerebrospinal fluid by capillary electrophoresis with laser-induced fluorescence detection. Anal. Chem. 66, 3512–3518.
103. Zhou, S. Y., Zuo, H., Stobaugh, J. F., Lunte, C. E., and Lunte, S. M. (1995) Continuous in vivo monitoring of amino acid neurotransmitters by microdialysis sampling with on-line derivatization and capillary electrophoresis separation. Anal. Chem. 67, 594–599.
104. Lada, M. W. and Kennedy, R. T. (1997) In vivo monitoring of glutathione and cysteine in rat caudate nucleus using microdialysis on-line with capillary zone electrophoresis-laser induced fluorescence detection. J. Neurosci. Meth. 72, 153–159.
105. Dawson, L. A., Stow, J. M., Dourish, C. T., and Routledge, C. (1995) Analysis of glutamate in striatal microdialysates using capillary electrophoresis and laser-induced fluorescence detection. J. Chromatogr. A 700, 81–87.
106. Chu, Q., Evans, B. T., and Zeece, M. G. (1997) Quantitative separation of 4-hydroxyproline form skeletal muscle collagen by micellar electrokinetic capillary electrophoresis. J. Chromatogr. B 692, 293–301.
107. Tucci, S., Pinto, C., Goyo, J., Rada, P., and Hernandez, L. (1998) Measurement of glutamine and glutamate by capillary electrophoresis and laser induced fluorescence detection in cerebrospinal fluid of meningitis sick children. Clin. Biochem. 31, 143–150.
108. Shihabi, Z. K. and Friedberg, M. A. (1997) Analysis of small molecules for clinical diagnosis by capillary electrophoresis. Electrophoresis 18,1724–1732.

109. Lehmann, R., Liebich, H. M., and Boelter, W. (1996) Application of capillary electrophoresis in clinical chemistry: developments from preliminary trials to routine analysis. J. Cap. Electrophoresis 3, 89–110.

110. Jellum, E., Thorsud, A. D., and Time, E. (1991) Capillary electrophoresis for diagnosis and studies of human disease, particularly metabolic disorders. J. Chromatogr. 559, 455–465.

111. Jellum, E., Dollekamp, H., Brunsvig, A., and Gislefoss, R. (1997) Diagnostic applications of chromatography and capillary electrophoresis. J. Chromatogr. B 689, 155–164.

112. Kang, S. H., Kim, J.-W., and Chung, S. S. (1997) Determination of homocysteine and other thiols in human plasma by capillary electrophoresis, J. Pharm. Biomed. Anal. 15, 1435–1441.

113. Jin, W. and Wang, Y. (1997) Determination of cysteine by capillary zone electrophoresis with end-column amperometric detection at a gold/mercury amalgam microelectrode without deoxygenation. J. Chromatogr. A 769, 307–314.

114. Lui, J., Dabrah, T. T., Matson, J. A., Klohr, S. E., Volk, K. J., Kerns, E. H., and Lee, M. S. (1997) Analysis of amino acid enantiomers derived from antitumor antibiotics using chiral capillary electrophoresis. J. Pharm. Biomed. Anal. 16, 207–214.

10
Organic Acids

Kern L. Nuttall and Norberto A. Guzman

1. INTRODUCTION

Organic acids are a heterogeneous class of low-mol-wt metabolites that contain at least one carboxylic acid group. Several hundred compounds may be included, depending on how expansive a definition is used. Normally, amino acids are not included, although some organic acids contain nitrogen. The wealth of clinical information obtained by analysis of organic acids has tended to be ignored for a number of reasons. The primary clinical application has been limited to the diagnosis of inborn errors of metabolism. Also, traditional analysis has been performed using gas chromatography-mass spectrometry (GC-MS), which is expensive and technically demanding. With the advent of less expensive methods of analysis such as capillary electrophoresis (CE), organic-acid analysis is finding many previously underutilized and unrecognized clinical applications. The current state of the art still requires organic acid profiling for inborn errors of metabolism by GC-MS analysis, however, this is unlikely to remain the case much longer. Already CE methods for the short-chain organic acids have been published and more comprehensive profiling methods are certain to be developed. The real promise of CE for organic acids, however, lies in fast and inexpensive assays for newer applications, several of which are discussed here.

Many of the CE applications for organic acids share a number of features to improve separation and detection. These include: 1) Flow reversal of the electroosmotic flow (EOF), 2) the use of indirect photometric detection or direct detection at short wavelengths, and 3) the need for specimen preparation, particularly at low concentrations of analyte. These features are discussed briefly in Sections 1.1.–1.3. below.

From: *Clinical and Forensic Applications of Capillary Electrophoresis*
Edited by: J. R. Petersen and A. A. Mohammad © Humana Press Inc., Totowa, NJ

1.1. Flow Reversal

In the standard configuration, cations pass the detector first, followed by neutral compounds and then anions. Reversal of the EOF produces much faster separations for anions such as organic acids. Although not all assays for organic acids use flow reversal, the majority do. Flow reversal is achieved by two basic methods, use of coated capillaries or uncoated fused-silica capillaries with a cationic surfactant added to the electrolyte. In general, coated capillaries require less conditioning and give more stable performance characteristics.

1.2. Detection Methods

Because commercially available instruments are equipped with photometric detection, many of the applications for organic acids use direct photometric detection at short wavelengths (185–200 nm) or indirect photometric methods. These detection methods are adequate and can be used for virtually any compound. One limitation is that identification depends entirely on the compound's characteristic migration time. Direct detection at longer wavelengths (>200 nm) offers more positive identification, but is limited to those organic acids that absorb strongly at these wavelengths. Other detection methods, such as fluorescence, have found fewer applications, mainly due to the limited number of organic acids that fluoresce or can be efficiently conjugated to a fluorogenic reagent *(11)*, in addition to the cost of the detector. Electrochemical methods are just beginning to be applied to organic acids *(2)*, and promise to provide good quality, sensitive, yet inexpensive detection methods in the future.

1.3. Specimen Preparation

Like many low-mol-wt compounds, organic acids may require specimen preparation to achieve adequate assay reproducibility *(3)*. This may be critical when detection of levels on the order of µmol/L is needed. To account for variation in sample recovery, addition of an internal standard is highly desirable. Internal standards also allow for the calculation of a relative migration index, increasing the precision of the assay. Currently specimen preparation for organic acids remains relatively unsophisticated, often relying on dilution, filtration, and simple forms of extraction prior to injection onto the capillary. More efficient methods such as on-line analyte concentration will undoubtedly prove useful in the future *(4)*.

2. APPLICATIONS FOR THE CLINICAL LABORATORY

The applications discussed in this chapter start with methylmalonic acid, since this is the one with which the authors have the most experience. An assay for urine methylmalonic acid has been operating on a routine basis in the first author's clinical laboratory since 1994. Several other applications share many characteristics with methylmalonic acid, and are discussed next, including succinic acid, oxalic and citric acids, and the simple short-chain organic acids. Most of these assays use either indirect detection or direct detection at short wavelengths. In contrast are the applications for orotic acid and xanthurenic acid, which rely on direct detection at longer wavelengths. Positive identification of these compounds can be enhanced by the use of diode array detection and spectral matching.

2.1. Methylmalonic Acid

Measurement of methylmalonic acid levels in urine or serum is an excellent way to assess vitamin B12 (cobalamin) status *(5,6)*. Vitamin B12 in the form of 5-deoxyadenosylcobalamin is an essential cofactor in the enzymatic conversion of methylmalonyl-CoA into succinyl-CoA. In vitamin B12 deficiency, methylmalonic acid rises early, often reaching 10–100 times the levels seen in normal individuals. In contrast, anemia and macrocytosis *(6)* and even serum vitamin B12 immunoassays are relatively insensitive markers. Because of cost and availability of automation, immunoassays are routinely used as the preferred screening method, although it is well-established that low normal vitamin B12 levels do not exclude vitamin B12 deficiency. In contrast, assays for methylmalonic acid, the most sensitive marker for vitamin B12 deficiency, is many times more expensive, particularly when using GC-MS. Because vitamin B12 deficiency is now recognized as being more common than previously thought *(5)*, an efficient and economic method for methylmalonic acid analysis is becoming increasingly important.

Methylmalonic acid is a deceptively simple dicarboxylic acid (HOOC-CH-CH3-COOH), but the analysis is challenging due to the number of closely related organic acids. Methylmalonic acid contains no strongly absorbing constituents, therefore, analysis by CE is currently based on two approaches, derivatization *(7)* or indirect detection *(8,9)*. Derivatization offers two advantages: 1) less specimen is required, and 2) the limit of detection is superior. Alternatively, indirect detection is faster and less expensive. Direct detection at ≤200 nm without derivatization is discussed further in Section 2.4. This method does not have adequate sensitivity to detect levels found in normal individuals. Its use, therefore, is limited to the detection of inborn errors of metabolism.

2.1.1. Methylmalonic Acid Derivatization

Schneede and Ueland *(7)* described a method using CE to quantitate levels of methylmalonic acid in serum. The assay used 1-pyrenyldiazomethane to react with acids present in serum producing a fluorescent 1-pyrenylmethyl monoester. After separation the products are detected by laser-induced fluorescence (LIF). Serum preparation requires addition of ethylmalonic acid as an internal standard, deproteinization with methanol, followed by a 12-h reaction with the derivatizing agent. Extensive dilution, needed to reduce matrix effects, is possible because of the sensitivity of the LIF method. Separation is based on a capillary (ID 75 μm) coated with a linear polyacrylamide to eliminate the EOF. The electrolyte consists of 30 mmol/L Tris-citrate buffer, pH 6.4. An organic modifier (50% dimethylformamide) and 0.1% hydroxypropyl methylcellulose are added to inhance separation and to suppress residual EOF. The specimen is introduced onto the capillary by pressure injection with a run time of about 26 min. The assay has a throughput of about 50 specimens per day. Reproducibility of the assay is acceptable with a coefficient of variation (CV) of 12% at 0.13 μmol/L and 5% at 4.3 μmol/L.

This method is adequate for routine analysis and the authors report having analyzed several thousand specimens at the time of publication. Although it represents a significant improvement over traditional GC-MS, the method requires a relatively lengthy specimen preparation and derivatization, in addition to an expensive method of detection. The HeCd laser is reported to be a major contributor to the cost. Use of ethylmalonic acid as an internal standard can also be problematic, since it can be found in some routine clinical specimens, although this is less of a problem for serum than for urine.

2.1.2. Methylmalonic Acid by Indirect Detection

Methods for the indirect detection of methylmalonic acid have been described in assays for urine *(9)*, and serum *(8)*. These assays are similar, employing phthalic acid as the indirect detection agent, electrolyte, and buffer. Because the serum and urine assays use the same basic technology, only the serum assay will be described in the following paragraph.

Specimen (0.5 mL) preparation begins with addition of a dimethyl-succinic acid as the internal standard, acidification, and extraction with ethylacetate. The solvent is then evaporated, reconstituted in water, filtered, and injected electrokinetically (5 kV for 25 s). Separation employs an uncoated fused silica capillary (ID 75 μm). Flow reversal is accomplished by addition of cetyltrimethylammonium bromide (CTAB), a cationic surfactant. The electrolyte is composed of 3.3 mmol/L phthalic acid at pH 6.0, 0.46 mmol/L CTAB, and 35% acetonitrile (v/v). The organic modifier, acetonitrile, is added to improve resolution. The phthalic acid background signal is monitored by a diode array detector at 210 nm against a reference signal at 320 nm. Run time is about 6–7 min, and a batch of 15 specimens can be prepared and run in about 4 h. The limit of detection (LOD) is 0.2 μmol/L with a CV of <10% at 0.3 μmol/L.

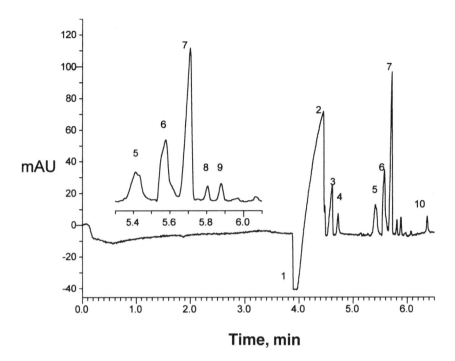

Time, min

Fig. 1. Indirect photometric detection of serum methylmalonic acid using phthalic acid at pH 6.0 and monitored at 210 nm (6); the signal has been reversed to make descreased phthalic acid absorbance appear as peaks. The numbered peaks correspond to: 1) bromide, 2) chloride, 3) nitrate and nitrite, 4) oxalate, 5) unidentified, 6) citrate and malate, 7) dibromosuccinate internal standard, 8) succinate, 9) methylmalonate (0.6 μmol/L), and 10) glutarate.

The LOD of 0.2 μmol/L using indirect detection and phthalic acid is close to the reference limit of 0.4 μmol/L, the upper limit seen in normal individuals. Because methylmalonic acid rises dramatically (10–100 times normal levels) in vitamin B12 deficiency, the assay is adequate for clinical purposes. Indirect detection, however, depends entirely on migration time for identification. There is always the possibility that a coeluting compound could be hidden in the methylmalonic acid peak, falsely elevating the value. When methylmalonic acid is elevated, dilution should be used to reduce the possibility of interference by coeluting compounds. Also plasma specimens collected with citric acid as the anticoagulant cannot be analyzed with this assay. The massive peak due to citric acid will overwhelm all other peaks in the vicinity, including the one for methylmalonic acid (*see* Fig. 1). EDTA plasma does not cause a similar problem. Specimen preparation is based on an organic phase extraction, representing a significant amount of the total assay time. Although the extraction method is acceptable, a more efficient method of specimen preparation would be a considerable improvement.

2.1.3. Indirect Methylmalonic Acid Assay Improvements

The assay of Franke et al. *(8)* has undergone a number of improvements to make it more robust for routine operation *(10)*. These include: 1) use of an amine-coated capillary rather than the combination of an uncoated capillary with surfactant, and 2) use of an electrolyte at pH 2.5 rather than the combination of an electrolyte at pH 6.0 with an organic modifier consisting of 35% acetonitrile. The reasons for these changes are discussed later, as are the advantages of using an instrument with a diode array detector and one with fluid-type cooling.

2.1.3.1. DIODE ARRAY FOR INDIRECT DETECTION

Most often indirect detection is used with a simple single-wavelength detector. This type of detector tends to be more sensitive in absolute terms than a diode array detector, in addition to being less expensive. However, it is the experience of the authors that a diode array produces better results when using indirect detection. In the assay described earlier, a single-wavelength detector (210 nm) produced a baseline that was relatively noisy giving a LOD of 1 µmol/L. Using the same conditions, a diode-array detector (210 nm against a reference wavelength of 300 nm), gave a baseline that was relatively flat with a LOD of 0.1 µmol/L. Because indirect detection operates in the setting of high background absorbance, noise may become the limiting factor for assay sensitivity as it is here.

2.1.3.2. CAPILLARY THERMOSTATING

Capillary thermostating to remove heat generated by the high voltage (Joule heating) used in CE is provided by two basic methods, air or fluid cooling. Air cooling is adequate for many purposes but it is not as efficient at removing heat as fluid cooling. It might be assumed that in a relatively low ionic-strength buffer, such as that used in the present assay (3.3 mmol/L phthalic acid), air cooling would be adequate. Direct comparison between commercially available air- and fluid-cooled instruments is difficult because instruments are configured differently. However, when this method was run in a fluid-cooled instrument, better overall assay performance was found. The clearest example of this was that larger samples could be introduced onto the capillary before broadening of the analyte peaks occurred. Presumably, this was due to inadequate heat-induced dispersion in the air-cooled instrument.

2.1.3.3. COATED CAPILLARIES

Replacing the uncoated capillaries with an amine-coated capillary and removing the surfactant from the electrolyte improved migration time stability considerably. It is known that surfactants are excellent at coating surfaces. However, they can also be difficult to keep in solution. Thus the use of a surfactant inevitably gives an electrolyte that tends to change composition with time, causing stability problems with the migration time. Using an amine-coated capillary (ID 50 μm) improved the reproducibility and durability of the methylmalonic acid assay.

2.1.3.4. pH

When investigating methods to separate anions, it is known that lowering the pH reduces the number of compounds that are ionized. These unionized compounds will be swept along with the EOF, thus, fewer anions will be present to cause potential interferences. For this reason, separation in acidic environment has the potential to reduce interfering compounds to a minimum. Although this approach has obvious limitations, it works well with methylmalonic acid (pK_{a1} 3.07). At pH 2.5, methylmalonic acid showed an electropherogram with significantly fewer interferences. Succinic acid (pK_{a1} 4.60), for example, is found in the EOF at this pH. Phthalic acid (pK_{a1} 2.89), used as electrolyte and indirect detection agent, still retains significant buffering capacity at this pH.

2.1.3.5. Organic Modiifiers

In the original assay *(11)*, an organic modifier consisting of 35% acetonitrile was added to the electrolyte to improve resolution between methylmalonic and succinic acids *(see* Fig. 1). Although organic modifiers can enhance resolution significantly, they can also cause unwanted side effects. One obvious problem is that the solution is prone to differential evaporation that can contribute to assay variability. When changing the pH from 6.0 to 2.5, succinic acid migrated with the EOF and an organic modifier was no longer required.

2.2. Succinic Acid

Succinic acid ($HOOC-CH_2-CH_2-COOH$) is a closely related isomer of methylmalonic acid, although clinically, the utility of these two organic acids is much different. Succinic acid is a major metabolite in the tricarboxylic acid cycle and can be used to monitor mitochondrial function *(12)*. Interestingly, succinic acid is also formed stoichiometrically as a product of the enzymatic synthesis of peptidyl hydroxyproline and it can be used to monitor increased collagen biosynthesis *(4)*. As with many of the organic acids, analysis has been performed with GC-MS and studies on the clinical significance has been limited by the relatively high cost and difficulty of the analysis.

As expected from the similarity of the assays, many of the applications developed for methylmalonic acid and other related short-chain organic acids can also be used to detect succinic acid (e.g., Fig. 1). The assay of Franke et al. *(8)* for methylmalonic acid required little modification for use for serum succinic acid *(12)*. Because the concentrations normally present are higher, succinic acid is a less demanding analyte. With the availability of a relatively easy and less expensive assay, increased investigations of the clinical utility of succinic acid can be expected in the future.

2.3. Oxalic and Citric Acids

Oxalic and citric acids are important analytes for the evaluation and treatment of urinary-tract calculi. The prevention of further stone formation is a major goal in the treatment of these individuals requiring an evaluation of the risk factors for calculi formation *(13)*. Elevated oxalic-acid excretion is a risk factor for the formation of calcium oxalate stones and treatment includes removing sources of oxalic acid from the diet. In contrast, elevated citric-acid excretion is a protective factor that tends to prevent urinary calcium from precipitating. Thus, recurrent stone formers with low urinary citric acid may benefit from treatments to increase urinary citric acid levels.

Holmes *(14)* describes an indirect detection method for oxalic and citric acid in 24 h urine collections. These compounds are also present on the electropherograms of many related assays (e.g., Fig. 1). Because oxalic and citric acids are present at relatively high concentrations in urine, specimen preparation is minimal, and consists of acidification, centrifugation, and dilution (100-fold). Dilution is required primarily to reduce the chloride concentration, which is also detected by the indirect method used for this assay. Separation employs an uncoated capillary (ID 75 μm), an electrolyte and indirect detection agent consisting of sodium chromate (10 mmol/L), and a flow reversal agent consisting of 0.5 mM tetradecylammonium bromide (TTAB). The detection limit was 7 mg/L for both oxalic and citric acids, which compares favorably to standard enzymatic assays. Although standard enzymatic methods test for oxalic and citric acids separately, the method of Holmes *(14)* measures both simultaneously. In addition, the assay can also be used to detect a number of related anions in urine, including chloride, sulfate, nitrate, phosphate, glycolate, and urate. All these components are potentially useful for the evaluation of the risks of urinary stone formation.

2.4. Profiling Short-Chain Organic Acids

The analysis of organic acids in urine is a well-established procedure for the diagnosis of inherited errors of metabolism *(15,16)*. The large number of organic acids and the complexity of the urine matrix makes separation and quantitation difficult. Currently, GC-MS is the most reliable technique for this purpose. However, GC-MS is also expensive, labor intensive, and generally limited to referral laboratories. On the other hand, CE can provide a simple and rapid alternative. The benefits of a method, such as CE, that is widely available and that provides rapid analysis, is apparent in such situations as the critically ill newborn presenting with coma and metabolic acidosis. In such cases, rapid diagnosis facilitates appropriate treatment. Although CE is limited at the present time to the analysis of the short-chain organic acids, this is changing rapidly.

The methods for the small short-chain organic acids, originally developed from applications in the food sciences *(9,17)*, share many characteristics, such as detection of similar compounds and migration orders. Both direct and indirect detection methods have been used. Direct detection is generally based on wavelengths from 200 to 185 nm, and are generally less sensitive than indirect methods.

2.4.1. Indirect Detection of Short-Chain Organic Acids

Chen et al. *(18)* described an indirect detection assay for 14 short-chain organic acids in serum and urine. The migration order was oxalic, citric, malonic, tartaric, methylmalonic, ketoglutaric, succinic, ethylmalonic, methylsuccinic, glutaric, adipic, methylglutaric, lactic, and pyruvic acids. Serum (0.5 mL) preparation consisted of deproteinization with methanol, centrifugation, drying the supernatant, and redissolving in water (250 µL) to provide concentration. Urine preparation consisted of filtration to remove particulates and a fivefold dilution. Ethylmalonic acid was used as an internal standard in both specimen types. Of the capillaries evaluated, polyacrylamide-coated capillaries showed superior performance. Phthalic acid was used as the indirect detection agent in a carbonate buffer; however to avoid interferences seen at shorter wavelengths, 230 nm was selected as the monitoring wavelength. The limit of detection was between 6 and 28 µg/mL for citric, methylmalonic, succinic, glutaratic, and lactic acids.

2.4.2. Direct Detection of Short-Chain Organic Acids

Shirao et al. *(19)* described an assay for 12 short-chain organic acids in urine based on direct detection at 185 nm. The migration order was: oxalic, formic, malonic, fumaric, succinic, α-ketoglutaric, citric, acetic, pyruvic, lactic, isovaleric, and hippuric acids. The limits of detection were given as 5 µg/mL for all but hippuric acid, which was 100 ng/mL. Urine was centrifuged and passed through a C18 column prior to hydrostatic injection. Separation was based on an uncoated capillary (ID 75 µm), with an electrolyte and buffer of 50 m*M* borate at pH 10.0 with addition of a commercial flow-reversal agent.

Hiraoka et al. *(20)* described a similar assay for cerebrospinal fluid based on direct detection at 185 nm. Compounds detected included (in migration order): oxalic, fumaric, acetic, pyruvic, lactic, and glutamic acids. However, unlike urine, ascorbic acid was also seen.

Jariego and Hernanz *(21)* also described an assay for 10 short-chain organic acids in urine based on direct detection at 185 nm. The migration order was methylmalonic, glutaric, 3-methylglutaric, *N*-acetylaspartic, 2-aminoadipic, propionic, lactic, 2-oxoisovaleric, isovaleric, and homogentisic acids. The limits of detection were between 5–15 μmol/L. Urine was prepared by passing through a centrifuge-type filter, and diluted to a creatinine concentration of about 1 mmol/L prior to introduction of the sample onto the capillary by pressure. Separation was accomplished using a polyimide-coated capillary (ID 75 μm). The electrolyte consisted of sodium sulfate, calcium chloride, and a commercial additive for flow reversal.

Barbas et al. *(22)* described an assay for 10 short-chain organic acids in urine employing direct detection at 200 nm. The migration order was: fumaric, malic, methylmalonic, citric, pyruvic, acetoacetic, propionic, lactic, butyric, and 3-hydroxybutyric acids. Urine preparation consisted of passing through a centrifuge-type filter, followed by introduction of the sample onto the capillary by pressure. Separation was achieved on a neutral-surface capillary (ID 75 μm) using an electrolyte of 200 mmol/L sodium phosphate buffer at pH 6.0 with 100 mL/L methanol. The organic modifier was added to resolve methylmalonic, propionic, and lactic acids. A variation on the method of Barbas et al. in which a total of 27 organic acids are identified in urine has been described by Garcia et al. *(15)*.

2.4.3. Orotic Acid

Orotic acid is an intermediate in the biosynthesis of pyrimidines and an important analyte in the examination of a number of inborn errors of metabolism *(23)*. The disorder most associated with elevated orotic acid is ornithine transcarbamylase deficiency, an inborn error of the urea cycle. In contrast, orotic acid is normal in the urea-cycle defect consisting of carbamoyl-phosphate synthase deficiency. Orotic acid can also useful for the evaluation of a number of other conditions including hereditary orotic aciduria and lysinuric protein intolerance.

Orotic acid has a distinctive absorbance signal in the region of 200–320 nm that makes direct detection possible. Unlike indirect photometric detection (and direct detection at very short wavelengths), direct detection in the mid-range UV offers the advantage of matching the obtained spectra with a spectral library for a more positive identification. Like fluorescence, this type of detection is obviously limited to compounds having a suitable absorbance.

Franke and Nuttall *(23)* describe an assay for orotic acid based on direct detection at 278 nm. Use of a diode-array detector allowed for automated spectral matching to monitor the purity of the orotic acid and internal standard peaks. Separation was on a polyvinyl alcohol-coated capillary (ID 50 μm), and an electrolyte consisting of 100 mM phosphate buffer at pH 3.0. Migration time at 20 kV was about 10 min at 35°C and about 14 min at 25°C. Above 20 kV, the Ohm's law plot deviated from linearity, although this was probably owing to the limitations of an air-cooled instrument. The migration time showed a coefficient of variation <1%. Urine-based control material showed a coefficient of variation <8% at 17 μmol/L (normal control).

2.4.3.1. SPECIMEN PREPARATION

Specimen preparation consisted of adding an internal standard (2,4-dinitrobenzoic acid) and barbituric acid buffer at pH 4.4 to the urine specimen, passing it through a single-use C18 reversed-phase column, and injecting the eluate. Although relatively complex, without preparation of the urine specimen, the migration time and assay precision did not have adequate reproducibility. Poor reproducibility resulting from minimal specimen preparation has been reported in a variety of circumstances *(24)*, particularly when the concentrations are in the μmol/L range.

2.4.3.2. COATED CAPILLARIES

A polyvinyl alcohol-coated capillary was used to provide flow reversal, and performed well in this application. The capillaries were easily conditioned in under 10 min, required no additional conditioning between specimen injections, and proved to be durable. It is worth emphasizing that the performance of coated capillaries far outstripped that of uncoated capillaries, which required lengthy pre-conditioning in addition to re-conditioning between specimens.

2.4.4. Xanthurenic Acid

Xanthurenic acid is a metabolite that can be used to evaluate vitamin B6 status *(25,26)*, much as methylmalonic acid can be used as a sensitive indicator of vitamin B12 status *(5,6)*. Xanthurenic acid is a metabolite of tryptophan via the kynurenine pathway. This is also referred to as the tryptophan-niacin pathway. Several enzymes in this pathway require vitamin B6 as a cofactor. As a result, high levels of several tryptohan metabolites, including xanthurenic acid, accumulate when vitamin B6 is deficient. Xanthurenic acid also has a strong absorbance signal making it suitable for direct photometric detection. Significantly, xanthurenic acid has limited solubility below pH 8.0. This requires operating at higher pH, increasing the potential for interfering anions. However, as with orotic acid, direct detection and spectral matching can be used for positive identification of the xanthurenic acid peak.

Separation of serum xanthurenic acid was based on a polyvinyl alcohol-coated capillary (ID 50 μm), similar to the orotic acid assay *(23)*. Instead of an acidic electrolyte, however, 200 m*M* glycylglycine was used to provide buffer capacity at pH 8.2. Specimen preparation started with 0.5 mL serum, addition of Tris acetate buffer at pH 9.0 (including an internal standard of 3-nitrobenzoic acid), and addition of urea and ethanol to completely solubilize xanthurenic acid. After mixing, this mixture was passed through a centrifuge-type filter, and pressure injected. A diode array detector was used to monitor peaks at 243 nm, and automated spectral matching was employed to monitor peak purity. The limit of detection for xanthurenic acid was 1 μmol/L with a coefficient of variation was < 9% at 10 μmol/L.

An assay that includes xanthurenic acid is described by Weber et al. *(27)*, and discussed briefly in Section 2.5.8.

2.5. Other Applications

Many organic acid assays can be found in the literature. Many are useful for applications in the food sciences *(17)* and for research purposes, but fewer have been developed with the specific needs of the clinical laboratory in mind. Reviews of biomedical applications are available *(3,16,28–30)*, but are inevitably incomplete by the time of publication.

2.5.1. Ascorbic Acid

Koh et al. *(24)* describe an assay for ascorbic acid (vitamin C) in fruit beverages using direct detection at 254 nm. Urine and plasma were also examined briefly.

2.5.2. Bile Acids

Yarabe et al. *(31)* describe an assay for the separation of 15 bile acids in serum based on indirect detection.

2.5.3. Electrochemical Detection

DeBacker and Nagel *(2)* describe a potentiometric method of detection for short-chain organic acids that may be useful for future studies.

2.5.4. Fatty Acids

Assays for saturated and unsaturated fatty acids in food products use indirect detection *(32,33)*.

2.5.5. Nicotinic Acid and Metabolites

Zarzycki et al. *(34)* describe an assay for nicotinic acid and its metabolites in human plasma. Nicotinic acid is related to the tyrptophan pathway, and the assay shows some similarities with that of Weber et al. *(27)* in that direct detection at 254 nm is used.

2.5.6. Phenylketonuria

Dolnik *(11)* described the separation of the acids of phenylketonuria based on direct detection at 260 nm. The specific organic acids identified were phenylpyruvate, 2-hydroxyphenylacetate, phenylacetate, mandelate, 4-hydroxyphenylpyruvate, and phenylalanine.

2.5.7. Profiling Organic Anions

Schoots et al. *(28)* described an assay based on direct detection at 254 nm for profiling organic anions in the serum of uremic patients. The quantitation of hippuric, p-hydroxyhippuric, and uric acids was emphasized. Specimen preparation consisted of deproteinization with centrifuge-type filtration, and dilution (10-fold). Separation was based on a Teflon capillary (ID 200 µm). Analysis required 8 min, which was a significant improvement over the 90 min required for similar HPLC methods. Petucci et al. *(35)* described an assay for profiling organic anions in serum and hemodialysate fluid from uremic patients using direct detection at 210 nm. Compounds identified included hippuric acid, tryptophan and tryptophan metabolites (indican, kynurenic acid, nicotinic acid), tyrosine, purine, and pyrimidine metabolites. Specimen preparation consisted of passing through a centrifuge-type filter to remove proteins. The filtrate was then pressure-injected. Separation was based on an uncoated capillary (ID 50 µm) and an electrolyte of 150 m*M* borate buffer at pH 9.0. Run time was about 16 min and did not use flow reversal. A similar assay based on micellar electrokinetic CE (MEKC) has also been described *(36)*.

2.5.8. Quinolinic Acid and Other Tryptophan Metabolites

Weber et al. *(27)* described an assay for tryptophan and 10 of its metabolites in urine using direct detection at 254 nm. Tryptophan metabolites are an interesting group of compounds that have not been fully exploited for their diagnostic potentials, and include xanthurenic acid (discussed in Section 2.4.4.) and quinolinic acid. Quinolinic acid appears to be toxic to neurons, and may have important implications for the development of some neurological diseases.

3. CONCLUSIONS

CE is a sensitive and versatile technique and represents an inexpensive and practical method for the determination of organic acids. Applications include far more than the traditional investigation of inborn errors of metabolism. From the applications discussed previously, several general conclusions can be drawn concerning organic-acid assays.

Given the complex nature of biological specimens and the stringent requirements of the clinical laboratory *(3)*, significant specimen preparation prior to injection is often needed to achieve stable migration times and good analytic precision, particularly when low concentrations are involved. The use of more sophisticated specimen preparation will undoubtedly make many applications more practical *(28)*.

The analysis of anions such as organic acids is faster when flow reversal is used. Flow reversal with coated capillaries performs better than uncoated fused silica capillaries in combination with cationic surfactants. Coated capillaries require less conditioning, and give more stable migration times. Relatively large-diameter capillaries (ID 75 μm) are being used in most applications, primarily to maximize the limits of detection. Air-cooled instruments are adequate for many applications, although fluid-cooled instruments dissipate heat more efficiently and may give better assay characteristics. This is particularly true when larger diameter capillaries are used to increase detection limits.

Assays for the organic acids also tend to be sensitive to small pH changes *(8,9,18)*, and may therefore be more reproducible when there is adequate buffering. When possible, operating at an acidic pH tends to reduce the number of potentially interfering anions.

REFERENCES

1. Mukherjee, P. S. and Karnes, H. T. (1996) Ultraviolet and fluorescence derivatization reagents for carboxylic acids suitable for high performance liquid chromatography: a review. Biomed. Chromatogr. 10, 193–204.
2. DeBacker, B. L. and Nagels, L. J. (1996) Potentiometric detection for capillary electrophoresis: determination of organic acids. Anal. Chem. 68, 4441–4445.
3. Lehmann, R., Voelter, W., and Liebich, H. M. (1997) Capillary electrophoresis in clinical chemistry. J. Chromatogr. B 697, 3–35.
4. Guzman, N. A. (1998) Prolyl 4-hydroxylase: an overview, in Prolyl Hydroxylase, Protein Disulfide Isomerase, and Other Structurally Related Proteins (Guzman, N. A., ed.), Marcel Dekker, New York, pp. 1–64.
5. Joosten, E., vanden Berg, A., Riezler, R., Naurath, H. J., Lindenbaum, J., Stabler, S. P., and Allen R. H. (1993) Metabolic evidence that deficiencies of vitamin B-12 (cobalamin), folate, and vitamin B-6 occur commonly in elderly people. Am. J. Clin. Nutr. 58, 468–476.
6. Lindenbaum, J., Healton, E. B., Savage, D. G., Brust, J. C. M., Garrett, T. J., Podell, E. R., et al. (1988) Neuropsychiatric disorders caused by cobalamin deficiency in the absence of anemia or macrocytosis. N. Engl. J. Med. 318, 1720–1728.
7. Schneede, J. and Ueland, P. M. (1995) Application of capillary electrophoresis with laser-induced fluorescence detection for routine determination of methylmalonic acid in human serum. Anal. Chem. 67, 812–819.
8. Franke, D. R., Marsh, D. B., and Nuttall, K. L. (1996) Serum methylmalonic acid by capillary zone electrophoresis using electrokinetic injection and indirect photometric detection. J. Cap. Electroph. 3, 125–129.

9. Marsh, D. B. and Nuttall, K. L. (1995) Methylmalonic acid in clinical urine specimens by capillary zone electrophoresis using indirect photometric detection. J. Cap. Electroph. 2, 63–67.
10. Franke, D. R. and Nuttall, K. L. (1998) An improved capillary electrophoresis assay for serum methylmalonic acid. J. Cap. Electrophor. (Submitted)
11. Dolnik, V. (1994) Capillary zone electrophoresis of pathological metabolites in phenylketonuria. J. Microcol. Sep. 6, 63–67.
12. Komaromy-Hiller, G., Sundquist, P. D., Jacobsen, L. J., and Nuttall, K. L. (1997) Serum succinate by capillary zone electrophoresis: marker candidate for hypoxia. Ann. Clin. Lab. Sci. 27, 163–168.
13. Coe, F. L., Parks, J. H., and Asplin, J. R. (1992) The pathogenesis and treatment of kidney stones. N. Engl. J. Med. 327, 1141–1152.
14. Holmes, R. P. (1995) Measurement of urinary oxalate and citrate by capillary electrophoresis and indirect ultraviolet absorbance. Clin. Chem. 41, 1297–1301.
15. Garcia, A., Barbas, C., Aguilar, R., and Castro, M. (1998) Capillary electrophoresis for rapid profiling of organic acidurias. Clin. Chem. 44, 1905–1911.
16. Jellum, E., Dollekamp, H., and Blessum, C. (1996) Capillary electrophoresis for clinical problem solving: analysis of urinary diagnostic metabolites and serum proteins. J. Chromatogr. B 683, 55–65.
17. Soga, T. and Wakaura, M. (1997) Determination of inorganic and organic anions in beer and wort by capillary electrophoresis. J. Am. Soc. Brew. Chem. 55, 44–46.
18. Chen, H., Xu, Y., Van Lente, F., and Ip, M. P. (1996) Indirect ultraviolet detection of biologically relevant organic acids by capillary electrophoresis. J. Chromatogr. B 679, 49–59.
19. Shirao, M., Furuta, R., Suzuki, S., Nakazawa, H., Fijita, S., and Maruyama, T. (1994) Determination of organic acids in urine by capillary zone electrophoresis. J. Chromatogr. A 680, 247–251.
20. Hiraoka, A., Akai, J., Tominaga, I., Hattori, M., Sasaki, H., and Arato, T. (1994) Capillary zone electrophoretic determination of organic acids in cerebrospinal fluid from patients with central nervous system diseases. J. Chromatogr. A 680, 243.
21. Jariego, C. M. and Hernanz, A. (1996) Determination of organic acids by capillary electrophoresis in screening of organic acidurias. Clin. Chem. 42, 477, 478.
22. Barbas, C., Adeva, N., Aguilar, R., Rosillo, M., Rubio, T., and Castro, M. (1998) Quantitative determination of short-chain organic acids in urine by capillary electrophoresis. Clin. Chem. 44, 1340–1342.
23. Franke, D. R. and Nuttall, K. L. (1996) Orotic acid in clinical urine specimens by capillary zone electrophoresis using polyvinyl alcohol coated capillaries. J. Cap. Electrophor. 3, 309–312.
24. Koh, E. V., Bissell, M. G., and Ito, R. K. (1993) Measurement of vitamin C by capillary electrophoresis in biological fluids and fruit beverages using a stereoisomer as an internal standard. J. Chromatogr. 633, 245–250.
25. Liu, M., Wang, G. R., Liu, T. Z., and Tsai, K. J. (1996) Improved fluorometric quantification of urinary xanthurenic acid. Clin. Chem. 42, 397–401.
26. Williams, S. A., Monti, J. A., Boots, L. R., and Cornwell, P. E. (1984) Quantitation of xanthurenic acid in rabbit serum using high performance liquid chromatography. Am. J. Clin. Nutr. 40, 159–167.

27. Weber, P. L., Malis, M., Palmer, S. D., Klein, T. L., and Lunte, S. M. (1997) Capillary zone electrophoresis separation of tryptophan and its metabolites, including quinolinic acid. J. Chromatogr. B 697, 263–268.

28. Guzman, N. A., Park, S. S., Schaufelberger, D., Hernandez, L., Paez, X., Rada, P., et al. (1997) New approaches in clinical chemistry: on-line analyte concentration and microreaction capillary electrophoresis for the determination of drugs, metabolic intermediates, and biopolymers in biological fluids. J. Chromatogr. B 697, 37–42.

29. Shihabi, Z. K. and Friedberg, M. A. (1997) Analysis of small molecules for clinical diagnosis by capillary electrophoresis. Electrophoresis 18, 1724–1732.

30. Xu, Y. (1997) Clinical chemistry: capillary electrophoresis. Anal. Chem. 69, 171R–179R.

31. Yarabe, H. H., Shamsi, S. A., and Warner, I. M. (1998) Capillary zone electrophoresis of bile acids with indirect photometric detection. Anal. Chem. 70, 1412–1418.

32. Collet, J. and Gareil, P. (1996) Capillary zone electrophoretic separation of C14-C18 linear saturated and unsaturated fee fatty acids with indirect UV detection. J. Cap. Electroph. 3, 77–82.

33. Heinig, K., Hissner, F., Martin, S., and Vogt, C. (1998) Separation of saturated and unsaturated fatty acids by capillary electrophoresis and HPLC. Am. Lab. May, 24–29.

34. Zarzycki, P. K., Kowalski, P., Nowakowska, J., and Lamparczyk, H. (1995) High-performance liquid chromatographic and capillary electrophoretic determination of free nicotinic acid in human plasma and separation of its metabolites by capillary electrophoresis. J. Chromatogr. A 709, 203–208.

35. Petucci, C. J., Kantes, H. L., Strein, T. G., and Veening, H. (1995) Capillary electrophoresis as a clinical tool: determination of organic anions in normal and uremic serum using photodiode-array detection. J. Chromatogr. B 668, 241–251.

36. Tran, T. C., Huq, T. A., Kantes, H. L., Crane, J. N., and Strein, T. G. (1997) Determination of creatinine and uremic toxins in human blood sera with micellar electrokinetic capillary electrophoresis. J. Chromatogr. B 690, 35–42.

11
Steroids

Cecilla Youh, Amin A. Mohammad,
and John R. Petersen

1. ADRENAL GLAND

1.1. Morphology

The adrenal glands are paired structures situated above the kidneys that are approx 2–3 cm wide and 6 cm long and weigh approx 5 g. The glands consists of a yellow, outer cortex that constitutes approx 80% of the adrenal gland and a gray, inner medulla *(1)*. The adrenal cortex consists of three distinct layers or zones of cells. The outermost layer, the zona glomerulosa, is the site of aldosterone synthesis, the principal mineralocorticoid produced by the human adrenal cortex, and corticosterone synthesis. The wider, middle zone is the zona fasciculata, and the innermost layer is the zona reticularis. The two inner zones of the adrenal cortex can be considered a single functional unit, where cortisol, along with some corticosterone, and dehydroepiandrosterone (DHEA) are synthesized. The glucocorticoids have widespread effects on carbohydrate and protein metabolism. Androgens secreted by the adrenal cortex pay a less important role than the androgens, which are secreted by the gonads.

1.2. Steroid Synthesis

The human adrenal cortex produces and secretes glucocorticoids (cortisol and corticosterone), a mineralocorticoid (aldosterone), biosynthetic precursors of three end products (progesterone, 11-deoxycorticosterone, and 11-deoxycortisol) and androgenic substances (DHEA and its sulfate ester). The synthesis of adrenal cortical steroids begins with cholesterol, which is converted to pregnenolone *(see* Fig. 1). A cholesterol hydroxylase and desmolase mediate this rate-limiting step. ACTH stimulates this conversion and also increases the uptake of lipoprotein, which is the major source of adrenal cholesterol, by the adrenal cortex and stimulates the hydrolysis of choles-

From: *Clinical and Forensic Applications of Capillary Electrophoresis*
Edited by: J. R. Petersen and A. A. Mohammad © Humana Press Inc., Totowa, NJ

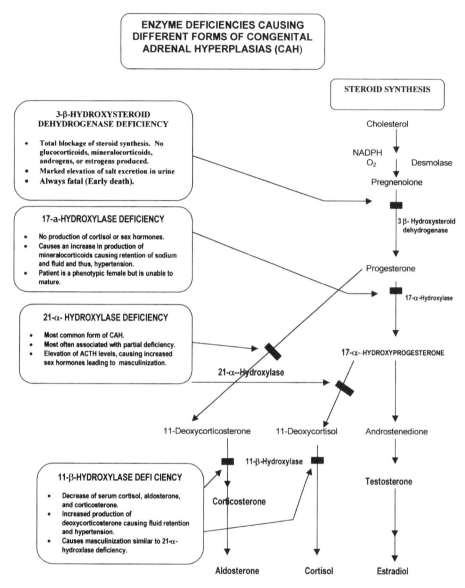

Fig. 1. Enzyme deficiencies causing different forms of congenital adrenal hyperplasias (CAH).

terol esters to free cholesterol. Many of the intermediates of steroid synthesis are secreted to some extent, but the steroids that are found in physiologically significant amounts are aldosterone, cortisol, corticosterone, DHEA, and androstenedione.

2. PHYSIOLOGICAL EFFECTS OF GLUCOCORTIOIDS

Of the naturally occurring steroids only cortisol, corticosterone, cortisone, and 11-dehydrocorticosterone have appreciable glucocorticoid activity. Cortisol, which is found in the highest concentration, accounts for most of this activity. About 75% of plasma cortisol is bound to cortisol binding globulin (CBG, an alpha globulin), 15% is bound to plasma albumin, and 10% is unbound (free), representing the physiologically active portion. CBG also has a high binding affinity for progesterone, deoxycorticosterone, and some synthetic analogs.

2.1. Anti-Inflammatory Effects

Glucocorticoids inhibit inflammatory and allergic reactions. They do this by stabilizing the lysosomal membranes, inhibiting the release of proteolytic enzymes, and by increasing capillary permeability. This in turn reduces diapedesis of leukocytes. Glucocorticoids also reduce the number of circulating lymphocytes, monocytes, eosinophils, and basophils. The decrease in the number of basophils accounts for the fall in blood histamine levels and the reduction of the allergic response. There is also an increase in the number of inflammatory cells (neutrophils) caused by a decrease in the migration from the capillaries and an accelerated release from bone marrow. Glucocorticoids also inhibit the ability of neutrophils to marginate to the vessel wall. In addition, they cause impairment of the lymph nodes, thymus, and spleen that directly leads to decreased antibody formation.

2.2. Antigrowth Effects

Large doses of cortisol have been shown to antagonize the effect of active vitamin D metabolites on the absorption of Ca^{2+} from the gut, inhibit mitosis of fibroblasts, and cause degradation of collagen. All of these effects can lead to osteoporosis, which is a reduction in bone mass per unit volume. Glucocorticoids can also delay wound healing because of the reduction of fibroblast proliferation. Connective tissue is reduced in quality and strength. In addition, chronic supra-physiologic doses of glucocorticoids will suppress growth secretion and inhibit somatic growth.

2.3. Vascular Effects

Cortisol in pharmacological doses will enhance the vasopressor action of catecholamines. Thus, corticosteroids have a role in maintenance of normal arterial systematic blood pressure and volume through their support of vascular responsiveness to vasoactive substances. Cortisol also enhances catecholamine synthesis via activation of the epinephrine-forming enzyme.

2.4. Other Effects

Glucocorticoids, unlike mineraldocorticoids, restore glomerular filtration rate (GFR) and renal plasma flow to normal following adrenalectomy. They also facilitate free-water excretion (clearance) and uric-acid excretion. Of Glucocorticoids have also been found to have psychoneural effects following chronic hyper- or hypo-cortisol secretion. In these cases patients may initially become euphoric and then psychotic, paranoid, and finally depressed. In addition, cortisol increases gastric flow and gastric secretion, while it decreases gastric mucosal-cell proliferation. The latter two effects can lead to peptic ulceration following chronic cortisol treatment.

2.5. Metabolic Effects

2.5.1. Carbohydrate Metabolism

Cortisol, the main glucocorticoid present in circulation, is a carbohydrate-sparing hormone exerting an anti-insulin effect, which can lead to hypoglycemia and insulin-resistance. In addition, glucocorticoids maintain blood glucose and the glycogen content of the liver by promoting the conversion of amino acids to carbohydrates and the storage of carbohydrate as hepatic glycogen.

2.5.2. Protein Metabolism

The most important gluconeogenic substrates are amino acids that are derived from proteolysis in skeletal muscle. Cortisol enhances the release of amino acids from proteins in skeletal muscles and other extra hepatic tissues including the protein matrix of bone. The amino acids released are transported to the liver and then converted to glucose. This increased in glucose production via gluconeogenesis causes an increased urea production because of the conversion of amino-acid nitrogen to urea, accounting for the increased urinary nitrogen excretion. The proteolysis in skeletal muscle brings about a negative protein balance since the amino acids taken up by the liver that would have been used in the synthesis of new protein are instead used to form glucose or glycogen. This anabolic effect is an important exception to the overall protein catabolic effect of cortisol.

2.5.3. Fat Metabolism

Glucocorticoids enhance the lipolytic actions of other hormones, such as growth hormone, catecholamines, glucagon, and thyroid hormone. Glucocorticoids also help in the mobilization of fatty acids from adipose tissues to the liver, where the metabolism of fatty acids inhibits glycolytic enzymes and promote gluconeogenesis. As a result of increased fatty acids oxidation, glucocorticoids may lead to increased ketosis, especially in patients with diabetes mellitus.

3. CONGENITAL ADRENAL HYPERPLASIA

Congenital adrenal hyperplasia (CAH) also known as the "adrenogenital syndrome" can be considered as a family of inborn error of steroidogensis (*see* Fig. 1). All CAH variants are inherited as autosomal recessive traits. Each member of this family is characterized by a specific enzyme deficiency that impacts cortisol production by the adrenal cortex, and if severe enough can lead to sexual ambiguity in both males and females. The enzymes usually affected are 21-hydroxylase (types I and II), beta hydroxylase (type III), 3 beta-hydroxylase (type IV), 17 hydroxylase (type V) and cholesterol 20-alpha hydroxylase (type VI). The most common syndromes are types I and II, which are caused by a 21-hydroxylase enzyme deficiency. The identification of the specific enzyme deficiency relies heavily on laboratory findings since all variants affect the glucocorticoid (cortisol) pathway in some manner. Although formation of cortisone and cortisol are blocked in type I and II CAH, precursors are still being manufactured, causing elevations of 17-hydroxyprogesterone. Normal basal serum 17-hydroxyprogesterone levels, however, cannot exclude late-onset CAH. Response to adrenocorticotrophic stimulation, however, clearly distinguishes this disorder from carriers of the classical disease *(2)*.

In addition to being precursors of cortisone, many of the early intermediates are also estrogenic compounds. In the presence of abnormally high production of androgens, secondary sexual characteristics are affected. If this condition is manifested in utero, pseudohermaphroditism (masculinzation) of external genitalia occur in girls and macrogentisomia praecox (accentuation of male genitalia) occurs in boys. If the condition is not manifested until after birth, virilism (masculinization) develops in girls and precocious puberty in boys. In CAH variants IV, V, and VI, there is also some degree of interruption of the adrenal pathway, so that the external appearance of the female genitalia is not significantly affected and subsequent virilization is minimal or absent.

In CAH, the adrenal glands themselves increase in size because of hyperplasia of the steroid-producing adrenal cortex. This is because the level of cortisone and hydrocortisone produced by the adrenal gland controls normal pituitary production of ACTH through a negative-feedback mechanism. In variants of congenital adrenal hyperplasia, cortisone production is partially or completely blocked, prompting the pituitary to produce more ACTH in an attempt to increase cortisone production. This continues until the adrenal cortex tissue becomes hyperplastic under the continual ACTH stimulation. Also when the mineralocorticoid pathway leading to aldosterone is blocked (CAH types II, IV, VI), salt losing crises similar to those of Addison's disease occur.

In CAH, the correct identification of the enzyme affected is achieved by observation of clinical symptoms reflecting distinct hormonal patterns leading to the measurement cortisol, which should be low, as well as increased levels of steroids proximal to the suspected blocked step.

Two rounds of polymerase chain reaction (PCR) and amplification-created restriction sites (ACRS) analysis may provide important information for genetic counseling, prenatal diagnosis, and management of families at risk for CAH *(3)*. The data from one study suggest that the steroidogenic acute regulatory protein amino acid replacement mutants that cause lipoid CAH are inactive because of fairly the inability of the enzyme to fold properly, which may be caused by the loss of salt bridges that stabilize the tertiary structure *(4)*.

Some governments have done studies to evaluate the benefits of neonatal screening for CAH. One such study was done in Sweden from January 1989 to December 1994. The study concluded that the main benefits of screening was avoidance of serious salt-losing crises, earlier correct gender assignment in virilized girls, and detection of patients who would otherwise have been missed in neonatal period *(5)*. Screening also prevented deaths due the decreased steroid production in the neonatal period.

4. USE OF CAPILLARY ELECTROPHORESIS (CE) IN THE SEPARATION AND DETECTION OF STEROIDS

Clinically the evaluation of steroid levels is of great interest. There are many disorders that have been identified as being caused either by under or over secretion of steroids, e.g., CAH, Cushing's syndrome, Addison's disease, acromegaly, hirsutism, and adenomas. The ability to simultaneously measure multiple steroids in the urine and/or serum of these patients would be helpful in making the diagnosis of their disorder. However, the structural similarity and low concentrations of steroids have made rapid, yet accurate, analysis a problem. Radioimmunoassay (RIA), although extremely sensitive, requires extraction and purification by high-performance liquid chromatography (HPLC) to provide the required specificity *(6–8)*. Thus, to analyze multiple steroids by RIA requires the same number of RIAs as steroids, limiting this application to specialized laboratories and, increasing the turnaround time. Other analytical methodologies based on chromatographic separation, such as gas chromatography (GC), gas chromatography-mass spectrometry (GC-MS), and HPLC, have also been used for steroid testing. These procedures also require extraction, concentration, and derivation to enhance sensitivity and specificity, limiting their routine use because they are time-consuming and expensive.

Ideally, methodologies suitable for determination of steroids in clinical samples should meet the following criteria *(9)* to be clinically justified. The methodology should:

1. Not require large sample volumes (typically <1 mL of plasma or serum should be used);
2. Have high sensitivity with detection limits in the 0.1–10 nmol/L range;
3. Be highly specific but retain the ability to detect and quantitate multiple steroids in the presence of other structurally similar compounds;
4. Have minimal derivation and/or prior sample preparation;
5. Provide a high sample throughput with a reasonable turnaround time;
6. Be relatively inexpensive; and
7. Be automatable.

In many ways capillary electrophoresis (CE) fit these criteria since it has the unique features high resolution, high mass sensitivity, low sample volume requirements, and over all versatility *(10)*.

4.1. Serum

Steroids are neutral compounds and therefore would not be mobilized or separated when subjected to electrophoretic conditions. To overcome this inherent problem of neutral compounds, micellar electrokinetic capillary chromatography (MEKC), which uses ionic micelles to effect separation, was developed by Terabe et al *(11)*. The separation principle of MEKC is similar to that of chromatography, except that MEKC utilizes electrokinetic phenomena to perform the chromatography instead of a liquid-delivery pump.

Using this technique, Abubaker et al. *(9)* succeeded in developing a method to separate rapidly steroids whose measurement gives clinically useful information (*see* Fig. 2). They found excellent resolution for eight steroids by using a buffer of sodium dodecyl sulfate (SDS) and acetonitrile with a neutral capillary. A similar resolution was achieved with a fused silica capillary using a dodecyl trimethylammonium bromide (DTAB) buffer, although the time required for separation was increased six- to seven-fold. The steroids separated were testosterone propionate, progesterone, 17-hydroxy progesterone, testosterone, 11-deoxycortisol, 21-deoxycortisol, hydrocortisone, and cortisone. Three of these hormones (11-deoxycortsol, 17-OH progesterone, and 21-deoxycortisol), are known to be important in helping to establish the diagnosis of CAH. Thus, using these methods to separate

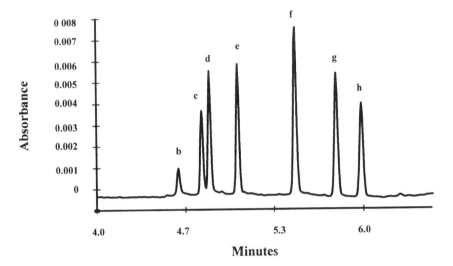

Fig. 2. Separation of testosterone propionate, progesterone, 17-hydroxy-progesterone, testosterone, 11-deoxycortisol, 21-deoxycortisol, cortisol, and cortisone (all at 10 μg/ mL) from a serum ultrafiltrate. All buffers and electrophoresis conditions are as stated in ref. *(9)*.

and quantitate these steroids could be very useful in screening newborns for CAH. However, the sensitivity was found to be inadequate without preconcentration.

The issue with sensitivity can potentially be overcome by using the on-line concentration techniques of stacking with reverse-migrating micelles or the field-enhanced sample injection with reverse migrating micelles developed by Quirino et al. *(12,13)*. Both techniques used the separation of ng/mL levels of testosterone and progesterone to demonstrate that this was a fast, effective, and easy way to concentrate neutral analytes inside the capillary. More work is still needed in this area to show its utility with serum.

4.2. Urinary-Free Cortisol

The total cortisol level in a 24-h urine represents the integrated or mean concentration of free cortisol in plasma over this 24-h period and provides an excellent diagnostic sensitivity and specificity for the detection of the increased secretion of cortisol by the adrenal glands (Cushing's syndrome) *(14)*. In contrast, total serum cortisol levels are not always an accurate measure of an overactive adrenocorticoid function and can be elevated in pregnancy, obesity, diabetes, or hyperthyroidism. Urinary free cortisol (UFC)

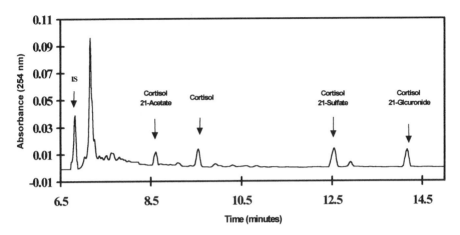

Fig. 3. Separation of Internal Standard (IS) (corticosterone) at 100 μg/dL and cortisol 21-acetate, cortisol, cortisol 21-sulfate, and cortisol 21-glucosidonate at 20 μg/dL in urine. The urine (15 mL) was spike with the various steroids and extracted using a 3M Empore disk cartridge. After washing with deionized water and 10% acetone/water, the steroids were eluted with acetonitrile followed by 10 m*M* SDS. All buffers and electrophoresis conditions were as stated in ref. *(15)*.

measurement is therefore the most reliable single approach for screening patients for Cushing's syndrome *(14)*. Currently the methods available for measuring UFC are associated with long turnaround times and interferences present in urine.

Lokinendi et al. *(15)* used solid-phase extraction in conjunction with MEKC as a method for the separation and detection of UFC. The addition of an internal standard was found to be necessary for accurate and reliable quantitation of the free cortisol in urine. The internal standard, corticosterone, was chosen because it did not coelute with the various compounds present in the extracted urine (*see* Fig. 3). The authors evaluated the overall performance and feasibility of the method. In addition, they also evaluated linearity, recovery, and lower limit of detection of free cortisol in human urine and compared the results with a commercially available immunoassay. They found an excellent correlation (R = 0.95 and slope = 0.934) with the immunoassay with little, if any, interference from endogenous urine substances.

4.3. Congenital Adrenal Hyperplasia

CAH as discussed earlier is a group of autosomal recessive disorders involving the adrenal glands, in which the primary defect is a deficiency of one or more enzymes involved in the biosynthesis. The main three steroids that are measured to help in making the differential diagnosis are 17-hydroxy progesterone, 21-deoxycortisol, and 11-deoxycortisol. In frank CAH the serum levels of these steroids can reach levels such that detection by CE is possible. The real challenge, however, is in the detection of normal levels in order to differentiate between patients who have a partial blockage and normals. The highest levels that these steroids are normally found in serum are 138 ng/dL and 155 ng/dL for 17-deoxy progesterone and 11-deoxy-cortisol, respectively *(16)*. MEKC can separate these structurally similar steroids rapidly, however, detection of normal serum levels is not currently possible with the conventional UV absorbance detectors available with most CE instruments *(17)*. Using UV absorbance, the lower limit of detection for these steroids by MEKC is 0.05 mg/dL *(17)*. Thus, a 3000-fold pre-concentration is needed to detect normal levels, which may be achieved using field-enhanced sample injection methods *(12,13)*.

5. CONCLUSION

It is possible to use CE to separate and detect steroids in body fluids (serum and urine). The problems (limitation in sensitivity and the sample matrix) associated with CE are similar to those outlined in the other chapters in this book. Bodily fluids represent a complex matrix with high levels of proteins and salt that can bind to or precipitate inside a capillary. This can result in variable migration times as the result of change in the capillary surface or actual blockage of the capillary. In addition to the problems associated with migration times and capillary occlusion, CE has the additional problem of sensitivity. Thus, preconcentration of samples, either by liquid-liquid or solid phase extraction becomes very important in the development of a CE assay for determination of steroids.

REFERENCES

1. Berne, R. M. and Matthew, N. (1988) in Physiology, 3rd ed. Mosby Year Book, St. Louis, MO.
2. Rumsy, G. and Avery, C. J. (1998) Genotype-phenotype analysis in late onset 21-hydroxylase deficiency in comparison to the classical forms. Clin. Endocrinol. 48, 707.
3. Ko, T. M. and Kao, C. H. (1999) Congenital hyperplasia. Molecular character-ization. J. Reprod. Med. 43, 379–386.
4. Bose, H. S., Baldwin, S., and Miller, W. L. (1998) Incorrect folding of ste-roidogenic acute regulatory protein (StAR) in cogenital adrenal hyperplasia. Biochem. 37, 9768–9775.
5. Nordenstrom, T. (1998) Benefits of neonatal screening for congenital adrenal hyperplasia (21-hydroxylase deficiency) in Sweden. Pediatrics 101, E11.

6. Fiet, J., Gosling, J. P., Galons, H., and Vexiau, P. (1994) Hirsutism and acne in woman: coordinated radioimmunoassays for eight relevant plasma steroids. Clin. Chem. 40, 2296–2305.
7. Bosworth, N. and Towers, P. (1989) Scintillation proximity assay. Nature 341, 167,168.
8. Gueux, B., Fiet, J., Pham-Huu-Trung, M. T., Villette, J. M., Gourmelen, M., Galons, H., et al. (1985) Radioimmunoassay for 21-deoxycortisol: clinical applications. Acta Endocrinol. 108, 537–544.
9. Abubaker, M. A., Bissell, M. G., and Petersen, J. R. (1995) Rapid profiling of clinically relevant steroids by micellar electrokinetic capillary chromatography. J. Cap. Electrophor. 2, 105–110.
10. Guzman, N. A. (1993) Capillary Electrophoresis Technology. Chromatographic Science Series, vol. 64.
11. Terabe, S., Otusuka, K., Ichikawa, K., Tsuchiya, A., and Ando, T. (1984) Electrokinetic separations with micellar solutions and open tubular capillaries. Anal. Chem. 56, 111–113.
12. Quirino, J. P. and Terabe, S. (1998) On-line concentration of neutral analytes for micellar electrokinetic chromatography. 3. Stacking with reverse migrating micelles. Anal. Chem. 70, 149–157.
13. Quirino, J. P. and Terabe, S. (1998) On-line concentration of neutral analytes for micellar electrokinetic chromatography. 5. Field-enhanced sample injection with reverse migrating micelles . Anal. Chem. 70, 1893–1901.
14. Vidal, T. G. Laudat, M. H., Thomopoulos, P., Luton, J. P., and Bricaire, H. (1983) Urinary free corticoids: an evaluation of their usefulness in the diagnosis of Cushing's syndrome. Acta Endocrinol. 103, 110–115.
15. Rao, L. V., Petersen, J. R., Bissell, M. G., Okorodudu, A. O., and Mohammad, A. A. (1999) Development of a urinary free cortisol assay using solid-phase extraction-capillary electrophoresis. J. Chrom. B 730, 123–128.
16. Tietz, N. W. (1995) Clinical Guide to Laboratory Tests, 3rd ed., W. B. Saunders Co., Philadelphia, PA.
17. Mohammad, A. A., Bissell, M. G., and Petersen, J. R. (1995) Micellar electrokinetic capillary chromatography steroids that are increased in congenital adrenal hyperplasia. Clin. Chem. 41, 1389–1390.

IV
Immunoassay

12

Capillary Electrophoresis Based Immunoassay

Bode Adesoji, Amin A. Mohammad,
and John R. Petersen

1. INTRODUCTION

Immunoassay is a procedure that involves an antigen–antibody reaction to estimate the concentration of an analyte in a sample. Over the years there has been a tremendous advancement in sensitivity and reliability of immunological assays. This was accomplished by the development of specific ultrasensitive antibodies along with automation to improve quality of results, precision, and efficiency. Initially, analytes were measured by agglutination, complement fixation, or neutralization. Focusing on the kinetics and stoichiometry of antigen–antibody reactions has allowed improvements on these basic methods. Because of these improvements, immunoassay has become a method of choice for a wide variety of clinical, pharmaceutical, environmental, and toxicological analysis.

1.1. Radioimmunoassay

The introduction of radioimmunoassay (RIA) led to the ability to quantitate low molecular weight analytes with an appreciable degree of sensitivity and precision. RIA also provided the needed template for numerous immunochemical studies. This increased our knowledge of the kinetics of solid-phase antigen–antibody interactions, the role of affinity, the half-life of the immune complexes, and the nature and liability of antigen epitopes.

1.2. Solid-Phase Immunoassay

The major constraint of RIA was the separation of the bound and unbound antigen. This led to the development of solid-phase immunoassays in which the analyte–antibody complex is bound to a solid matrix allowing the free (unreacted) analyte to be easily removed (e.g., by simply decanting the solution). The solid-phase matrix could be the surface of plastic ware, mem-

From: *Clinical and Forensic Applications of Capillary Electrophoresis*
Edited by: J. R. Petersen and A. A. Mohammad © Humana Press Inc., Totowa, NJ

branes, beads (e.g., microparticles), microtiters plates, and so on. The use of microparticles as a solid phase has subsequently gained widespread use in clinical laboratory because of easy automation, precision, shorter turnaround tine (TAT) and most importantly, increased sensitivity.

Immobilization of reactants on a solid-phase occurs in one of three ways: 1) adsorption to hydrophobic surfaces; 2) covalent attachment to activated surface groups; or 3) non-covalent, electrostatic, and hydrophilic bonds between another molecule immobilized using method 1 or 2. Immobilization of reactants, however, is a heterogenous system and can vary with the analyte, type of matrix surface, and also the conditions used during the immobilization. The major drawback of solid-phase immobilization is the potential for conformational changes of the proteins (specifically antibodies) following immobilization on the solid phase. This can be reflected as a decrease in affinity or avidity of the antibody depending on the type of solid-phase, concentration, and method of immobilization resulting in a loss of assay sensitivity. Additionally, a number of variables, such as pH, types of binding forces involved, concentration of reactants, and so on, can affect the adsorptive capacity of the solid-phase matrix. Even after all of these factors have been minimized, separation of bound and free antigen is still required.

1.3. Types of Immunoassay

The types of immunoassay range from homogenous to heterogenous immunoassays. Homogenous assays require no physical separation of bound and unbound antigen, making them readily adaptable to existing clinical analyzers. A greater efficiency is achieved by the avoiding the use of a dedicated immunoassay analyzer along with a shorter TAT. The main limitation of homogenous assays is the size of analytes that can be detected. Only low molecular weight analytes that are found in relatively high concentrations (>μM) can be detected.

Heterogenous assays, on the other hand, can measure both small and large analytes. With this type of assay, unbound antigen is physically separated, eliminating many of the interference's plaguing homogenous assays. Although much more sensitive than homogenous assays, heterogenous assays are more labor-intensive, time-consuming, and usually require a dedicated immunoassay analyzer. The need for an effective yet fast separation technique on instruments that have multiple uses has led to the investigation of capillary electrophoresis (CE)-based immunoassay.

2. CE-BASED IMMUNOASSAY

CE evolved from the investigation of column electrophoresis by Hjerten *(1)* and Castimpoolas *(2)*. Later, Martin and Everaets developed a capillary isotachophoresis system that became commercially available in the mid-1970s. Subsequently, Jorgen and coworkers demonstrated the analytical potential of CE using 75-μm fused silica capillaries *(3–5)* leading to the adaptation and modification of CE for specific applications. The main advantage of CE when used as a separation technique is the small sample-size requirement, minimal sample preparation, rapid TAT, and the potential for automation *(6)*. Currently, nonimmunological CE-based assays are increasingly being used in toxicological drug screening and confirmation for drugs of abuse in urine *(7–10)*. Preliminary confirmation is by on-column, multiwave length UV detection of the solutes with comparison to normalized standard spectra with final confirmation by gas chromatography-mass spectrometery (GC-MS). These CE-based methods rely mainly on capillary zone electrophoresis (CZE) and micellar electrokinetic capillary chromatography (MEKC). Separation of enantiomers can also be achieved by addition of a chiral selector such as cyclodextrin *(11,12)*. This is important in the detection of banned substances having therapeutic enantiomers such as anabolic steroids and ephedrine/norephedrine *(13)*. However, the level for many drugs, such as tacrolimus and digoxin, fall far below the detection limits of CE without extraction and preconcentration. This lack of sensitivity has increased the need for better and more sensitive methods of detection.

Responding to this issue, Chen and Evangelista *(14)* described an immunoassay that used CE as the separation method. By coupling immunoassay, CE, and laser-induced fluorescence (LIF), they were able to separate and detect simultaneously several drugs *(see* Fig. 1). As with other immunoassays, this method involves the reaction of antibodies of known specificity with antigens in the presence of a labeled tracer. Because of the ability of CE to separate multiple components in a mixture, it is now possible to simultaneously detect multiple analytes using small amounts of samples (20–50 μL). When combined with fluorescence, extremely sensitive CE-based immunoassays can now be developed. The advantages include highly efficient separation, small quantity of sample required per analysis, minimal nonspecific interference, and, when screening for multiple constituents in a single sample, a reduced TAT. Usually CZE is used as the separation medium for CE-based immunoassay. The format can either be in a competitive or a direct-binding format. In all cases, CE- based immunoassays are used as a screen, complementing other chromatographic methods, such as CG-MS *(7)* or high-performance liquid chromatography (HPLC) with multiwavelength detection *(8)* that are typically used for confirmatory testing.

The long-term success of CE immunoassay will depend on the ability to automate the method by using multicapillary instruments or microchips.

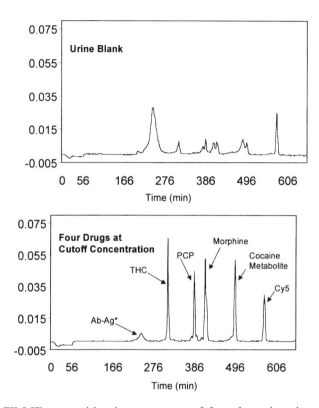

Fig. 1. CE-LIF competitive immunoassay of four drugs in urine. This figure refers to the separation of four drugs in urine. A fused silica capillary 27 cm × 20 μ, was used for separation. Buffer was 200 m*M* borate, pH 10.2, with LIF detection (633 mn excitation an 665 nm detection), voltage was 15 kV. The top figure is blank urine and the bottom figure is a urine spiked with the four drugs of interest. Cy5 is a negatively charged fluorescent cyanine dye. The drug concentrations were 73 n*M* (25 ng/mL) for THC-COOH, 100 n*M* (243 ng/mL) for PCP, 1 m*M* (285 ng/mL) for morphine, and 860 n*M* (248 ng/mL) for benzoylecgonine. Reproduced with permission from A. Chen, Beckman Coulter, Inc.

Although both of these methods will probably be developed, the underlying principle will be the same. Thus this chapter will focus only on the principles behind the technique along with examples of how it has been used.

2.1. Competitive Binding Immunoassay

The competitive binding assay is the most widely used immunoassay format used with CE. In this method, the sample containing the analyte, antibody or antibody fragment, and fluorescent-labeled tracer are mixed and incubated. The tracer competes with the analyte in the sample for a limited number of antibody binding sites. After equilibrium is reached, the mixture is injected onto a column, where the free tracer and the Ab-Ag complexes (including fluorescent Ab-Ag complexes) are electrophoretically separated and detected by on-column LIF. For this type of immunoassay, the concentrations of tracer and antibody injected onto the CE column are essential for valid quantitation of the analyte *(15)*.

The immunoassay of insulin was the first reported competitive CE-based immunoassay using an antibody fragment (fab) *(16,17)*. However, the microheterogeity of the fab fragments produced two peaks during separation, making it difficult to interpret the assay results. In addition, the detection limit (3 nmol) could not be improved because the covalent attachment of the label to the amino acid on insulin reduced the affinity of the antibody for the tracer. Optimization of the assay subsequently led to the development of an on-line CE immunoassay device. This allowed for analysis of the insulin content of single islets of Langerhans in addition to the quantitation of glucose-stimulated insulin release *(18)*. For this assay, three independent channels were used, one each for the labeled insulin, intact monoclonal antibody (MAb), and sample containing unknown levels of insulin. The contents of the channels were mixed where the channels intersect. The mixture was then directed to the reaction capillary through a stopper to a flow-gated interface. Incubation took place at the reaction capillary and the samples injected onto the column. The electropherogram typical of competitive immunoassays was obtained for insulin with a clear separation of the Ab-Ag peak and the fluorescent-labeled insulin peak. Because of the competition between the insulin in the sample and the labeled insulin for a limited number of antibody binding sites, quantitation of the insulin was possible. This assay generated a standard curve typical of a competitive binding immunoassay where high insulin levels produce a small Ab-Ag peak, whereas low insulin levels generate a large Ab-Ag peak.

In a manner similar to insulin, multianalyte drug assays have been developed using the competitive- based CE immunoassay format. In this type of assay, clear separation of free and bound tracer was observed *(14)* (*see* Fig. 1). Similar to the insulin immunoassay, the peak heights of the free tracers were also found to be concentration-dependent. Most of these assays have used the fluorescein-labeled tracer from fluorescence-polarization assay kits. Employing equal volumes of urine, tracer, and antibody CE-based immunoassays for methadone *(19)*, benzoylecgonine, and amphetamine/methamphetamine *(20)* have been developed. An immunoassay that can separate the four analytes (methadone, morphine, benzoylecgonine and D-amphetamine) with sensitivity comparable to Abbott's TDx FLx FPIA assays has also been developed *(21)*.

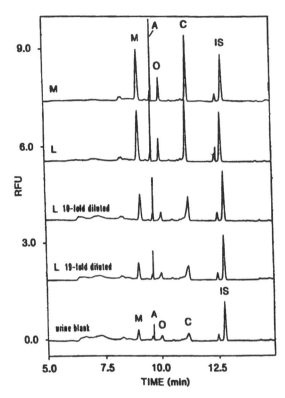

Fig. 2. MOCA multianalyte immunoassay. This figure refers to the separation of methadone (M), morphine (O), benzoylecgonine (C), and D-amphetamine (A). The L and M refer to low- and medium-level multiconstituent controls, respectively. A fused silica capillary, 47 cm (40 cm to detector) × 75 μ, was used for the separation. Buffer was 50 m*M* borate, pH 9.3, with LIF detection (488 nm excitation and 520 nm emission), voltage was 13 kV, and the capillary was kept at 20°C. Reproduced with permission from ref. *(22)*.

Caslavka et al. *(22)* developed a CE-based immunoassay using 50 m*M* borate buffer, pH 9.3, for the simultaneous detection and quantitation of methadone (M), morphine (O), benzoylecgonine (C), and D-amphetamine (A). Using the fluorescein tracer from a tricyclic antidepressant FPIA assay kit (Abbott Diagnostics) as the internal standard (I.S.), the electrophero-grams in Fig. 2 were obtained for a blank urine, low-level control urine (19-fold dilution), low-level control urine (10-fold dilution), low-level control urine, and medium-level control urine (from bottom to top). These data reveal that peak heights for all free tracers increase with increasing drug concentration. The ratios of the tracer peak heights with peak height of the I.S were used for multilevel internal calibration. The typical calibration

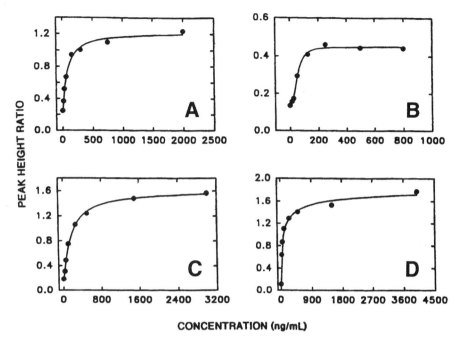

Fig. 3. Calibration graph of the MOCA multianalyte immunoassay. Data are based on peak height ratios divided by the peak height of the internal standard. Reproduced with permission from ref. *(22)*.

curves are shown in Fig. 3. This assay was found to be more sensitive than the enzyme multiplied immunoassay technique (EMIT) d.a.u. assay used in the authors' routine drug-assay laboratory.

Other examples of CE-based multianalyte immunoassay include analysis of urinary morphine, PCP, THC, benzoylecgonine *(23)*, salicylate and paracetamol *(24)*, theophylline and quinidine in serum *(24)*, morphine and PCP in urine. The main limitation in multianalyte assays is the ability of CE to separate labeled antigen from each other and from the antibody–antigen complex. Using Abbott's TDxFLx FPIA reagents, as in the MOCA assay, a significantly increased response for free tracer was obtained. Ninefold dilution of all mixed fluids showed decreased responses when compared to threefold dilution.

2.2. Direct CE

For direct CE-based immunoassay, fluorescent- or enzyme-labeled antibody or antibody fragments are added in excess to a sample. After incubation, a small aliquot of mixture is injected onto the CE column and the fluorescent complex (antigen-antibody) is separated from excess-labeled antibody with detection by LIF. Only the signal for the complex (Ab-Ag) is used for quantitation and total amount of antigen present is determined by comparing the peak height and or peak area of complex to the linear range of the calibration curve. Interferences have been found to be minimal since CE separates the potential interfering substances from the Ab-Ag complex. In addition, the different spectroscopic properties of the components relative to the Ab-Ag complex allow interfering substances to be separated and identified *(25)*. A variant of the sandwich format was also introduced to improve the separation. This involves using a matched pair of antibodies to perform independent binding to the analyte and subsequent mobility tailoring *(26)*. The first antibody is the tracer (fluorescent- or enzyme-labeled) is for detection whereas the second is to modify mobility (highly charge modified). After equilibrium is reached the complex (Ab-Ag-Ab) is quantitated. Another version of the direct assay uses fluorescein-labeled protein G to quantitate IgG in human serum *(27)*.

2.3. Microchip-Based CE

Microchip-based CE was developed by Manz and Harrison in 1992 *(28,29)*. The procedure is based on micro-machining technology and involves chemical etching, photolithography, and water binding to build channels in glass or fused silica substrates. The chip can then be used to electrophoretically separate analytes. This is faster, more flexible, and can have an enormous sample throughput relative to conventional CE. The first adaptation of immunoassay on the microchip was by Koutny et al. *(30)*. Using microchips, the authors developed an assay that could quantitate the levels of serum cortisol. Microchips provide have many performance-enhancing features (such as lower reagent consumption), faster separations, integrated sample handling steps (such as on-chip mixing, dilution, and labeling), as well as parallel multianalyte analysis by microfabrication of a multichannel device *(31)*. High performance on-chip separations by CE have also been readily achieved using glass substrates *(32,33)*. With the microchip, it is possible to control the flow of fluid at channel intersections using the electrokinetic and electroosmotic flow (EOF). Electrical and reagent leakages at intersections were also eliminated by application of bias voltages *(34,35)*. Complex biochemical quantitations and reactions can be affected with microchips. Various modifications have been made in an attempt to adapt the microchip CE technology to the clinical laboratory including interfacing multiple-channel glass chips to an electrospray ionization mass spectrometer *(36)*.

3. CONCLUSION

The use of CE in combination with immunoassay opens up some interesting avenues of investigation, specifically in the ability simultaneously to screen and detect multiple analytes. The development of CE-based multianalyte immunoassays is limited only by the ability to separate the analytes from each other and from the Ab-Ag complex. As with other CE methods, the multianalyte CE-based immunoassay is rapid, sensitive (if using LIF), and reliable for screening purposes. In addition, custom-made reagents, such as antibodies and tracers that have specific, yet different, mobilities, can be prepared and used to detect a variety of antigens. The method can also be extended to the simultaneous detection of a variety of fluorescent tracers, e.g., fluorescein in combination with rhodamine, along with LIF detection using multiple laser lines. This, along with wavelength resolved fluorescence detection as proposed by Thormann et al. represents some interesting approaches to the simultaneous separation and detection of multiple analytes.

Finally, microchips made from inexpensive materials, such as glass or plastic, will make the device inexpensive. This could be an area where CE in combination with immunoassay will fit into the clinical laboratory. It is quite conceivable that in the future microchips will be adapted to point-of-care uses.

REFERENCES

1. Hjerten, S. (1967) Free-zone electrophoresis. Chromatogr. Rev. 9, 122–219.
2. Castimpoolas, N. (1971) Scanning density gradient isoelectric separation of proteins on a mole scale. Sep. Sci. 6, 435.
3. Jorgenson, J. W. and Lukacs, K. D. (1981) Zone electrophoresis in open-tubular glass capillaries. Anal. Chem. 53, 1298.
4. Jorgenson, J. W. and Lukacs, K. D. (1981) High resolution separations based on electrophoresis and electro-osmosis. J. Chromatogr. 218, 209.
5. Jorgenson, J. W. and Lukacs, K. D. (1981) Capillary zone electrophoresis in glass capillaries. Clin. Chem. 27, 1551–1553.
6. Thormann, W., Aebi, Y., and Caslavska, J. (1998) Capillary electrophoresis in clinical toxicology. Forensic Sci. Int. 92, 157–183.
7. Maurer, H. H., Arlt, J. W., Kraemer, T., Schmitt, C. J., and Weber, A. A. (1997) Analytical development of low molecular weight xenobiotic compounds. Arch. Toxicol. Supp. 19, 189–197.
8. Binder, S. R. (1996) Analysis of drugs of abuse in biological fluids by liquid chromatography. Adv. Chromatogr. 35, 201–271.
9. Wernly, P. and Thormann, W. (1991) Analysis of illicit drugs in human urine by micellar electrokinetic capillary chromatography with on-column fast scanning polychron absorption detection. Anal. Chem. 63, 2878–2882.

10. Wernly, P. and Thormann, W. (1992) Drug of abuse confirmation in human urine using stepwise solid-phase extraction and micellar electrokinetic capillary chromatography. Anal. Chem. 64, 2155–2159.
11. Foret, F., Krivankova, L., and Bocek, P. (1993) Capillary Zone Electrophoresis. VCH Publishers, Weinheim, Germany.
12. Engelhard, H., Beck, W., and Schmitt, T. (1996) Capillary Electrophoresis: Methods and Potentials. Springer-Verlag, Heidelberg, Germany.
13. Chicharro, M., Zapardiel, A., and Bermejo, E. (1993) Direct determination of ephedrine and norephedrine in human urine by capillary zone electrophoresis. J. Chromatog. 622, 103–108.
14. Chen, F.-T. and Evangelista, R. A. (1994) Feasibility studies for simultaneous immunochemical multianalyte drug assay by capillary electrophoresis with laser-induced fluorescence. Clin. Chem. 40, 1819–1822.
15. Odell, W. D. and Franchimont, P. (1993) Principles of Competitive Binding Assays, John Wiley, New York
16. Schultz, N. M. and Kennedy, R. T. (1993) Rapid immunoassays using capillary electrophoresis with flourescence Detection. Anal. Chem. 65, 3161–3665.
17. Schultz, N. M., Huang, L., and Kennedy, R. T. (1995) Capillary electrophoresis-based immunoassay to determine insulin content and insulin secretion from single Islets of Langerhans. Anal. Chem. 67, 924–929.
18. Tao, L. and Kennedy, R. T. (1996) On-line competitive immunoassay for insulin based on capillary electrophoresis with laser-induced fluorescence detection. Anal. Chem. 68, 3899–3906.
19. Thormann, W., Lanz, M., Caslavska, J., Siegenthale, P., and Portmann, R. (1998) Screening for urinary methadone by capillary electrophoretic immunoassays and confirmation by capillary electrophoresis-mass spectrometry. Electrophoresis 19, 57–65.
20. Ramseier, A., Caslavska, J., and Thormann, W. (1989) Screening for urinary amphetamine and analogs by capillary electrophoretic immunoassays and confirmation by capillary electrophoresis with on-column multiwavelength adsorbance detection. Electrophoresis 19, 2956–2966.
21. TDx-TDxFLx Testanleiting Drogentests Tests und Toxikologische Test, No. B4D241 82-4441/R1, Abbott, Wiesbaden-Delkenheim, Germany.
22. Caslavska, J., Allermann, J., and Thormann, W. (1999) Analysis of urinary drugs of abuse by a multianalyte capillary electrophoretic immunoassay. J. Chromatogr. A. 838, 237–249.
23. Chen, F.-T. and Evangelista, R. A. (1997) Handbook of CE Applications. Blackie Academic and Professional, London, pp. 219–239.
24. Steinmann, L. and Thormann, W. (1996) Characterization of competitive binding, flourescent drug immunoassays based on micellar electrokinetic capillary chromatography. Electrophoresis 17, 1348–1356.
25. Schmalzing, D. and Nashabeh, W. (1997) Capillary electrophoresis based immunoassays: a critical review. Electrophoresis 18, 2184–2893.
26. Lidosky, III S. D., Hinsberg, W. D., and Zare, R. N. (1981) Proc. Natl. Acad. Sci. USA, 78, 1901–1905.

27. Reif, O. W., Lausch, R., Schepner, T., and Freitag, R. (1994) Flourescein isothiocyanate-labeled protein G as an affinity ligand in affinity/immuno capillary electrophoresis with flourescence detection. Anal. Chem. 66, 4027–4033.

28. Manz, A., Harrison, D. J., Verpoorte, M. J., Feltinger, J. C., Paulus, A., Ludi, H., and Widmer, H. M. (1992) Planar chips technology for miniaturization and intergration of separation techniques into monitoring systems: capillary electrophoresis on a chip. J. Chromator. 593, 253–258.

29. Harrison, D. J., Manz, A., Fan, Z., Ludi, H., and Widmer, H. M. (1992) Capillary electrophoresis and sample injection systems integrated on a planar glass chip. Anal. Chem. 64, 1926–1932.

30. Koutny, L. B., Schmatzing, D., Taylor, T. A., and Fuchs, M. (1996) Microchip electrophoresis immunoassay for serum cortisol. Anal. Chem. 68, 18–22.

31. Coyler, C. L., Tang, T., Chiem, N., and Harrison, D. J. (1997) Clinical potential of microchip capillary electrophoresis systems. Electrophoresis 18, 1733–1741.

32. Seiler, K., Harrison, D. J., and Manz, A., (1993) Planar glass chips for capillary electrophoresis: repetitive sample injection, quantitation, and separation efficiency. Anal. Chem. 65, 1481–1488.

33. Fan, H. and Harrison, D. J. (1994) Micromachining of capillary electrophoresis injectors and separators on glass chips and evaluation of flow at capillary intersections. Anal. Chem. 66, 177–184.

34. Manz, A., Fettinger, J. C., Verpoote, E., Widmer, H. M., and Harrison, D. J. (1991) Trends Anal Chem. 10, 144–149.

35. Harrison, D. J, Fluri, K., Seiler, K., Fan, Z., Effenhauser, C. S., and Manz, A. (1993) Science 261, 895–897.

36. Xue, Q. F., Foret, F., Dunayevskiy, Y. M., Zavracky, P. M., McGruer, N. E., and Karger, B. L. (1997) Multichannel microchip electrospray mass spectrometry. Anal. Chem. 69, 426–430.

V
Molecular Diagnostics

13
Quantitation of Viral Load

Jill M. Kolesar

1. INTRODUCTION

Viruses, the world's smallest organisms, are a large group of single cell organisms comprised of nucleic acid surrounded by a protein coat. Pathogenic viruses play an important role in many human diseases, including hepatitis, cancer, and AIDS, as well as the common cold. These viruses are of particular concern for patients who are immune compromised, those undergoing transplant procedures with donor organs, and/or those receiving blood from human sources.

Because of the intracellular nature of viral diseases, it was very difficult to diagnose and monitor disease progress. With modern immunological techniques, which rely on detection of the host response to the virus, by production of specific antibodies, it is now possible to detect viral infection. With the advent of molecular biology, it is now possible to detect viral particles (also called viral load) present in the host. Measurement of viral loads is an emerging technique for the diagnosis and monitoring of viral disease. Although treatment options currently are limited for many virally mediated diseases, improved diagnostic and monitoring techniques may lead to improved treatment options in the near future.

Current methods for assessing viral loads generally rely on an amplification step followed by detection of a fluorescent, chemiluminescent, or radioactive label. Capillary electrophoresis (CE) with laser induced fluorescence (LIF) is a method that allows for sensitive, reliable, rapid and automated quantitation of nucleic acids. Although not currently used for routine analysis of viral loads, further research may reveal it to be an important advance in the diagnosis and monitoring of viral disease.

From: *Clinical and Forensic Applications of Capillary Electrophoresis*
Edited by: J. R. Petersen and A. A. Mohammad © Humana Press Inc., Totowa, NJ

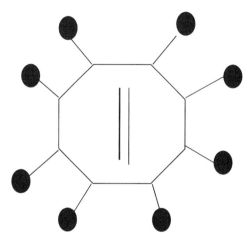

Fig. 1. Schematic representation of a adenovirus made up of a icosohedral proteins surrounding a dsDNA genome. Viruses are obligate intracellular parasite comprised of a DNA or RNA genome surrounded by a protein coat. Immunoassays detect a host response toward a viral protein or antigen. Viral loads measure the quantity of virus present by detecting viral nucleic acid.

2. CLINICAL VIROLOGY

2.1. DNA and RNA Viruses and Human Disease

Viruses are infectious particles generally composed only of nucleic acid surrounded by a protein coat (*see* Fig. 1). Viruses survive by infecting a host cell, where viral proteins take over host cellular machinery to produce viral progeny. The host cell may be killed in the process, as in the case of most adenoviral infections, or harbor a latent viral infection, such as herpes simplex virus (HSV), for many years. The type of nucleic acid and the presence or absence of an envelope categorizes viruses (*see* Table 1). The nucleic acids may be DNA or RNA and double-stranded, single-stranded, sense, or antisense.

Analysis of viral loads, which estimates the virus particles present in the host serum at a given time, may be very important in diagnosing, treating, and monitoring viral illness. In particular, viral loads may be very useful in detecting the presence of latent infections, when low copy numbers of virus are present (as in early viral illness) and to determine response to antiviral therapy.

2.2. Clinical Utility of Viral Loads

2.2.1. DNA Viruses: CMV

Human cytomegalovirus (CMV) is a DNA virus associated with significant human disease. CMV is a pathogen in immunocompromised *(1)* indi-

Table 1
Classification of Viruses Associated with Human Disease

Virus family	Nucleic acid	Sense	Envelope	Example of human disease
Picornaviridae	RNA	+	–	Polio
Calciviridae	RNA	+	–	Gastroenteritis
Togaviridae	RNA	+	+	Rubella
Flaviviridae	RNA	+	+	Hepatitis C
Coronaviridae	RNA	+	+	Avian infectious bronchitis
Rhabdoviridae	RNA	–	+	Rabies
Paramyoxoviridae	RNA	–	+	Mumps, measles, pneumonia,
Orthomyxoviridae	RNA	–	+	Influenza
Filoviridae	RNA	–	+	Ebola
Bunyaviridae	RNA	–	+	Hantaan
Arenaviridae	RNA	–	+	Lassa fever
Reoviridae	RNA	ds	+	Diarrhea, encephalitis
Retroviridae	RNA	–	+	AIDS (HIV)
Hepadnaviridae	DNA	–	+	Hepatitis B
Papovaviridae	DNA	ds	–	Genital warts
Adenovirus	DNA	ds	–	Colds
Herpesviridae	DNA	ds	+	Cold sores (HSV1), shingles, Chicken pox (HSV3), Genital ulceration (HSV2)
Poxviridae	DNA	ds	+	Smallpox

viduals, especially those with end-stage AIDS *(2)*, solid organ *(3)*, and allogeneic bone marrow transplant recipients. Risk factors associated with serious CMV infection include; 1) degree of immunosuppression, and 2) the presence of CMV viremia.

Quantitative nucleic acid detection methods, including polymerase chain reaction (PCR), branched-DNA assay, and the DNA hybrid capture assay for CMV, have been developed in recent years. The DNA hybrid assay is able to detect viral particles present in the pg/mL range, corresponding to 675 copies for the lower limit of detection and 1446 copies for the lower limit of quantitation *(4–8)*.

Due to their high sensitivity, these assays can detect CMV early, and quantitation may be able to predict disease risk and monitor the effect of antiviral therapy. Generally, a high systemic viral load is correlated with CMV disease *(9,10)*. This correlation is strong in the HIV-infected population and in solid-organ transplant recipients but less clear in allogeneic marrow transplant recipients *(11)*.

Alternatively, viral loads may be measured at specific anatomic sites *(12)*. This may be a more accurate method to assess disease activity in clinical situations where the systemic viral load does not correlate with disease activity. A reduction of the systemic CMV load also correlates with a response to antiviral treatment. Quantitative CMV detection techniques are used widely to direct and monitor antiviral treatment, however, reproducibility and standardization of the various assays needs further analysis. In addition, the FDA has not approved to date a viral load assay for CMV.

2.2.2. DNA Viruses: Hepatitis B

Hepatitis B is a blood-borne disease representing a serious, worldwide public health problem. More than 1 million individuals in the United States alone are infected the virus. Hepatitis B is endemic in China, Southeast Asia, and the Middle East as well as parts of Africa and South America. In addition to the acute manifestations of hepatitis, individuals infected with hepatitis B may develop chronic hepatitis and are at increased risk of liver cancer. The risk of liver cancer appears to be higher for patients with higher viral loads, indicating actively replicating virus, whereas viral titers (indication of the host immune response to the virus) are not predictive of progression to liver cancer *(13)*.

In the United States, the primary routes of transmission are through direct contact with infected blood and body secretions and the clinical use of infected blood products. Routine screening of the blood supply for the hepatitis B surface antigen (HbsAg) has virtually eliminated post-transfusion hepatitis B infection. However, other blood products, such as clotting factors produced from blood concentrates, can still transmit infection. Currently, viral loads are not used routinely to screen blood, blood products, or donated organs. Analysis of viral loads may, however, be useful in decreasing transmission of infection *(14,15)*. Viral loads are also often quantified to assess response to therapy with interferon (IFN) or lamivudine. Lower viral loads are associated with an increased rate of seroconversion for patients, which lowers the risk for clinical disease progression *(12,16)*. Lower viral titers are also associated with a decreased frequency of mutations associated with resistance.

2.2.3. RNA Viruses: Hepatitis C

Hepatitis C is an RNA virus and like hepatitis B is transmitted via contact with infected blood or other body fluids. Infection with hepatitis C results in chronic hepatitis in up to 70% of individuals and cirrhosis in approx 50% of those developing chronic hepatitis. Currently, the only treatment of patients with hepatitis C is with IFN and more recently IFN in combination with ribavirin. In chronic hepatitis C infection, a high viral load per liver cell predicts long-term response to therapy. Loss of viremia at the second week of therapy is the strongest predictor for a long-term IFN response, followed by the initial viral load and loss of viremia at the fourth week of therapy. It may be possible to predict a long-term response as early as at the second and fourth weeks after the start of therapy by screening for HCV-RNA. Patients unlikely to respond to therapy could be discontinued after 2 wk, decreasing the adverse effects and associated cost of prolonged therapy *(12)*.

2.2.4. RNA Viruses: HIV

Primarily infection with the human immunodeficiency virus type 1 (HIV-1) and less frequently by HIV-2 cause acquired immune deficiency syndrome (AIDS). AIDS, first identified as a clinical syndrome in 1981, is currently a worldwide epidemic *(17,18)*. The CDC estimates that 1.2 million individuals are infected in the United States and the WHO reports 2.5 million cases of AIDS worldwide.

Viral loads are routinely assessed in AIDS patients and are the single best predictor of disease progression *(19–23)*. A major advance in monitoring has been development of plasma HIV RNA assays of increased sensitivity, which have a detection range of approx 20–50 to approx 50,000 copies/mL of plasma. These assays are suitable for monitoring the majority of patients on anti-retroviral treatment. Assay precision at lower limits is usually poor with CVs approaching 90% making quantitation at these levels questionable. Current methodology, however, can be viewed as a detection tool at the 50-copies/mL lower limit. Assays will likely improve even further regarding lower limits of sensitivity, reliability, and quantitation as described in the following sections on capillary electrophoresis (CE).

The International AIDS Society-USA panel recommends anti-retroviral therapy for any patient with established HIV infection and a confirmed plasma HIV-1 RNA level greater than 5000–10,000 copies/mL and willingness to undergo the complex, long-term therapy *(24,25)*. Viral load is a strong, independent predictor of clinical outcome. Degree and durability of viral response correlates directly with plasma HIV-RNA level and CD4+ cell count at diagnosis. For asymptomatic patients with low (e.g., <5000–10,000 copies/mL) plasma HIV-RNA level and high CD4 counts, deferral of therapy with close follow-up may be recommended. These individuals may be categorized as potential long-term nonprogressors. For those with low HIV RNA level and low CD4+ cell count, initiation of therapy is recommended, since the CD4 count gives independent prognostic information and data from clinical trials document the benefit of initiating therapy when the CD4 count is low.

The goal of antiretroviral therapy is to reduce plasma HIV-RNA below the detection limit of the most sensitive assays. Even modest reductions in viral load (e.g., 0.5–1 log reductions) provide clinical benefit, therefore regimens that provide maximal suppression of HIV replication are expected to improve survival and decrease morbidity via continuous suppression of HIV replication. A combination of three drugs, including a nucleoside reverse transcriptase inhibitor (nRTI) (zidovudine, didanosine, zalcitabine, lamivudine, and stavudine), a nonnucleoside reverse transcriptase inhibitor (nnRTI) (nevirapine and delavirdine), and protease inhibitor (PI) (ritonavir, indinavir, nelfinavir, and saquinavir) is commonly used as initial therapy. These regimens result in virologic success rates of 60–90% in anti-retroviral naive patients, as determined by plasma HIV-1 RNA level <500 copies/mL at 24 wk or beyond. Currently, the combination of a potent PI and 2 nRTIs should remain the primary consideration, based on clinical trials documenting the efficacy and durability of responses.

Since clinical outcome clearly correlates with disease activity and antiretroviral treatment is made based on viral-load determinations, the most sensitive assays available are recommended with viral-load monitoring every 2 mo for patients treated with antiviral therapy. Ongoing viral replication is reported for patients with a consistent viral load between 50 and 500 copies/mL. For patients with levels <50 copies/mL, development of resistance is decreased, although low levels of viral replication may persist. The strictest definition of treatment failure is that of confirmed detectable plasma HIV RNA (i.e., >50 copies/mL) in an compliant patient who had achieved a viral-load level below the detection limit and has not experienced a recent acute infectious illness.

Clearly, viral diseases play a significant role in the health of individuals worldwide. Currently, viral loads are used to monitor disease progression and response to therapy for patients with HIV. Viral loads may also play an emerging role in assessing the response to therapy for patients with hepatitis B, hepatitis C, and CMV. Other potential applications include instances where early and very low-level detection is required. Examples of these include screening of donor blood, organs for transplant, and very early infection after exposure to an infected individual.

3. METHODS OF VIRAL-LOAD ASSESSMENT

Current methods for assessing viral loads generally rely on amplification reactions of either the viral nucleic acid (PCR) and reverse-transcription (RT-PCR) or the signal (bDNA) and are labeled with fluorescence or chemiluminescence probes for analysis in plate readers or by slab gel electrophore-

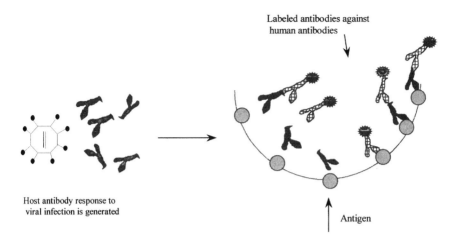

Fig. 2. Schematic representation of an immunoassay. When infected with a virus, the host will produce antibodies directed against the virus. These antibodies are then detected by ELISA or similar assay, indicating indirectly the presence of a viral infection.

sis. Quantification by current assays is relative and quantitative results obtained by different methods are not interchangeable.

3.1. Immunoassays

Many viral diseases are routinely diagnosed by immunological testing *(26)*. These tests screen for an antibody generated by the infected host against the viral pathogen *(see* Fig. 2). As such, immunological-based tests are evaluating a host response to an infection, rather than the infectious organism itself. This type of testing was initially developed because isolation and culture of the infecting virus was very difficult. Antibody tests have the advantages of being relatively inexpensive, rapid and accurate with specificities often in excess of 99%. For the HIV-enzyme-linked immunosorbent assay (ELISA) reported sensitivities range from 93 to 97%.

The limitations of antibody testing are:

1. Inability to detect early infection when the virus is present while the immune response is still being generated. Patients have a viral load but will test negative by antibody testing. Since most diseases are more curable at an early stage, diagnosis at this stage would be advantageous.
2. When there are low levels of infection or immunological response indicating that the level of infection may be inadequate to stimulate a host immunological response, or if a patient is immunosuppressed, they may not be able to mount an immunological response. In both these situations, the patient may test negative by antibody testing, while still having an active disease process.

Cycle 1

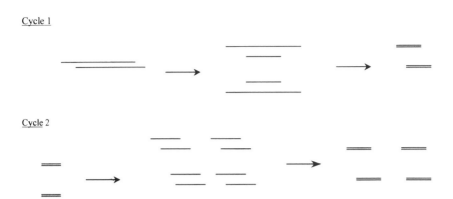

Cycle 2

Fig. 3. The PCR process. Target nucleic acid is amplified by primers directed towards the region of interest, generating sufficient DNA for analysis. After one cycle of PCR there are two copies of the target gene. The second cycle generates four copies and the third eight copies. Because each subsequent cycle produces a copy of each target DNA, amplification is exponential.

3. When quantitative results are required. Since an antibody test measures a host response to an infection, it does not give a quantitative measure of virus present.

3.2. Nucleic Acid-Based Assays

3.2.1. PCR and RT-PCR

The primary limitation to genetic analysis prior to the conception of PCR was the small quantity of nucleic acid available for analysis. PCR is in essence a nucleic acid xerox machine, making many genetic analyses routine. Initially, primers flanking the region of interest are designed and synthesized (*see* Fig. 3). The PCR reaction is set-up in a microcentrifuge tube with the reaction components consisting of the template DNA, primers, nucleotide bases, TAQ polymerase, and the appropriate buffer and salt concentration. The tube is heated to approx 95°C, allowing denaturation of the target DNA and attachment of the primers. TAQ polymerase then uses the nucleotide building blocks to fill in the space between the primers, creating an exact replica of the target DNA and doubling the amount of target DNA strands. This process is repeated again and again, making a large number of fragments, all which contain the DNA region of interest.

PCR requires DNA for a template, however, RNA can also be used. RNA isolated by standard methods is reverse-transcribed into cDNA by the enzyme reverse transcriptase. The cDNA can then be amplified by PCR as described earlier. PCR and RT-PCR can also be used to increase the quan-

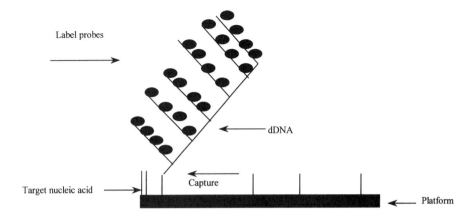

Fig. 4. bDNA assay. Target nucleic acid is hybridized to the capture probe attached to the platform, which is then hybridized to the label. The label probe is very large and contains a large quantity of fluorophor, allowing for signal amplification.

tity of nucleic acid present to amounts that are easily detectable. PCR products are then run on a gel matrix, which separates by molecular size and are visualized by ultraviolet (UV), radiolabeled, or fluorescence detection *(27)*.

3.2.2. Other Nucleic Acid-Based Detection Techniques Relying on Amplification

Branched DNA (bDNA) is a technique that relies on the amplification of the signal rather than the amplification of the target nucleic acid (*see* Fig. 4). Target nucleic acid is hybridized to a probe that is attached to a platform. Bound probe is then hybridized to additional probes, with a fluorescent or chemiluminescent label, which amplifies the signal. This approach is commercially available as the Quantiplex assay. This technique relies on amplification to detect very low levels (50 copies/mL plasma) of HIV virus (*see* Table 2). The DNA hybrid capture assay is an alternative approach using an RNA probe directed towards a DNA virus. An antibody with a chemiluminescent label then recognizes the resulting DNA/RNA hybrid (*see* Fig. 5). Since a large portion of the genome is probed, there are multiple sites for antibody attachment. The long probe, which increases the number of antibody binding sites serves as the signal amplification step in this technique.

3.2.3. Direct Detection

In direct detection, target viral DNA or RNA is hybridized with a specific fluorescent-labeled probe. Excess single stranded RNA or DNA is then digested away. Because this method does not rely on amplification of target or signal, variability resulting from amplification is eliminated. The method does require separation of the hybridized target and since viral

Table 2
Selected Commercially Available Assays for Assessment
of Viral Loads in Human Disease

Assay (manufacturer)	Test basis	Detection limits	Clinical use
DNA Hybrid Capture Assay (Digene/Murex)	Molecular hybridization with chemiluminescent detection of DNA/RNA complexes	675 copies/mL- detection limits 1146 copies/mL- quantitation limits	Monitoring antiviral therapy for CMV and HepB
AMPLICOR (Roche)	RT-PCR for HIV	50 copies/mL	Monitoring therapy for HBV, HCV, HIV
Quantiplex HCV-RNA (Chiron)	Hybridization with amplification of chemiluminescent signal	50 copies/mL for HIV	Monitoring therapy for HCV, HBV, HIV

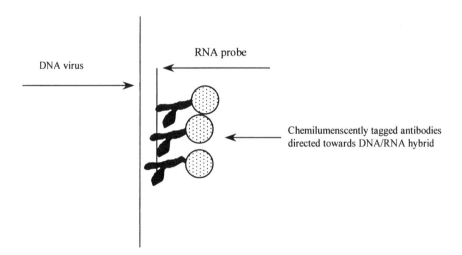

Fig. 5. Molecular hybridization assay. An RNA probe is directed toward the DNA virus. An antibody with a chemeluminscent tag against DNA/RNA hybrids is used to visualize the hybrid. The probe is large in relationship to the target, allowing for multiple binding sites for the antibody and signal amplification.

nucleic acids are often present in very small quantities, a highly sensitive method for detection, such as CE with laser induced fluorescence (CE-LIF) is required *(28).*

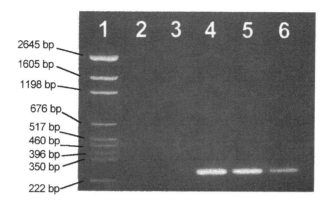

Fig. 6. Example of agarose gel electrophoresis of PCR products. The band present at 269 in lanes 4, 5, and 6 indicates the presence of the gene. Lane 1, pGEM Markers (2. 6, 1. 6, 1. 2 kb, 676, 517, 460, 396, 350, and 222 bp); Lane 2, Negative control; Lane 3, CHO; Lane 4, CHO-812; Lane 5, CHO-815; Lane 6, MCF-7.

4. DETECTION METHODS FOR VIRAL-LOAD ASSESSMENT

A number of assays are currently commercially available for the analysis of viral loads and are used in clinical laboratories. These include RT-PCR (Amplicor-Roche), bDNA (Chiron), and molecular hybridization (Digene), although the FDA has only approved RT-PCR for HIV viral-load assessment, These assays are able to detect as few as 50 copies/mL in serum and represent an important advance in the diagnosis and monitoring viral disease. Since most of these assays rely on amplification, variability is introduced and CVs are often high. As such, advances in technology, i.e., CE-LIF, that improve reliability, quantitation, and detection are needed. CE-LIF detection that is able to detect attomolar concentrations is highly reproducible and fully automatable has the potential for improving viral-load analysis.

4.1. Slab Gel Electrophoresis

PCR products are commonly analyzed by slab gel electrophoresis (SGE) (*see* Fig. 6), where an agarose gel containing ethidium bromide acts as the separation medium and products are visualized directly with UV light. Visualization by SGE is a rapid and inexpensive method for the analysis of PCR products. The major limitation of SGE is a relatively high detection limit, usually on the order of nanograms. Slab gel electrophoresis with radiolabeled probes is able to detect 1–5 pg of target DNA with an overnight exposure. Radioactive-detection methods, however, have significant disadvantages with respect to safety, stability of the labeled nucleic acids, and automation *(29).*

4.2. Capillary Electrophoresis with Laser-Induced Fluorescence

High pressure liquid chromatography (HPLC) was initially studied as a replacement for slab gel electrophoresis, although restricted intraparticle diffusion of biopolymers resulted in only limited improvement of resolution and speed *(30,31)*. Alternatively, electrophoretic separations (CE) can be performed in narrow-bore tubes or capillaries and may be viewed simply as another mode of electrophoresis *(32–34)*. Originally, CE utilizing hydroxyethylcellulose and ethidium bromide was shown to have increased resolving power when compared to HPLC for dsDNA, however, the detection level still remained in the nanogram range.

CE has since been used successfully in the research setting to separate and quantitate PCR products of HIV-1, HBV, CMV, and HCV *(35–39)*. The introduction of CE with LIF and intercalating dyes improved detectability to the attomole level with sample volumes as little as a few picoliters *(40–43)*. CE represents a safe and automatable assay system for quantitative analysis and routine laboratory analysis may soon be the norm.

Capillary gel electrophoresis (CGE) initially used either a fixed or immobilized polymerized matrix which acts as a "molecular sieve" within the capillary to separate DNA based on size and charge *(44–46)*. Since the mass to charge ratio of DNA remains constant with increasing mass, separations are made based on differences in molecular weight. As charged solutes migrate through the polymer network, they are retarded with larger molecules being retarded, more than smaller ones, allowing for separation based on molecular weight. Initially, CE used crosslinked agarose and polyacrylamide for the separation of DNA. However, polymerization of gels within the capillary is difficult and time-consuming. Polymerization that occurs too rapidly, use of impure chemicals and solutions that are not degassed can lead to bubble formation and unstable gels. Additionally, these capillaries are very rigid, making hydrodynamic injections impossible and the capillary susceptible to breakage. Linear polymer solutions are more flexible and pressure can be used to refill the capillary *(47,48)*. Additionally, they are much less susceptible to bubble formation and breakage. Although the polymer structure of the cross-linked gel is much different than the linear polymer solution, the mechanism of separation is identical and the ease of use with the replaceable polymer networks have made these the capillary system of choice for most laboratories *(49,50)*. CGE is used most frequently for the analysis of nucleic acids and will be the focus of this discussion.

4.2.1. CE-LIF Analysis of RT-PCR Products

To quantitate viral load, the measured concentration must be a reliable gauge of the amount of nucleic acid present in the original sample. This is usually a two-part process; amplification followed by detection. RNA

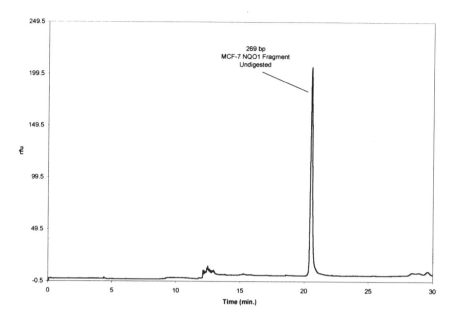

Fig. 7. Electropherogram of PCR products analyzed by CE-LIF. RNA obtained from MCF-7 cells is amplified by RT-PCR and analyzed. DNA elutes at 21 min, indicating the presence of the target gene in the sample.

samples are usually amplified by RT-PCR. In this process an internal standard that will amplify under the same conditions as the target sequence is introduced prior to amplification. The internal standard is used to control for variability within the PCR reaction as well as to provide a reference to calculate the initial concentration of unknown *(51)* *(see* Fig. 7).

To ensure peak areas reported by CE-LIF are an accurate measure of the amount of RT-PCR product present in the sample, a calibration curve is generated by injecting known concentrations DNA. The same solution of standard DNA fragments can also be used to calibrate the capillary and determine the molecular weight of fragments based on retention times. In addition to being an additional step towards the accurate quantitation of gene expression, this technique offers several advantages. Sample volumes are small (1–5 µL), sensitivity is high (attomolar), and the hazards associated with isotopic storage, use and disposal are eliminated. This technique can also be automated, used for fraction collection, and validated. There are, however, drawbacks to CE-LIF, including expense. Initially, there is an investment in equipment, CE, laser, computer and application software that must be made. In addition, consumable supplies, primarily intercalating dyes and capillaries can also be expensive and in the case of capillaries, fragile.

With current CE-LIF technology, samples are analyzed individually *(52)*. Each sample usually has a 15–45 min run time, whereas multiple samples can be analyzed simultaneously by SGE. For analysis of a single sample, CE-LIF may be faster, but when multiple analyses are required, SGE may be more time efficient. With the multicapillary instruments currently under development, analysis of multiple samples simultaneously by CE-LIF will be possible. In addition to requiring a longer time, individual sample processing also means that each sample is analyzed separately increasing risk of bias. Of the steps involved in analyzing PCR products, injection bias is the most frequent source of error, although this can be minimized by using hydrodynamic injections. Interassay variation can also be minimized by the addition of a reference of known concentration into each of the samples after PCR amplification. DNA fragments of similar, but not identical molecular weight to the unknown sample are best used as a reference. Although not currently used for commercial analysis of viral loads, CE-LIF represents an important avenue for exploration. CE-LIF has been used to analyze HIV, HBV, HCV, and CMV, in addition to many other PCR-generated fragments *(53,54)*.

4.2.1.1. EXPERIMENTAL CONDITIONS AND REAGENTS: RNA PURIFICATION

Total cellular RNA and RNA obtained from human tissue samples including tumor biopsies and whole blood can be obtained by standard procedures. Alternatively, commercially available system such as Ultraspec II RNA isolation system (Biotecx, Houston, TX) may be used. This system isolates total RNA by disruption and homogenization of samples with 14 *M* guanidine salts and urea followed by chloroform extraction. The sample is centrifuged and the upper aqueous phase containing the RNA is isolated followed by isopropanol precipitation. A proprietary RNATack resin that specifically binds RNA and then eluted with TE (Tris-EDTA, pH 7.4) buffer purifies the RNA. The RNA concentration is quantitated spectrophotometrically. The entire isolation can be completed in approx 1 h, which is a significant advantage over standard methods. RNA can also be extracted directly from lymphocytes obtained from whole blood. Concentrations of 10–15 ng of RNA are routinely obtained from 10 mL of whole blood comparing favorably to standard methods *(55)*.

4.2.1.2. EXPERIMENTAL CONDITIONS AND REAGENTS: DESIGN OF INTERNAL STANDARD

An internal standard may be designed by purifying, using SGE, the desired PCR product and identifying restriction sites 30–70 base pairs apart that will generate compatible ends. Digestion with the appropriate enzymes and re-ligation generates a DNA fragment that is identical to the target DNA, but 30–70 base pairs smaller. The primer recognition sites and the sequence are identical and the internal standard should amplify under identical conditions. After gel purification and elution in TE, the internal standard is quantified spectrophotometrically and stored at –20°C. The internal standard concentration is then titrated to determine what concentration is optimal for amplification, usually 10^{-6} ng/PCR reaction.

Using a DNA standard has the benefit of ease of preparation and storage, amplification under identical conditions, and low expense. It does not, however, control for variability present within the RT step. Thus, RNA standards are usually introduced prior to reverse transcription to control for variability throughout the RT-PCR process *(51)*.

4.2.1.3. Experimental Conditions and Reagents: RT-PCR

To improve reproducibility, all RT and PCR steps are done with master mixes that contain all components except the target nucleotides and Taq polymerase. Since PCR is by nature prone to contamination and false-positive results, precautions must be taken to ensure the validity of results. All reagents should be aliquotted into single use portions and separate pipets should be set aside to be used only for PCR. Reactions can be set-up in a biological hood and all surfaces exposed to UV light between reactions. Adequate controls (both positive and negative) should be used for all reactions *(27)*.

4.2.1.4. Experimental Conditions and Reagents: Instrument Parameters

Separations are performed on a CE-LIF system, with the temperature held constant at 20°C. PCR products are detected by LIF in the reversed polarity mode (anode at the detector site) with excitation at 488 nm and emission at 520 nm. Samples are introduced hydrodynamically using 10-s injections at 0.5 psi into a 100 mm i.d. × 65 cm coated (neutral) capillary filled with TBE containing replaceable linear polyacrylamide. No sample preparation of PCR products is required. The capillary is conditioned with buffer containing 60 μg thiazole orange (an intercalator) per 20 mL and rinsed at high pressure for 3 min. Separations are performed under constant voltage at 7.0–9.0 kV for 15–50 min. The capillary is rinsed with gel buffer for 3 min prior to each injection *(51)*.

4.2.2. Direct Detection of Nucleic Acids

Reliance on an amplification step is the major problem associated with PCR based methodology *(56)*. Despite the incorporation of internal standards, quantitation is still problematic, particularly when the target template is small. To decrease the variability associated with PCR-based assays and to take advantage of the exquisite sensitivity of CE-LIF, the direct detection of nucleic acids has been developed.

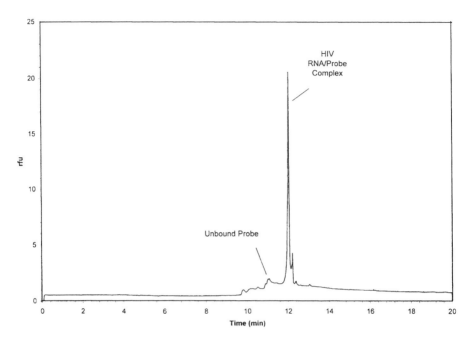

Fig. 8. Electropherogram analysis of hybridization products. RNA samples obtained from a HIV seropositive patient were hybridized with a HIV specific probe and analyzed. HIV RNA/Probe complex elutes at 12 min, indicating the presence of HIV RNA in the patient's serum.

A report has attempted to quantify HIV-1 RNA directly from the plasma by assuming that all plasma RNA is due to HIV-1. However, without specific HIV-1 probes, plasma samples may contain non-HIV-1 viral RNA including HTLV-1 (human T-cell leukemia virus Type-1), and hepatitis A, C, D, and E, which reduces the specificity for HIV-1. Additionally, contamination of plasma with leukocytes or other cells would result in the presence of nonspecific human RNA.

In an alternative approach, cellular RNA is hybridized with a HIV-1 specific probe that has been labeled with fluorescene. A complex is formed if HIV-1 RNA is present and unbound RNA is digested with RNAase I. Samples are then analyzed by CE-LIF with thiazole orange or other intercalators present in the buffer system. Two peaks elute if HIV-1 RNA is present; the first is the DNA/DNA unbound probe complex, followed by the DNA/RNA hybrid. Although the complexes are the same lengths, the DNA/RNA complex has a different secondary structure and slightly higher molecular weight and a subsequently longer retention time (*see* Fig. 8).

Thiazole orange present in the buffer intercalates into 1 out of 2 bp for DNA and 1 out of 10 bp for RNA. Although the intercalation parameters of thiazole orange into a DNA/RNA complex is unknown, it is assumed to be between 10 and 50%, providing a 10–50% enhancement in sensitivity over the RNA/RNA complex. The addition of a fluorescein label to the probe provides a double-detection system over the intercalator alone, also enhancing sensitivity.

The double-detection system is linear from 0.072–21.46 pg, the migration time precision is <1% and the peak-area precision ranges from 1–11%. The minimal detectable level is 36 atg, which corresponds to 4 equivalents (4 copies/mL) of HIV. As little as 19 fg (1710 copies per 1 mL of starting plasma) of HIV-RNA can be reliably and quantitatively detected. Although still a research tool, direct detection of nucleic acids may be an important improvement in assay reliability.

5. VALIDATION AND QUANTITATION ISSUES

5.1. Standardization and Validation Methodology

5.1.1. Determination of the Injection Volume (28)

The injection volume is an important parameter in quantitating samples by CE-LIF. Based on literature values, the calculated injection volume is 7. 1 nL when a sample is injected onto a 100 μm i.d. capillary at 0.34 Pa for 10 s. The injection volume can be verified for each system by measuring the mass difference after injection by placing 20 mcL of hybridization sample in a microcuvet and weighing on a Sartorius BP 210D balance. After weighing, the microcuvette containing the sample is transferred to the auto-sampler tray and injected hydrodynamically at 0.34 Pa for 990 s (99 s × 10 injections, 99 s maximum injection time). The microcuvet is then re-weighed with a mean decrease in weight after injection of 707 ng ($n = 3$). Since the hybridization solution was very dilute, it was assumed to have the specific gravity of water (1.00 g/L), corresponding to a mean volume of 706. 86 nL/990 s injection or 7.14 nL/10 s injection ($n = 3$).

5.1.2. Calibration of CE-LIF: Preparation of DNA Solution for Standard Curve

A commercially available DNA ladder, ranging from 36 to 2645 bases at a concentration of 1. 0 mg/mL, can be used to calibrate the CE-LIF (Fig. 9). The DNA standard is aliquotted in 10 μL portions and stored at –20°C. The solution contains a 222 bp fragment present in a concentration of 129 μg/mL initially. This solution is diluted 1:10 with DEPC-treated water and injected for 5–20 s. To generate a standard curve, 10 μL of diluted DNA standard solution is placed in a microcuvet and six pressure injections at 0.5 psi are

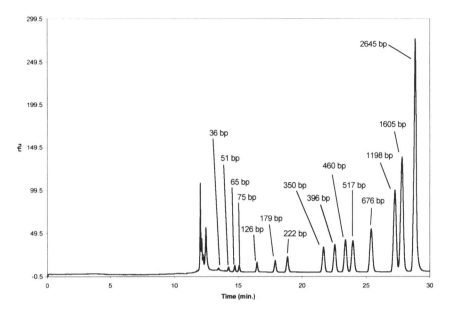

Fig. 9. Electropherogram of DNA standards.

made from the vial for 5, 10, 12.5, 15, 17.5, and 20 s. Separations are performed based on the parameters detailed under instrument parameters.

To determine the linear range, the peak area reported on the electropherogram vs the concentration of the 222 bp fragment injected is plotted. With this assay, a linear relationship between the peak area and concentration exists for the 222 bp fragment over the range 0.5–183 pg. The concentration of unknown samples can be determined in this range by comparison of the peak areas obtained to the standard curve.

The same solution of standard DNA fragments can also be used to determine the molecular weight of fragments based on retention times. Plot the migration time for each peak vs the known molecular weights and determine the linear range. The linear range will not be over the entire range of molecular weights since intercalating dyes such as thiazole orange can affect migration times at higher (>1000 bp) molecular weights. With this assay, a linear relationship exists between retention time and molecular weights of the standard fragments between 126 bp and 460 bp ($r^2 = 0.996$). This standard can then be used to determine the molecular weights of unknown samples.

5.1.2. Validation of RT-PCR CE-LIF Assay (51)

To validate the assay, cDNA from two different sources is amplified in triplicate and analyzed on three separate days generating 18 data points. The ratio of the peak area of the internal standard to the peak area of the gene of interest is calculated. The linear range is then determined by plotting the ratio vs the starting amount of cDNA. We have found a linear relationship ($r^2 = 0.991$) over the range of 0–312.5 ng of starting cDNA, (the RNA is quantitated spectrophotometrically and the RT process is assumed to be 100%). The PCR is no longer linear when more than 400 ng of cDNA is amplified. This is consistent with data reported by Rossomondo and colleagues, who also showed a linear relationship between peak area and starting amount of RNA at low concentrations and a nonlinear relationship when higher concentrations were amplified.

The mean retention time for the reference peak is determined (we commonly analyze the internal standard fragment as well as the target sequence) and used to calculate interday precision and the intraday precision, a measure of the method reproducibility. With this assay, we have interday and intraday migration-time precision of <1.0%. The same samples can also be used to determine the peak-area precision, a measure that represents the reproducibility of both the CE and PCR aspects of this assay. The ratio of the peak area of the gene of interest to internal standard is calculated and compared. Because PCR with an internal standard is competitive, the peak area of one or the other product is not representative. This assay has a peak area intraday precision of 12–15% and interday precision of 10–16%. Strategies to improve assay precision should target the RT-PCR portion and could include automation and use of RNA standards.

The major limitations to accurate quantitation in the assay are: 1) the inability of spectophotometric analysis to predict accurately RNA concentration, 2) the assumption that the reverse transcription step was 100% efficient, and 3) the need for accurate calibration of the RNA internal standard. To overcome these limitations a calibrated RNA internal standard could be added prior to reverse transcription.

6. CONCLUSION

Viral diseases play a significant role in the health status of individuals worldwide. Viral loads are used routinely to monitor disease progression and response to therapy of patients with HIV. Viral-load analysis also plays an emerging role in assessing the response to therapy of patients with hepatitis B, hepatitis C, and CMV. Other potential applications include instances where early and very low-level detection is required.

A variety of assays are currently commercially available for the analysis of viral loads and are used in clinical laboratories including RT-PCR, bDNA, and molecular hybridization. Able to detect as few as 50 copies/mL of serum, these assays represent an important advance in the diagnosing and monitoring viral disease. However, since most assays rely on amplification, variability is introduced and CVs are often high. As such, advances in technology, such as CE-LIF, that improve reliability, quantitation, and detection are needed.

Capillary electrophoresis may be an important step in improving viral-load analysis. CE-LIF offers several advantages over current detection techniques. Required sample volumes are small (1–5 µL), sensitivity is high (attomolar) and the hazards associated with isotopic storage, use, and disposal are eliminated. Additionally, CE-LIF can be readily automated, used for fraction collection, and the assay can be validated. Combining CE-LIF with existing assays for viral-load analysis may improve the reliability, speed, and sensitivity of viral-load analysis. In addition, CE-LIF can be applied to the analysis of gene expression, gene therapy, single-stranded oligonucleotide, and point mutations *(57–60)*.

REFERENCES

1. Zaia, J. A., Gallez-Hawkins, G. M., Tegtmeier, B. R., ter Veer, A., Li, X., Niland, J. C., and Forman, S. J. (1997) Late cytomegalovirus disease in marrow transplantation is predicted by virus load in plasma. J. Infect. Dis. 176, 72–75.
2. Boivin, G., Handfield, J., Toma, E., Murray, G. Lalonde, R., and Bergeron, M. G. (1998) Comparative evaluation of the cytomegalovirus DNA load in polymorphonuclear leukocytes and plasma of human immunodeficiency virus-infected subjects. J. Infect. Dis. 177, 355–360.
3. Cope, A. V., Sabin, C., Burroughs, A., Rolles, K., Griffiths , P. D., and Emery, V. C. (1997) Interrelationships among quantity of human cytomegalovirus (HCMV) DNA in blood, donor-recipient serostatus, and administration of methylprednisolone as risk factors for HCMV disease following liver transplantation. J. Infect. Dis. 176, 1484–1490.
4. Boeckh, M. and Boivin, G. (1998) Quantitation of cytomegalovirus: methodologic aspects and clinical applications. Clin. Microbio. Rev. 11, 533–554.
5. Chatellard, P., Sahli, R., Iten, A., von Overbeck, J., and Meylan, P. R. (1998) Single tube competitive PCR for quantitation of CMV DNA in the blood of HIV+ and solid organ transplant patients. J. Virol. Meth. 71, 137–146.
6. Gerna, G., Sarasini, A., Baldanti, F., Percivalle, E., Zella, D., and Revello, M. G. (1997) Quantitative systemic and local evaluation of the antiviral effect of ganciclovir and foscarnet induction treatment on human cytomegalovirus gastrointestinal disease of patients with AIDS. Italian Foscarnet GID Study Group. Antiviral Res. 34, 39–50.
7. Lazzarotto, T., Campisi, T., Dal Monte, P., Galli, S., Spezzacatena, P., Guglielmi, P., and Landini, M. P. (1996) A quantitative test (HCMV-hybrid-capture(TM)) to detect human cytomegalovirus DNA in the blood of immunocompromised patients compared with antigenemia and polymerase chain reaction. New Microbiol. 19, 193–201.

8. Poirier-Toulemonde, A. S., Imbert-Marcille, B. M., Ferre-Aubineau, V., Besse, B., Le Roux, M. G., Cantarovich, D., and Billaudel, S. (1997) Successful quantification of cytomegalovirus DNA by competitive PCR and detection with capillary electrophoresis. Mol. Cell. Probes. 11, 11–23.

9. Boivin, G., Gilbert, C., Morissette, M., Handfield, J., Goyette, N., and Bergeron, M. G. (1997) A case of ganciclovir-resistant cytomegalovirus (CMV) retinitis in a patient with AIDS: longitudinal molecular analysis of the CMV viral load and viral mutations in blood compartments. AIDS 11, 867–873.

10. Gerna, G., Percivalle, E., Baldanti, F., Sarasini, A., Zavattoni, M., Furione, M., et al. (1998) Diagnostic significance and clinical impact of quantitative assays for diagnosis of human cytomegalovirus infection/disease in immunocompromised patients. New Microbiol. 21, 293–308.

11. Hebart, H., Schroder, A., Loffler, J., Klingebiel, T., Martin, H., Wassmann, B., et al. (1997) Cytomegalovirus monitoring by polymerase chain reaction of whole blood samples from patients undergoing autologous bone marrow or peripheral blood progenitor cell transplantation. J. Infect. Dis. 175, 1490–1493.

12. de Jong, M. D., Boucher, C. A., Danner, S. A., Gazzard, B., Griffiths, P. D., Katlama, C., et al. (1998) Summary of the international consensus symposium on management of HIV, CMV and hepatitis virus infections. Antiviral Res. 37, 1–16.

13. Evans, A. A., O'Connell, A. P., Pugh, J. C., Mason, W. S., Shen, F. M., Chen, G. C., et al. (1998) Geographic variation in viral load among hepatitis B carriers with differing risks of hepatocellular carcinoma. Cancer Epidemiol. Biomarkers Prevention 7, 559–565.

14. Huang, X., Gordon, M. J., and Zare, R. N. (1988) Bias in quantitative capillary zone electrophoresis caused by electrokinetic sample injection. Anal. Chem. 60, 375–377.

15. Simpson, P. R., Yu, X. H., Redza, Z. M., Anson, J. G., Chan, S. H., and Lin, Y. (1997) Quantification of hepatitis B virus DNA using competitive PCR and a scintillation proximity assay. J. Virol. Methods 69, 197–208.

16. Dienstag, J. L., Perrillo, R. P., Schiff, E. R., Bartholomew, M., Vicary, C., and Rubin, M. (1995) A preliminary trial of lamivudine for chronic hepatitis B. New Engl. J. Med. 333, 1657–1661.

17. Perelson, A. S., Neumann, A. U., Markowitz, M., Leonard, J. M., and Ho, D. D. (1996) HIV-1 dynamics in vivo: virion clearance rate, infected cell lifespan, and viral generation time. Science 271, 1582–1586.

18. Piatak, M., Saag, M. S., and Yang, L. C. (1993) High levels of HIV in plasma during all stages of infection determined by competitive PCR. Science 259, 1749–1754.

19. Ho, D. D., Neumann, A. U., Perelson, A. S., Chen, W., Leonard, J. M., and Markowitz, M. (1995) Rapid turnover of plasma virions and CD4 sup + lymphocytes in HIV-1 infection. Nature 373, 123–126.

20. Marschner, I. C., Collier, A. C., and Coombs, R. W. (1998) Use of changes in plasma levels of human immunodeficiency virus type 1 RNA to assess clinical benefit of antiretroviral therapy. J. Infect. Dis. 177, 40–47.

21. Mellors, J. W., Munoz, A. M., and Giorgi, J. V. (1997) Plasma viral load and CD4 sup + lymphocytes as prognostic markers of HIV-1 infection. Ann. Intern. Med. 126, 946–954.

22. Montaner, J., DeMasi, R., and Hill, A. (1997) Validation of HIV-1 RNA and CD4 count as surrogate markers in the CAESAR trial, in: Program and abstracts of the 6th European Conference on Clinical Aspects and Treatment of HIV Infection; October 11–15, 1997. Hamburg, Germany, Abstract 207.

23. Wei, X., Ghosh, S. K., and Taylor, M. E. (1995) Viral dynamics in HIV-1 infection. Nature 373, 117–122.

24. Carpenter, C. C. J., Fischl, M. A., and Hammer, S. M. (1997) Antiretroviral therapy for HIV infection in 1997: updated recommendations of the International AIDS Society-USA panel. JAMA 277, 1962–1969.

25. US Department of Health and Human Services and the Henry J. Kaiser Family Foundation. (1998) Guidelines for the use of antiretroviral agents in HIV-1 infected adults and adolescents. MMWR Morb. Mortal. Wkly. Rep. 47 (RR-05), 43–82.

26. Brandsma, J. and Miller, G. (1980) Nucleic acid spot hybridization: rapid quantitative screening of lymphoid cell lines for Epstein-Barr virus. Proc. Natl. Acad. Sci. USA 77, 6851–6855.

27. Ferre, F., Marchese, A., and Pezzoli, P. (1994) Quantitative PCR: an overview, in PCR. The Polymerase Chain Reaction (Mullis, K. B., Ferre, F., and Gibbs, R. A., eds.), Birkhauser, Boston, MA.

28. Kolesar, J. M., Allen, P. A., and Doren, C. M. (1997) Direct quantification of HIV-1 RNA by CE-LIF. J. Chrom. B 697, 189–194.

29. Dieguez-Lucena, J. L., Ruiz-Galdon, M., Morell-Ocana, M., Garcia-Villanova, J., Flores-Polanco, F. J., and Reyes-Engel, A. (1994) Capillary electrophoresis compared with silver staining of polyacrylamide gels for quantification of pcr products. Clin. Chem. 40, 493,494.

30. Haupt, W. and Pingoud, A. (1983) Comparison of several high performance liquid chromatography techniques for the separation of oligodeoxynucleotides according to their chain lengths. J. Chromatogr. 260, 419–423.

31. Oefner, P. J., Bonn, G. K., Huber, C. G., and Nathakarnkitkoll, S. (1992) Comparative study of capillary zone electrophoresis and high performance liquid chromatography in the analysis of oligonucleotides and DNA. J. Chromatogr. 625, 331–340.

32. Karger, B. L., Chu, Y. H., and Foret, F. (1995) Capillary electrophoresis of proteins and nucleic acids. Annu. Rev. Biophys. Biomol. Struct. 24, 579–610.

33. Kuhr, W. G. and Monnig, C. A. (1992) Fundamental reviews: capillary electrophoresis. Anal. Chem. 62, 403R–414R.

34. Landers, J. P. (1995) Clinical capillary electrophoresis. Clin. Chem. 41, 495–509.

35. Gelfi, C., Leoncini, F., Righetti, P. G., Cremonsei, L., di Blasio, A. M., Carniti, C., and Vignali, M. (1995) Separation and quantitation of reverse transcriptase polymerase chain reaction fragments of basic fibroblast growth factor by capillary electrophoresis in polymer networks. Electrophoresis 16, 780–783.

36. Lu, W., Han, D. S., Yuan, J., and Andrieu, J. M. (1994) Multi-target PCR analysis by capillary electrophoresis and laser induced fluorescence. Nature 368, 269–271.

37. Rossomando, E. F., White, L., and Ulfelder, K. J. (1994) Capillary electrophoresis: separation and quantitation of reverse transcriptase polymerase chain reaction products from polio virus. J. Chromatogr. B 656, 159–168.

38. Schwartz, H. E. and Ulfelder, K. J. (1991) Analysis of DNA restriction fragments and polymerase chain reaction products towards detection of the AIDS (HIV-1) virus in blood. J. Chromatogr. 559, 267–283.

39. Stalbom, B. M., Torven, A., and Lundberg, L. G. (1994) Application of capillary electrophoresis to the post polymerase chain reaction analysis of rat mRNA for gastric H+, K+-ATPase. Ann. Biochem. 217, 91–97.

40. Schwartz, H. E. and Ulfelder, K. J. (1992) Capillary electrophoresis with laser induced fluorescence detection of PCR fragments using thiazole orange. Ann. Chem. 64, 1737–1740

41. Schwarz, H. E., Ulfelder, K. J., Chen, F. T. A., and Pentoney, S. L. (1994) The utility of laser induced fluorescence detection in applications of capillary electrophoresis. J. Cap. Electrophor. 1, 36–54.

42. Srinivasan, K., Girard, J. E., and Williams, P. (1993) Electrophoretic separations of polymerase chain reaction-amplified DNA fragments in DNA typing using a capillary electrophoresis-laser induced fluorescence system. J. Chromatogr. 652, 83–91.

43. Srinivasan, K., Morris, S. C., and Girard, J. E. (1993) Enhanced detection of PCR products through use of TOTO and YOYO intercalating dyes with laser induced fluorescence-capillary electrophoresis. Appl. Theoret. Electrophor. 3, 235–239.

44. Hjerten, S. (1985) High performance electrophoresis: elimination of electro-endosmosis and solute absorption. J. Chromatogr. 347:191–198.

45. Schmalzing, D., Piggee, C. A., Foret, F., Carrilho, E., and Karger, B. L. (1993) Characterization and performance of a neutral hydrophilic coating for the capillary electrophoretic separation of biopolymers. J. Chromatogr. A 652, 149–159.

46. Tsuda, T. (1987) Modification of electroosmotic flow with cetyltrimethyl-ammonium bromide in capillary electrophoresis. J. High Resolut. Chromatogr. 10, 622–624.

47. Hwang, S. J., Leem S. D., Lu, R. H., Chan, C. Y., Lai, L., Co, R. L., and Tong, M. J. (1996) Comparison of three different hybridization assays in the quantitative measurement of serum hepatitis B virus DNA. J. Virol. Methods 62, 123–129.

48. Kleparnik, K., Garner, M., and Bocek, P. (1995) Injection bias of DNA fragments in capillary electrophoresis with seiving. J. Chromatogr. A 698, 375–383.

49. Heller, C. (1995) Capillary electrophoresis of proteins and nucleic acids in gels and entangled polymer solutions. J. Chromatogr. A 698, 19–31.

50. Pariat, Y. F., Berka, J., Heiger, D. N., Schmitt, T., and Vilenchik, M. (1993) Separation of DNA fragments by capillary electrophoresis using replaceable linear polyacrylamide matrices. J. Chromatogr. A 652, 57–66.

51. Kolesar, J. M., Rizzo, J. D., Kuhn, J. G. (1995) Quantitative analysis of NQO1 gene expression by RT-PCR and CE-LIF. J. Cap. Electrophor. 2, 287–290.

52. Kunkel, A., Degenhardt, M., and Watzig, H. (1996) Precise quantitative results by capillary electrophoresis (CE): instrumental aspects (an update) Proceedings from the 8th International Symposium on High Performance Capillary Electrophoresis 17, 140 (Abstract).

53. Butler, J. M., McCord, B. R., and Jung, J. M. (1994) Quantitation of polymerase chain reaction products by capillary electrophoresis using laser fluorescence. J. Chromatogr. B 658, 271–280.

54. Fasco, M. J., Treanor, C. P., Spivack, S., Figge, H. L., and Kaminsky, L. S. (1995) Quantitative RNA-polymerase chain reaction-DNA analysis by capillary electrophoresis with laser induced fluorescence. Anal. Biochem. 224, 140–147.

55. Glasel, J. (1995) Validity of nucleic acid purities monitored by 260nm/280nm absorbance ratios. Biotechniques 18, 62,63.

56. Kuypers, A., Meijerink, J. P., Smetsers, T., Linssen, P., and Mensink, E. (1994) Quantitative analysis of DNA aberrations amplified by competitive polymerase chain reaction using capillary electrophoresis. J. Chromatogr. B 660, 271–277.

57. Kolesar, J. M., Burris, H., and Kuhn, J. G. (1995) Detection of a point mutation in NQO1 (DT-diaphorase) in a patient with colon cancer. J. Natl. Cancer Inst. 87, 1022–1024.

58. Khrapko, K., Hanekamp, J. S., Thilly, W. G., Belenkii, A., Foret, F., and Karger, B. L. (1994) Constant denaturant capillary electrophoresis (CDCE): a high resolution approach to mutational analysis. Nucleic Acids Res. 22, 364–369.

59. Kumar, R., Hanekamp, J. S., Louhelainen, K., Burvall, K., Onfelt, A., Hemminki, K., and Thilly, W. G. (1995) Separation of transforming amino acid-substituting mutations in codons 12, 13, and 61 of the n-ras gene by constant denaturant capillary electrophoresis (CDCE). Carcinogenesis 16, 2667–2673.

60. Mitchell, C. E., Belinsky, S. A., and Lechner, J. F. (1995) Detection and quantitation of mutant K-ras codon 12 restriction fragments by capillary electrophoresis. Ann. Biochem. 224, 148–153.

14

The Application of Capillary Electrophoresis in the Analysis of PCR Products Used in Forensic DNA Typing

Bruce R. McCord and John M. Butler

1. INTRODUCTION

The development of methods for the amplification and detection of specific regions of the DNA molecule using the polymerase chain reaction (PCR) has resulted in rapid and dramatic advances in biochemical analysis *(1)*. With the advent of the PCR it is now possible to easily produce analytically significant amounts of a specified DNA product. A typical PCR reaction can produce microgram quantities of target DNA, allowing rapid and efficient screening of genetic defects, cancer susceptibility, and low level bacterial contamination *(2)*. The sensitivity of the technique has freed biochemists from the many laborious processes necessary to isolate and examine small quantities of DNA. In the forensic arena, PCR methods have permitted rapid and specific tests of evidence produced in a crime *(2)*.

The impact of PCR has also resulted in a need for efficient and automated procedures to analyze the reaction products. For many years it has been recognized that capillary electrophoresis (CE) has had the potential to fill this requirement. The capillary system can produce rapid and efficient separations of DNA, as a result of the efficient heat dissipation of the capillary when compared to standard slab gel methods. Additionally, the capillary can be easily manipulated for efficient and automated injections. Despite these advantages, it has been only recently that dedicated commercial systems for PCR product analysis have begun to appear.

The slow development of CE systems for PCR analysis has been because of the scarcity of efficient methods for injection, separation, and detection of DNA fragments. For example, the high ionic strength of the PCR reaction mixture is incompatible with CE injection methods. Gel-based separations

From: *Clinical and Forensic Applications of Capillary Electrophoresis*
Edited by: J. R. Petersen and A. A. Mohammad © Humana Press Inc., Totowa, NJ

are difficult to implement in the capillary format, and commonly utilized ultraviolet (UV) detection techniques have poor sensitivity. These problems have been overcome as a result of better understanding of the nature of the CE procedure.

This review will focus on the development of capillary systems for the analysis of PCR products. Advancements in separation, sample preparation, and detection will be emphasized, and the chapter will conclude with a discussion of forensic applications.

2. POLYMERASE CHAIN REACTION

In the PCR process, a thermostable DNA polymerase (Taq) is used to copy small amounts of DNA template by means of a temperature dependent reaction. The PCR reaction mixture is prepared by combining the target DNA, oligonucleotide primers, the polymerase and a mixture of four deoxyribonucleotide triphosphates (dNTPs) in a Tris-HCl buffer containing approx 50 mM KCl and 1.5 mM MgCl. The primers consist of two short 20–30 oligomer (mer) segments that are selected to bracket a specific location of interest on the target DNA. The reaction is initiated using a three-step temperature program in which the two strands of DNA template are separated (melted) by heating at 95°C. The primers are then annealed to the template at approx 60°C. The enzyme then extends the primer sequence at approx 72°C by incorporating the individual deoxyribonucleotide using the target DNA as a template. By cycling through these temperatures using an oven that rapidly and precisely alters the reaction temperature, it is possible to double the amount of target DNA with each cycle. Theoretically, 30 cycles of heating and cooling the mixture can produce up to a billion copies of the target DNA from one copy of template *(3)*. In situations where the quantity of sample is limited, it is also possible to perform amplifications of multiple loci by simultaneously targeting different regions of the genome in a single reaction. Such multiplexed reactions are carefully balanced by optimizing the reaction conditions and primer sequences in order that one locus with its respective set of primers does not preferentially amplify over the others. The result of a multiplex amplification is the production of a series of DNA fragments that must be optimally separated over a specific size range.

3. SEPARATION TECHNIQUES

3.1. Polymer Matrix

One of the earliest efforts to use CE to separate DNA fragments was carried out by Kasper et al. *(4)*, who concluded that effective separation of large, linear DNA must either be carried out using affinity or gel electrophoresis. DNA fragments have proved difficult to separate because all DNA fragments have virtually the same charge-to-mass ratio. The logical solution was to perform sieving experiments by filling the capillary with an agarose or polyacrylamide gel similar to those used in slab gel electrophoresis *(5)*. However, it was clear from the beginning that at the high field strengths and temperatures used in CE, the stability of these "chemical gels" would be a problem *(4)*. One solution was to attach chemically (cross-link) the gel to the capillary wall *(6)*. Separations using this procedure with polyacrylamide gels produced exceptional separations of PCR products with analysis times typically <30 min. These capillaries can still be purchased from a number of commercial manufacturers. The problem with the chemical gels is that even when manufactured under well-controlled conditions, they are still susceptible to such problems as bubble formation and contamination from the sample matrix. In addition, sample injections were only possible using the electrokinetic mode. For the CE technique to be truly automated, a replaceable sieving matrix was required.

The development of replaceable "physical gels" was initiated by Zhu and coworkers *(7)*. Experiments carried out using hydroxy propylmethyl cellulose, methyl cellulose, and polyethylene glycol (PEG) showed that it was not necessary to use crosslinked gels in the capillary format. Additionally, with these physical gels, a variety of injection techniques could be utilized, and capillaries could be flushed and chemically etched between each analysis. The disadvantage of these gels was that early experimental systems could not achieve the separation efficiency of cross-linked polyacrylamide. Since then a large amount of research has been carried out in order to understand the theory of electrophoresis in physical gels. As a result of this research it has been shown that at least three different mechanisms have been found to be responsible for the separation of DNA in these physical gels, transient entanglement coupling *(8)*, Ogston sieving *(9)*, and reptation *(10)*. The three different modes of separation in CE are illustrated in Fig. 1. At low polymer concentrations, separation takes place through a frictional interaction between the DNA and the polymer strands known as transient entanglement coupling *(8)*. As the polymer concentration increases, the strands of different polymer molecules begin to interact producing a solution of entangled polymers. The polymer concentration at which this occurs is known as the entanglement threshold *(11)*. Above the entanglement threshold, DNA fragments separate by sieving through transient pores created in the polymer mesh. Fragments that are larger than the average pore size reptate or move in a snakelike manner through the mesh *(11)*. The key to producing an acceptable separation is to determine a polymer concentration at which the size of these virtual pores approximates the radius of the DNA in solution.

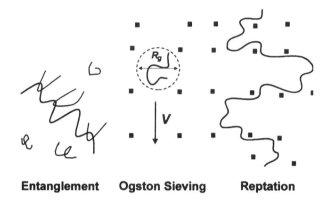

Entanglement   Ogston Sieving   Reptation

Fig. 1. Three different mechanisms for the separation of DNA: at low concentrations of polymer, DNA migration is inhibited through transient interactions with free polymer strands. As the polymer concentration increases to the point of entanglement, the DNA then is sieved through transient pores created in the polymer mesh. Larger strands of DNA reptate, passing through multiple pores simultaneously.

Additionally, the polymer length must not be too great or the solution will become too viscous.

Other characteristics that have been found to be of importance include the relative stiffness and polydispersity of the polymer *(12)*. With these characteristics in mind, a number of water-soluble polymers have been found to be particularly useful for DNA separations including linear polyacrylamide *(13)*, Methyl cellulose *(14–19)* hydroxyethylcellulose *(20–23)*, hydroxy propyl methyl cellulose *(19,24–27)* polyethylene oxide *(28)*, and poly(*N*-acryloylaminoethoxyethanol) *(29)*. In addition, a commercial polymer known as POP4 has also been described *(30)*. Thus, the key to producing an acceptable separation is to optimize the polymer molecular weight and concentration relative to the DNA fragment size and desired resolution.

3.2. Capillary

In uncoated capillary columns, residual charges on the silica surface induce a flow of the bulk solution toward the negative electrode. This is known as electroosmotic flow (EOF). The magnitude and direction of the EOF is dependent of the number and type of active sites on the capillary surface and the pH of buffer. EOF is generally considered a detriment to stable DNA separations because its velocity can change from run to run, making peak migration times irreproducible.

To control the EOF, capillary columns must be coated to mask charged sites. Two different approaches have been used: 1) dynamic coatings that must be periodically replenished or 2) static coatings that are chemically bonded to the capillary walls. One such method is to periodically rinse the capillary with acid, which protonates the active silanols on the walls of the capillary *(31)*. This effectively neutralizes the negative charges on the column surface, reducing or eliminating the EOF. Recently a novel polymer POP4, polydimethyl acrylamide has been developed that performs a dual function, dynamically coating the capillary as well as sieving the DNA *(31a)*. With such systems, capillaries can routinely last over 100 runs.

A second method of eliminating EOF is to coat the column walls with an inert substance that masks the charged sites on the capillary walls. Such coatings must be stable at the pH of analysis and free from contamination. These coatings include hydrophilic substances such as polyacrylamide and polyvinyl alcohol, as well as more hydrophobic coatings such as the phenyl methyl and C18 coatings adapted from gas chromatography (GC) and high-performance liquid chromatography (HPLC). The key factor in selecting a coating is its stability and its ability to last under the conditions used in the separation. With periodic rinsing, coated capillaries can last for months before needing to be replaced. Continued development in this area is necessary as periodic replacement of capillaries limits the ability of large multicapillary systems to run unattended.

3.3. Buffer

Buffers commonly used in DNA analysis by CE include Tris-borate, Tris-acetate, and TAPS in a pH range of 7.0–9.0. These buffers have the advantage of low conductivity, minimizing Joule heating and allowing higher buffer concentrations to be used. High buffer concentrations also can help minimize interactions between the DNA and the capillary wall and stabilize DNA conformation *(32)*. Other buffers have also been examined *(24,33)*. For example, residual primers and dNTPs are separated better at low pH, presumably due to differences in charge between the four bases under these conditions *(24)*.

The choice of buffer additives for PCR analysis is dependent on whether single-stranded (ssDNA) or double-stranded DNA (dsDNA) is to be analyzed. In general, ssDNA separations yield higher resolution and are less complicated by PCR artifacts such as heteroduplex formation and variations in sequence. Detection of ssDNA requires labeling the DNA through the use of fluorescent primers or other means *(35)*. The DNA solution is denatured prior to analysis by dilution in a formamide solution and heating to 95°C prior to analysis. To prevent reannealing, urea or formamide is added to the buffer, and the temperature of the separation is increased to greater than 50°C *(35)*. Problems with the use of these additives include the limited shelf life of urea solutions, the tendency of urea solutions to sublimate, and the toxic nature of formamide.

Double-stranded DNA requires less treatment prior to analysis. For both UV and fluorescence detection, intercalating dyes can be added to the buffer to enhance resolution *(25,36)*. These dyes have also been shown to minimize the effects of sequence variations on migration time *(25,37–39)*. In addition, EDTA can be added to the buffer to chelate excess magnesium from the PCR reaction, and alkaline salts can be used to alter the ionic strength of the buffer and minimize osmotic flow *(20)*. The use of such salts may also aid in preventing the formation of secondary structures, as the formation of ion pairs will help to stabilize the DNA molecule in solution.

3.4. Injection and Sample Preparation

One of the major advantages of a CE system is its capability to perform automated injections. In general, there are two modes of injection: hydrodynamic and electrokinetic. Hydrodynamic injections are performed using pressure to force the sample solution into the capillary. This injection technique can only be carried out using soluble polymer buffers, as pressure injections into crosslinked gels would disrupt the interior of the capillary. Hydrodynamic injections are particularly well suited for quantitative analyses. When properly initiated, reproducible quantities of sample may be introduced onto the capillary. Standard deviations (SD) of injection volume have been shown to be approx 3% *(40)*. However, the broad injection bands produced in this technique tend to limit resolution.

Electrokinetic injections are performed using an applied voltage to induce the sample to migrate into the capillary. Unlike hydrodynamic injections, this process is a function of the injection voltage, injection time, and sample matrix. Sample ions with a higher charge-to-mass ratio than DNA will tend to be injected selectively into the capillary. Thus, the ionic strength of the sample may alter the applied field. Figure 2 illustrates the difference between the two injection modes in CE.

The injection of PCR products into a capillary is particularly difficult because the products are contained in a salt matrix (>50 mM Cl$^-$), which inhibits the injection. To overcome these problems, PCR samples are purified by means of dialysis *(41)*, spin columns *(42,43)*, or ethanol precipitation *(20)*. The dialysis step appears to be the most effective for removing excess salt, whereas the spin columns are more effective at removing primer peaks, enzyme, and dNTPs. Dilution of the sample in water or deionized formamide is another technique for eliminating injection interferences *(22,44)*.

These steps greatly improve the injection by removing interferences, and by enhancement of a process known as stacking *(32)*. Stacking, also called

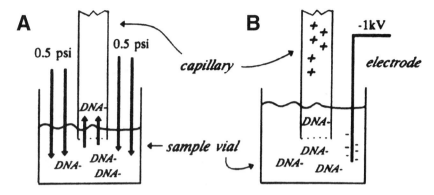

Fig. 2. The two injection modes of CE. (**A**) In hydrodynamic injection pressure is used to force sample into the capillary. There is no matrix effect in this injection mode. (**B**) In electrokinetic injection, the electric field induces sample ions to migrate into the capillary. Injection is dependent on the charge-to-mass ratio of the sample and matrix ions.

field amplified injection, occurs when the ionic strength of the sample zone is lower than that of the buffer. Because the current through the system is constant, the lack of charged carriers in the sample zone produces a strong electric field that ends abruptly at the interface between the sample zone and the buffer inside the capillary. DNA molecules mobilized by this field move rapidly towards the capillary as the injection voltage is applied and "stack" in a narrow zone at the interface. Stacking allows a large sample zone to be loaded onto the capillary with a minimum of band broadening. Stacking also aids in producing efficient separations. The sharper the injection zone, the less gel media is required to effect a separation. Extremely short columns and microchips have exploited this fact to produce rapid and efficient separations of PCR products *(45,46)*. Figure 3 illustrates the 45-s separation of two PCR products overlaid on a 20 bp ladder. The effective length of the capillary was 2 cm.

4. DETECTION AND DATA ANALYSIS

In early separations of PCR products by CE, UV absorbance was the method of detection. PCR products analyzed by this procedure required extensive deionization and concentration prior to analysis *(20,41,42)*. The relatively short path length and the dispersion produced by the capillary walls limited sensitivity. Laser-induced fluorescence (LIF) solved the problem of sensitivity by focusing the light beam directly onto the capillary window *(36,47,48)*. Detection enhancements of 400-fold or more have been achieved using LIF as compared to UV detection *(36)*.

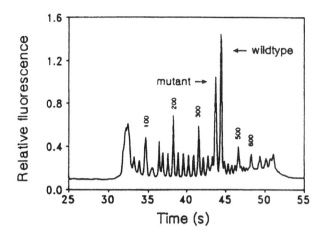

Fig. 3. An illustration of the 45-s separation of two PCR products coinjected with a 20 basepair sizing ladder. The analysis was performed on a 2-cm coated capillary at 260 v/cm. The DNA was detected using an intercalating dye and laser-induced fluorescence *(45)*.

Fluorescence detection of dsDNA is primarily achieved through the use of intercalating dyes. These dyes bind to the DNA molecule by inserting themselves into the DNA helix, affecting the configuration of the aromatic rings of the dye and enhancing the fluorescence signal *(38,49)*. Additionally, intercalating dyes help to minimize effects of DNA structure on migration rate, resulting in better estimates of fragment lengths *(39,50)*. The low background fluorescence of the uncomplexed dyes allows them to be added directly to the CE buffer. Monomeric intercalating dyes such as ethidium bromide, thiazole orange, and oxazole yellow have proven to be the most useful, providing precise and reproducible estimates of DNA size and quantity *(40,51)*.

Fluorescent dye molecules may also be covalently bound to the DNA fragments *(34)*. Labeling one or both of the primers prior to the amplification step can perform this most efficiently. After completion of the PCR, all of the target DNA molecules are labeled with a fluorophore. By labeling a series of different primers with a number of different dyes, several loci may be targeted, amplified, and labeled in a single multiplexed reaction. These dyes absorb at similar wavelengths but emit at different wavelengths. A multichannel analyzer can then identify the specific PCR product by detecting the various emission wavelengths of the bound dye *(52)*.

The development of methods for data analysis by CE is of particular importance in the examination of PCR products. Precise and reliable meth-

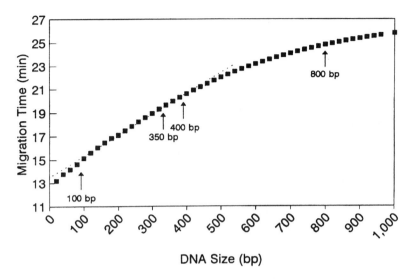

Fig. 4. The relationship between DNA size and migration time for native DNA. The figure illustrates that a linear relationship exists up to 400 basepairs.

ods must be developed for product analysis. Slab gel methods permit the analysis of multiple samples run concurrently. At present, CE is a serial technique and samples can only be run one at a time. Thus, comparison of multiple samples requires the addition of internal standards to correct for the inevitable variations in injection, temperature, and current *(22)*. This observation is particularly relevant in quantitative methods where variations in sample injection can limit the usefulness of the technique *(40)*.

When adding internal standards for quantitation, it is important that they do not interfere with the detection of the PCR product. When intercalating dyes are used in the analysis, peak intensity is a function of the length of the PCR product, and corrections for product length may be necessary *(53)*. A further concern in PCR analysis using these dyes is the effect of buffer depletion on the sample fluorescence intensity and migration time *(40,50)*. For this reason, buffer vials must be periodically replenished to avoid depletion of the intercalating dye and pH variations.

Size estimates of PCR products can be performed by interpolation of size based on the migration of one or more internal standards *(22)*. For products in the size range from 100–400 bp, a linear relationship exists between size and migration time (Fig. 4) *(54)*. The size of larger products may also be estimated using nonlinear, curve-fitting algorithms *(50)*. Specialized instrumentation has been developed specifically for DNA analysis utilizing internal standards that have been labeled with a fluorescence dye different than that of the product *(52)*. For such systems, interferences between sample and standard are much less of a problem, and specific algorithms have been developed to deconvolute the fluorescence signals and perform size estimates *(55)*.

5. APPLICATIONS

Most applications of CE for the analysis of PCR products have been adapted from slab gel assays. A number of current reviews have discussed many of these applications *(56–59)*. Recently, studies have begun to appear in which the advantages of CE, such as high speed, low sample requirement, and automation, have been exploited. These advantages, which aid in tracking of large databases and permit easy setup and operation of the equipment, match the needs of the forensic community. They are also responsible for the increasing acceptance of the technique.

In the next section, the two main applications of the technique, DNA sizing and quantitation, will be covered. The section will conclude with a discussion of future applications including DNA sequencing, in-line PCR, and microchip based separations.

5.1. DNA Sizing/Genetic Analysis

DNA fragments above a certain minimum length have roughly the same charge to mass ratio, making them migrate at approximately the same rate in free solution. As mentioned earlier, the addition of a sieving agent permits a separation of the DNA as a function of its size. By correlating migration time with the molecular weight of the fragments, an estimate of the DNA size is produced. Conformational differences can create some variations in this result, especially for dsDNA *(39)*. However, the analysis of DNA used in forensic analysis has shown precise correlations between DNA size and migration time *(22,54)*.

Most applications of CE involving DNA sizing utilize PCR to amplify specific regions in the genome in which changes in length or sequence can occur. Highly variable, polymorphic sites are located that contain repetitive DNA in which a particular sequence of bases is repeated multiple times. This type of polymorphism is known as a variable number tandem repeat (VNTR). The different alleles, which are produced by the VNTRs used in forensic testing, are distributed randomly through a population. The frequency of occurrence of a particular allele in a population potentially can be used to identify the perpetrator of a crime *(60)*. A useful subset of VNTRs known as short tandem repeats (STRs)contains repeat motifs that are typically four bases in length. An example of an STR might be the sequence ATTGC $(AATG)_n$ AAGTG. STRs are typically produced with sizes ranging from 100–400 base pairs in length depending on the primers used.

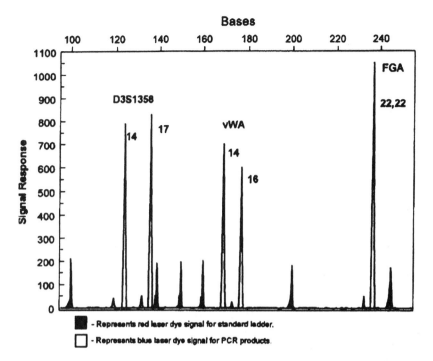

Fig. 5. Dual wavelength detection of a multiplex amplified PCR product consisting of three genetic loci, D3S1358, vWA, and FGA. Conditions: 3% HEC, 7 m*M* urea, 100 m*M* Tris-borate, pH 8.4, 375 V/cm. The amplified product is labeled with a blue emitting dye, and the internal sizing standard is labeled with a red emitting dye.

Recently, CE has been used to detect STR fragments resulting from reactions in which several sets of primers are combined. These multiplexed amplifications allow a series of genetic markers to be probed simultaneously. In situations where the amount of available DNA is limited, multiplexed amplifications also allow a larger amount of information to be gathered from a single sample.

The development of commercial CE with multichannel fluorescence detection has extended such applications by enabling the user to track the positions of different amplified products individually labeled with specific fluorescent dyes. The dyes that are used are excited by one or more laser lines and contain emission maxima that are sufficiently separated to allow deconvolution of overlapped peaks. Kits have been developed that allow amplification of 10 or more STR systems simultaneously, which allow identification of a unique person with probabilities of 1 in 10^{11} or greater *(44)*. For these reasons, multiplexed amplification of STRs using multiwavelength fluorescence is currently being implemented in many forensic laboratories worldwide *(35,60,61)*. Figure 5 illustrates the separation of a sample obtained from the multiplex amplification of four different loci labeled with a blue-emitting dye. The sample is diluted in purified formamide and denatured. An internal standard labeled with a red-emitting dye is added to each sample to estimate fragment size *(30,62)*. The samples are then analyzed using a viscous buffer containing a soluble polymer in addition to 7 *M* urea to keep the sample DNA denatured. The analysis temperature is kept at 60°C to melt out (eliminate) secondary structures that can cause problems with reproducibility.

5.2. Analytical Aspects in Developing a CE Separation

Among the instrumental factors that are important in developing a CE assay for genetic typing, precision and resolution are perhaps the most important. These two issues, however, are not dependent on each other. Precision is determined by the run to run reproducibility of the migration time of the peak apex, whereas resolution is a function of band broadening and column efficiency.

The precision of the assay is important because it defines the minimum difference in allele size that can be determined. For example, if the size of a particular allele is 200 bases with a standard deviation of 0.17 bases, then 99.3% of the time that allele will be given a size of 200 bases, assuming a normal distribution of the data. Such precision is important given the existence of variant alleles that can differ from the normal 4 base repeat motif by 1–3 bases. In addition, many forensic samples are mixtures of more than one donor.

The mixture problem also can be a factor when resolution is considered. In the aforementioned example, the precision of 0.17 bases permits us to distinguish between a peak at 200 and 201 bases. However if the resolution,

$$R = \frac{(t_2 - t_1)}{0.5 \ (w_2 - w_1)} ,$$

between the two peaks is 0.67 or less, it will be difficult to resolve these two peaks. If the area of peak 1 is more than three times that of peak 2, the two peaks will appear to co-elute, as the system will not have the capacity to separate the two peaks *(63)*. This is illustrated in Fig. 6.

Thus, when developing a protocol for the analysis of mixtures by CE, it is important to consider both precision and resolution. As mentioned earlier, the

---

Fig. 6. *(opposite page)* The analysis of a mixture of two samples of PCR amplified DNA. The large peak at the right is a mixture of two DNA samples, which measure 185 and 186 bases in length. At a ratios from 20:1 to 3:1 the software is unable to distinguish the fact that two peaks exist. At ratios of 1.4:1 and 1:1, the peak to right can be distinguished and is colored gray. Conditions: ABI310 Capillary electrophoresis system, POP4 buffer system 15 kV.

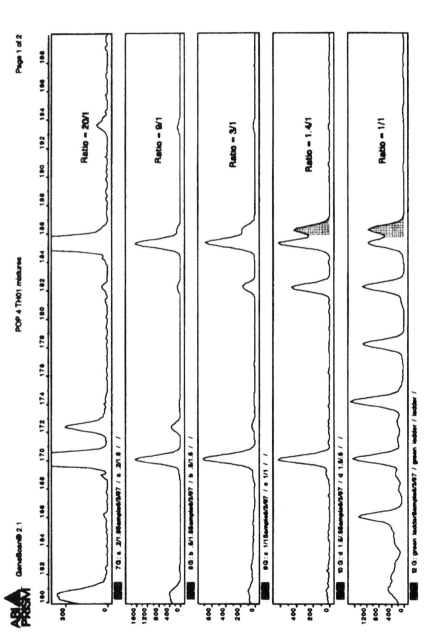

Fig. 6

precision is determined by factors that affect the stability of the measurement; temperature, injection, and sample conformation. The resolution is primarily affected by the polymer concentration and by the effects of sample stacking on injection. Both factors must be characterized to achieve optimum results.

A third issue that can be of importance is the determination of peak area. In situations where mixtures are present, the peak area can help define which samples are related. With proper control of the PCR conditions, the areas of related sample alleles will be consistent from one locus to the next, allowing the user to determine major and minor contributors to the electrophoretic profile. There are, however, important exceptions to this rule, which arise from the nature of the PCR reaction and from the injection process. Issues in the PCR process include artifacts such as stutter, in which a minor product band is produced one repeat unit shorter than the main allele. Values of stutter of 4–9% were reported for the vWA locus *(64)*. The presence of stutter can affect the areas of peaks by decreasing the efficiency of amplification of the main peak, and by interfering with the areas of nearby peaks. PCR efficiency can also be affected by low quantities of template and improper reaction conditions. Another factor to consider is matrix effects on sample injection. The sample matrix can influence the overall peak area from one run to the next, however, this effect can be corrected through proper reference to the internal standard.

At present there have been a number of reports in the literature regarding the analytical capability of capillary systems for typing STRs *(30,62,65,66)*. At least three different polymer systems have been reported for multiplex PCR analysis: hydroxyethyl cellulose, polydimethyl acrylamide, and linear polyacrylamide. Resolution varies between 1 and 2 bases depending on the size of the allele and the concentration and type of the polymer. Reported precision of the estimated allele size as measured by standard deviation ranges from 0.16–0.23 bases. These results clearly show that 2 base differences will be easily distinguished by these systems and depending on the allele size and polymer type, single-base differences may also be distinguished. In an extensive forensic validation study, Wallin and coworkers demonstrated and compared the results on the validation of the AmpliSTR Blue locus using both slab gels and CE *(80)*. In this work, population samples from different racial groups were examined as well as studies on the effect of environment, sample matrix, and sample mixtures. Figure 7 illustrates results from this paper in which two nonprobative sexual assault cases were analyzed by CE using the POP4 polymer. The results portray an exclusion of the suspect in the first case: however, in the second case suspect 2 is a potential contributor of the sample DNA.

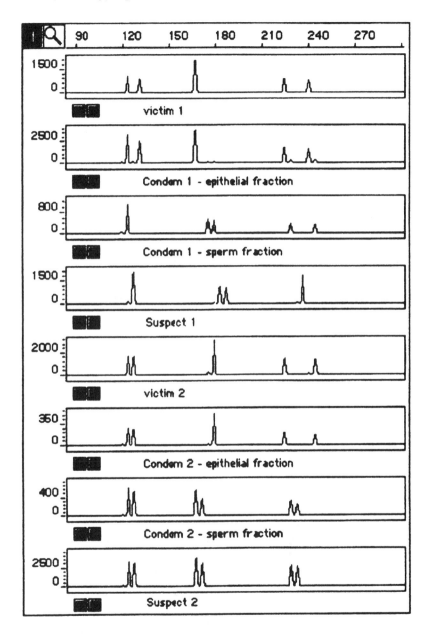

Fig. 7. Two nonprobative sexual assault cases analyzed by CE. In case 1, suspect one is excluded as his DNA profile does not match that extracted from the condom. In case 2, suspect two cannot be excluded as a potential donor of the extracted DNA. Conditions: PE/ABI 310 Genetic Analyzer, POP4 polymer, laser-induced fluorescence detection using the AmpFlSTR Blue (Perkin-Elmer) multiplex PCR amplification kit *(80)*.

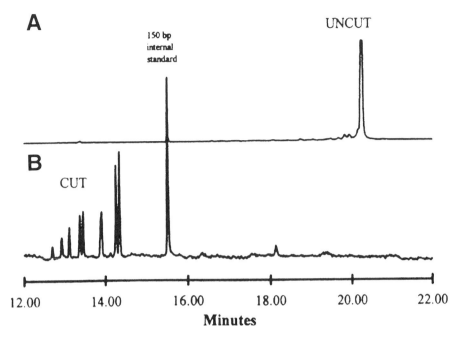

Fig. 8. The analysis of an amplified mitochondrial DNA fragment. (**A**) The uncut fragment. (**B**) The fragment following digestion. The presence of point mutations can be detected by differences in size of the digested fragments. Conditions: 27-cm coated capillary at 185 v/cm. Detection conditions as shown in Fig. 3 *(68)*.

5.3. Other Applications for CE in Forensic DNA Analysis

In certain situations, such as the analysis of hair or highly degraded DNA, there is insufficient nuclear DNA to yield an amplified product of sufficient quantity to type. In this situation, there may still be enough mitochondrial DNA to provide genetic information *(43)*. The DNA present in mitochondria is approx 16,000 bases long and contains a section known as the control region that contains a number of polymorphic sites, which are usually point mutations. Amplifying the region of interest and sequencing the product DNA can identify these polymorhic sites. CE is used in this process to determine if the amplified product is present in sufficient quantity and purity to be sequenced *(40,67)*. CE has also been used to identify these mutations by subjecting the amplified mitochondrial fragments to restriction enzymes. Point mutations present in these products will affect the fragment patterns produced by the digestion *(68)*. Figure 8 illustrates the analysis of mitochondrial DNA using CE and restriction fragment digestion. Finally, as CE sequencers become more widespread, both the product quantitation and the sequence analysis will be performed via CE.

6. FUTURE TRENDS FOR CE AND DNA ANALYSIS

6.1. Capillary Array Electrophoresis

Because CE is by nature a serial operation, a single capillary system cannot match the sample throughput available in a multi-lane slab gel experiment. Higher throughput, however, is available with capillary array electrophoresis (CAE), where multiple capillaries are run in parallel *(69)*. Separation times are on the order of 15–50 min, but up to 96 samples can be analyzed simultaneously. Each DNA sample is analyzed in an individual capillary and migration times are adjusted using an internal lane standard. A recent demonstration of the throughput capabilities of CAE included the generation of over 8000 genotypes on a 48-capillary instrument in a matter of days *(61)*. This type of CAE instrument will probably find application in laboratories which genotype a large number of samples.

6.2. Automation and CE

Automation of the entire process from extracted DNA to analyzed PCR product is an important issue for large laboratories. The potential of coupling CE analysis to the previous sample preparation steps of DNA extraction, PCR amplification, or restriction digestion has already been demonstrated with robotics *(70,71)* and microchip fluidics *(46,71)*. The rapid speed of CE separations cannot be translated into sustainable high-throughput operations until the entire process, including sample preparation and data analysis, is fully automated.

6.3. Microchip CE Assays

The advent of photolithography has permitted micromachining of capillary channels in glass *(73)*. Because of the small dimensions of the separation channels, separations may be performed even more rapidly than with conventional CE equipment. DNA restriction fragments have been separated in a matter of seconds using channels that are only a few centimeters in length *(46,72,74,75,78,79)*. One of the major challenges in microchip CE analysis is sample preparation on a scale that is compatible with the small device. Integration of sample preparation steps with the separation portion is one solution to this dilemma *(76,77)*. The recent integration of PCR and CE on a microchip *(46)* illustrates that such devices may soon be available. Figure 9 gives an example of the separation of a 4 locus multiplex on a microchip containing a 3-cm channel *(78)*.

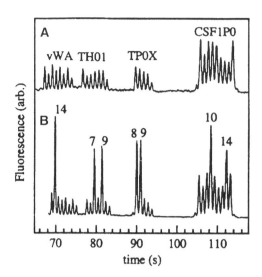

Fig. 9. Microchip separation of a multiplex of 4 STRs: (**A**) allelic ladder (**B**) allelic ladder spiked with amplified sample. Conditions: 3-cm separation channel, 200 v/cm. Laser induced fluorescence detection was used with fluorescein labeled PCR products *(78)*.

7. CONCLUSIONS

The advantages of CE, including single-sample analysis speed and automation, have resulted in its increasing visibility in molecular biology and forensic DNA laboratories. Multichannel fluorescence CE systems have become the instrument of choice for STR analysis in many DNA typing laboratories, primarily because of the appealing aspect of unattended operation, a fact that frees busy forensic scientists to work on other tasks. Recently developed commercial 96-capillary array instruments promise to improve dramatically sample throughput capabilities. CE is reliable and reproducible when performed carefully, and as the number and variety of applications increase, a greater role for CE in the future of DNA separations can be anticipated.

8. ACKNOWLEDGMENTS

Major funding for this work was provided by the National Institute of Justice under grants #93-IJ-0030 and 1999-IJ-CX-KO14. The authors would also like to thank Dr. Alice Isenberg for many helpful discussions.

REFERENCES

1. Mullis, K. B. and Faloona, F. A. (1987) Specific synthesis of DNA in vitro via a polymerase-catalyzed chain reaction. Methods Enzymol. 155, 335–350.

2. Erlich, H. A. (ed.) (1989) PCR Technology. Stockton Press, New York, NY.
3. Gibbs, R. A. (1990) DNA Amplification by the polymerase chain reaction. Anal. Chem. 62, 1202–1214.
4. Kasper, T. J., Melera, M., Gozel, P., and Brownlee, R. G. (1988) Separation and detection of DNA by capillary electrophoresis J. Chromatogr. 458, 303–312.
5. Cohen, A. S., Paulus, A., and Karger, B. L. (1987) High-performance capillary electrophoresis using open tubes and gels. Chromatographia 24, 15–24.
6. Cohen, A. S. and Karger, B. L. (1987) High performance sodium dodecyl sulfate polyacrylamide gel capillary electrophoresis of peptides and proteins. J. Chromatogr. 409, 697.
7. Zhu, M., Hansen, D. L., Burd, S., and Gannon, F. (1989) Factors affecting free zone electrophoresis and isoelectric focusing in capillary electrophoresis. J. Chromatogr. 480, 311–319.
8. Barron, A. E., Blanch, H. W., and Soane, D. S. (1994) A transient entanglement coupling mechanism for DNA separation by capillary electrophoresis in ultra-dilute polymer solutions. Electrophoresis 15, 597–615.
9. Ogston, A. G. (1958) The spaces in a uniform random suspension of fibres. Tran. Faraday Soc. 54, 1754–1757.
10. Lerman, L. S. and Frisch, H. L. (1982) Why does the electrophoretic mobility of DNA in gels vary with the length of the molecule? Biopolymers 21, 995–997.
11. Grossman, P. D. and Soane, D. S. (1991) Capillary electrophoresis of DNA in entangled polymer solutions. J. Chromatogr. 559, 257–266.
12. Barron, A. E., Sunada, W. M., and Blanch, H. W. (1996) The effect of polymer properties on DNA separations by capillary electrophoresis in uncrosslinked polymer solutions. Electrophoresis 17, 744–757.
13. Heiger, D. N., Cohen, A. S., and Karger, B. L. (1990) Separation of DNA restriction fragments by high performance capillary electrophoresis with low and zero crosslinked polyacrylamide using continuous and pulsed electric fields. J. Chromatogr. 558, 33–48.
14. Srinivasan, K., Morris, S. C., Girard, J. E., Kline, M. C., and Reeder, D. J. (1993) Use of TOTO and YOYO intercalating dyes to enhance detection of PCR products with laser induced fluorescence-capillary electrophoresis. Appl. Theor. Electrophoresis 3, 235–239.
15. Clark, B. K., Nickles, C. L., Morton, K. C., Kovac, J., and Sepaniak, M. J. (1994) Rapid separation of DNA restriction digests using size selective capillary electrophoresis with application to DNA fingerprinting. J. Microcol. Sep. 6, 503–513.
16. Kim, Y. and Morris, M. D. (1994) Separation of nucleic acids by capillary electrophoresis in cellulose solutions with mono- and bis-intercalating dyes. Anal. Chem. 66, 168–174.
17. Strege, M. and Lagu, A. (1991) Separation of DNA restriction fragments by capillary electrophoresis using coated fused silica capillaries. Anal. Chem. 63, 1233–1236.
18. MacCrehan, W. A., Rasmussen, H. T., and Northrop, D. M. (1992) Size-selective capillary electrophoresis (SSCE) separation of DNA fragments. J. Liq. Chromatogr. 15, 1063–1080.

19. Baba, Y., Ishimaru, N., Samata, K., and Tsuhako, M. (1993) High-resolution separation of DNA restriction fragments by capillary electrophoresis in cellulose derivative solutions. J. Chromatogr. 653, 329–335.

20. Nathakarnkitkool, S., Oefner, P. J., Bartsch, G., Chin, M. A., and Bonn, G. K. (1992) High-resolution capillary electrophoretic analysis of DNA in free solution. Electrophoresis 13, 18–31.

21. Kleemiss, M. H., Gilges, M., and Schomburg, G. (1993) Capillary electrophoresis of DNA restriction fragments with solutions of entangled polymers. Electrophoresis 14, 515–522.

22. Butler, J. M., McCord, B. R., Jung, J. M., Lee, J. A., Budowle, B., and Allen, R. O. (1995) Application of dual internal standards for precise sizing of polymerase chain reaction products using capillary electrophoresis. Electrophoresis 16, 974–980.

23. Barron, A. E., Soane, D. S., and Blanch, H. W. (1993) Capillary electrophoresis of DNA in uncrosslinked polymer solutions. J. Chromatogr. 652, 3–16.

24. Pearce, M. J. and Watson, N. D. (1993) Rapid analysis of PCR components and products by acidic non-gel capillary electrophoresis, in DNA Fingerprinting: State of the Science (Pena, S. D. J., Chakraborty, R., Epplen, J., and Jeffreys, A. J., eds.), Birkauser Verlag, Basel, Switzerland, pp. 117–124.

25. Schwartz, H. E., Ulfelder, K., Sunzeri, F. J., Busch, M. P., and Brownlee, R. G. (1991) Analysis of DNA restriction fragments and polymerase chain reaction products towards detection of AIDS (HIV-1) virus in blood. J. Chromatogr. 559, 267–283.

26. Kim, Y. and Morris, M. D. (1994) Separation of nucleic acids by capillary electrophoresis in cellulose solutions with mono- and bis-intercalating dyes. Anal. Chem. 66, 1168–1174.

27. Chan, K. C., Whang, C. W., and Yeung, E. S. (1993) Separation of DNA Restriction fragments using capillary electrophoresis. J. Liq. Chromatogr. 16, 1941–1962.

28. Chang, H.-T. and Yeung, E. S. (1995) Poly(ethyleneoxide) for high-resolution and high-speed separation of DNA by capillary electrophoresis. J. Chromatogr. B, 669, 113.

29. Chiari, M., Nesi, M., and Righetti, P. G. (1994) Capillary zone electrophoresis of DNA fragments in a novel polymer network: poly (N-acryloylaminoethoxyethanol). Electrophoresis 15, 616–622.

30. Lazaruk, K., Walsh, P. Oaks, F., Gilbert, F., Rosenblum, D., Barnett, B., Menchen, S. et al. (1998) Genotyping of forensic short tandem repeat (STR) systems based on sizing precision in a capillary electrophoresis instrument. Electrophoresis 19, 86–93.

31. Fung, E. N. and Yeung, E. S. (1995) High speed DNA sequencing by using mixed poly(ethyleneoxide) solution in uncoated capillary columns. Anal. Chem. 67, 1913–1919.

31a. Rosenblum, B. B., Oaks, F., Menchen, S., and Johnson, B. (1997) Improved single-strand DNA sizing accuracy in capillary electrophoresis. Nucleic Acids Res. 25(19), 3925–3929.

32. Weinberger, R. (1993) Practical Capillary Electrophoresis. Academic, San Diego, CA.

33. Muth, J., Williams, P. M, Williams, S. J., Brown, M. D., Wallace, D. C., and Karger, B. L. (1996) Fast capillary electrophoresis-laser induced fluorescence analysis of ligase chain reaction products: human mitochondrial point mutations causing Leber's hereditary optic neuropathy, Electrophoresis 17, 1875–1883.

34. Mansfield, E. S. and Kronick, M. N. (1993) Alternative labeling techniques for automated fluorescence based analysis of PCR products. BioTechniques 15, 274–279.

35. McCord, B. R., Budowle, B., Isenberg, A. R., and Allen, R. O. (1996) Capillary electrophoresis for the automated analysis of multiplexed STRs using multiwavelength detection, Proceedings of the Seventh International Symposium on Human Identification. Promega Corporation, pp. 116–122.

36. Schwartz, H. E. and Ulfelder, K. J. (1992) Capillary electrophoresis with laser-induced fluorescence detection of PCR fragments using Thiazole Orange. Anal. Chem. 64, 1737–1740.

37. McCord, B. R., McClure, D. M., and Jung, J. M. (1993) Capillary electrophoresis of PCR-amplified DNA using fluorescence detection with an intercalating dye. J. Chromatogr. 652, 75–82.

38. Zhu, H., Clark, S. M., Benson, S. C., Rye, H. S., Glazer, A. N., and Mathies, R. A. (1994) High-sensitivity capillary electrophoresis of double-stranded DNA fragments using monomeric and dimeric fluorescent intercalating dyes. Anal. Chem. 66, 1941–1948.

39. Berka, J., Pariat, Y. F., Müller, O., Hebenbrock, K., Heiger, D. N., Foret, F., and Karger, B. (1995) Sequence dependent migration behavior of double-stranded DNA in capillary electrophoresis. Electrophoresis 16, 377–388.

40. Butler, J. M., McCord, B. R., Jung, J. M., Wilson, M. R., Budowle, B., and Allen, R. O. (1994) Quantitation of polymerase chain reaction products by capillary electrophoresis using laser fluorescence. J. Chromatogr. 658, 271–280.

41. Marino, M. A., Turni, L. A., Del Rio, S. A., and Williams, P. E. (1994) Molecular size determinations of DNA restriction fragments and polymerase chain reaction products using capillary gel electrophoresis. J. Chromatogr. A, 676, 185–189.

42. McCord, B. R., Jung, J. M., and Holleran, E. A. (1993) High resolution capillary electrophoresis of forensic DNA using a non-gel sieving buffer. J. Liq. Chromatogr. 16, 1963–1981.

43. Wilson, M. R., Polanskey, D., Butler, J. M., DiZinno, J. A., Replogle, J., and Budowle, B. (1995) Extraction, PCR amplification and sequencing of mitochondrial DNA from human hair shafts. BioTechniques, 18, 662.

44. Perkin Elmer Applied Biosciences Division protocols for ABD 310 Genetic Analyzer and AmpFlSTR Profiler Plus (1995) Foster City, CA.

45. Chan, K. C., Muschik, G. M., and Issaq, H. J. (1997) High-speed electrophoretic separation of DNA fragments using a short capillary. J. Chromatogr. B 695, 113–115.

46. Woolley, A. T., Hadley, D., Landre, P., DeMello, A. J., Mathies, R. A., and Northrup, M. A. (1996) Functional integration of PCR amplification and cap-

illary electrophoresis on a microfabricated DNA analysis device. Anal. Chem. 68, 4081.

47. Clark, B. K. and Sepaniak, M. J. (1993) Evaluation of on-column labeling with intercalating dyes for fluorescence detection of DNA fragments separated by capillary electrophoresis. J. Microcol. Sep. 5, 275–282.

48. Schwartz, H. E., Ulfelder, K. J., Chen, F. A., and Pentoney, S. L., Jr. (1994) The utility of laser-induced fluorescence detection in applications of capillary electrophoresis. J. Cap. Elec. 1, 36–54.

49. Lee, L. G., Chen, C. H., and Chiu, L. A. (1986) Thiazole Orange: a new dye for reticulocyte analysis. Cytometry 7, 508–517.

50. Isenberg, A. R., McCord, B. R., Koons, B. W., Budowle, B., and Allen, R. O. (1996) DNA typing of a polymerase chain reaction amplified D1S80/amelogenin multiplex using capillary electrophoresis and a mixed entangled polymer matrix. Electrophoresis 17, 1505.

51. Lu, W., Han, D. S., Yuan, J., and Andrieu, J. M. (1994) Multi-target PCR analysis by capillary electrophoresis and laser-induced fluorescence. Nature 368, 269–271.

52. Wang, Y., Ju, J., Carpenter, B., Atherton, J. M., Sensabaugh, G. F., and Mathies, R. A. (1995) High-speed, high-throughput TH01 allelic sizing using energy transfer fluorescent primers and capillary array electrophoresis. Anal. Chem. 67, 1197–1203.

53. Pariat, Y. F., Berka, J., Heiger, D. N., Schmitt, T., Vilenchik, M., Cohen, A. S., Foret, F., et al. (1993) Separation of DNA fragments by capillary electrophoresis using replacable linear polyacrylamide matrices. J. Chromatogr. 652, 57–66.

54. Butler, J. M. (1995) Sizing and quantitation of polymerase chain reaction products by capillary electrophoresis for use in DNA typing. University of Virginia, Ph. D. dissertation.

55. ABI Prism 310 Genescan Chemistry Guide, Perkin Elmer, Foster City, CA (1995).

56. Righetti, P. G. and Gelfi, C. (1997) Recent advances in capillary electrophoresis of DNA fragments and PCR products in poly(N-substituted acrylamides). Anal. Biochem. 244, 195–207.

57. Cheng, J., Kasuga, T., Watson, N. D., and Mitchelson, K. R. (1995) Enhanced Single-stranded DNA conformation polymorphism analysis by entangled solution capillary electrophoresis. J. Cap. Elec. 2, 24–29.

58. Ulfelder, K. J. and McCord, B. R. (1996) Separation of DNA by capillary electrophoresis, in Handbook of Capillary Electrophoresis, (Landers, J. P., ed.), CRC, New York.

59. Butler, J. M. (1997) Separation of DNA restriction fragments and PCR products, in Analysis of Nucleic Acids by Capillary Electrophoresis (Heller, C., ed.), Vieweg, Germany, Chapter 8, pp. 195–217.

60. Hammond, H. A., Jin, L., Zhong, Y., Caskey, C. T., and Chakraborty, R. (1994) Evaluation of 13 short tandem repeat loci for use in personal identification applications. Am. J. Hum. Genet. 55, 175–189.

61. Mansfield, E. S., Vainer, M., Enad, S., Barker, D. L., Harris, D., Rappaport E., and Fortina, P. (1996) Sensitivity, reproducibility and accuracy in short tandem repeat genotyping using capillary array electrophoresis. Genome Res. 6, 893.

62. Isenberg, A. R., Allen, R. O., Keys, K. M., Smerick, J. B., Budowle, B., and McCord, B. R. (1998) Analysis of two multiplexed short tandem repeats using capillary electrophoresis with multiwavelength fluorescence detection. Electrophoresis 19, 94–100.

63. McCord, B. R., Budowle, B., Isenberg, A. R., and Allen, R. O. (1997) Precision and resolution studies utilizing capillary electrophoresis: investigations of the effect of polymer type and concentration, Proceedings from the Eighth International Symposium on Human Identification, p. 192.

64. Walsh, P. S., Fildes, N. J., and Reynolds, R. (1996) Sequence analysis and characterization of stutter products at the tetranucleotide repeat locus vWA. Nucleic Acids Res. 24(14), 2807–2812.

65. Dimo-Simonin, N., Grange, F., Kratzer, A., Brandt-Casadevall, C., and Mangin, P. (1998) Forensic validation of the short tandem repeat HUMACTBP2 using capillary electrophoresis. Electrophoresis 19, 256–261.

66. Mansfield, E. S., Robertson, J. M., Vainer, M., Isenberg, A. R., Frazier, R. R., Ferguson, K., et al. (1998) Analysis of multiplexed short tandem repeat (STR) systems using capillary array electrophoresis. Electrophoresis 19, 101–107.

67. Marchi, E. and Pasacreta, R. J. (1997) Capillary electrophoresis in court: the landmark decision of the people of Tennessee versus Ware. J. Cap Electr. 4(4),145–156.

68. Butler, J. M., Wilson, M. R., and Reeder, D. J. (1998) Rapid mitochondrial DNA typing using restriction enzyme digestion of polymerase chain reaction amplicons followed by capillary electrophoretic separation with fluorescence detection. Electrophoresis 19, 119–124.

69. Clark, S. M. and Mathies, R. A. (1993) High-speed parallel separation of DNA restriction fragments using capillary array electrophoresis. Anal. Biochem. 215, 163–170.

70. Belgrader, P., Del Rio, S. A., Turner, K. A., Marino, M. A., Weaver, K. R., and Williams, P. E. (1995) Automated DNA purification and amplification from blood stained cards using a robotic workstation. BioTechniques 19, 427.

71. Belgrader, P., Devaney, J. M., Del Rio, S. A., Turner, K. A., Weaver, K. R., and Marino, M. A. (1996) Automated polymerase chain reaction sample preparation for capillary electrophoresis. J. Chromatogr. B Biomed. Appl. 683, 109.

72. Jacobson, S. C. and Ramsey, J. M. (1996) Integrated microdevice for DNA restriction fragment analysis. Anal. Chem. 68, 720.

73. Manz, A. (1997) Ultimate speed and sample volumes in electrophoresis. Biochem. Soc. Trans. 25, 278.

74. Effenhauser, C. S., Paulus, A., Manz, A., and Widmer, H. M. (1994) High-speed separation of antisense oligonucleotides on a micromachined capillary electrophoresis device. Anal. Chem. 66, 2949–2953.

75. Woolley, A. T. and Mathies, R. A. (1994) Ultra-high-speed DNA fragment separations using microfabricated capillary array electrophoresis chips. Proc. Natl. Acad. Sci. USA 91, 11,348–11,352.

76. Burns, M. A., Mastrangelo, C. H., Sammarco, T. S., Man, F. P., Webster, J. R., Johnson, B. N., et al. (1996) Microfabricated structures for integrated DNA analysis. Proc. Natl. Acad. Sci. USA 93, 5556.
77. Service, R. F. (1995) Genomics: DNA chips survey an entire genome. Science 268, 26.
78. Schmalzing, D., Koutny, L., Adourian, A., Matsudiara, P., Ehrlich, D., and Belgrader, P. (1998) Ultrafast STR analysis by microchip gel analysis. Proceedings from the Eighth International Symposium on Human Identification, Promega Corp., Madison, WI.
79. Schmalzing, D., Koutny, L., Adourian, A, Belgrader, P., Matsudiara, P., and Ehrlich, D. (1997) DNA typing in thirty seconds with a microfabricated device. Proc. Natl. Acad. Sci. USA 94, 10,273–10,278.
80. Wallin, J. M., Buoncristiani, M. R., Lazaruk, K., Fildes, N., Holt, C. L., and Walsh, P. S. (1998) Validation of the AmpFlSTR bluePCR amplification kit for forensic casework analysis. J. Forensic Sci. 43, 854–870.

15
Combining Capillary Electrophoresis with Electrospray Ionization Mass Spectrometry

Samir Cherkaoui

1. INTRODUCTION

Since its first introduction in 1981 by Lucaks and Jorgenson *(1,2)*, capillary electrophoresis (CE) has become a rapidly expanding analytical technique that has been successfully employed in a wide range of analytical areas, including pharmaceutical, agrochemical, and environmental fields and in clinical, pharmacological, and drug metabolism studies *(3)*. The reasons for this fast breakthrough are the high efficiency, short analysis time, rapid method development, and simple instrumentation. Other advantages include the very small sample quantities (e.g., femtomoles) that can be analyzed. This is particularly important for studies in which sample size is limited. In addition, exotic and/or expensive background electrolyte (BGE) solutions can be used with minimal cost and disposal problems because of the low usage associated with CE compared to liquid chromatography. Because of the numerous publications in peer-reviewed journals, CE has been established as a method that is complementary to the more conventional separation techniques, such as high-performance liquid chromatography (HPLC) and gas chromatography (GC).

Ultraviolet-visible (UV-VIS) spectrophotometry has been found to be one of the better methods for the on-line detection of compounds after separation by CE *(4)*. (However, the CE-UV bottleneck is a relatively low sensitivity due to the short optical path-length afforded by the small internal diameters of capillaries.) Several approaches, such as extended path-lengths in Z-shaped detection cells, bubble cells, or rectangular capillaries, have been used to enhance sensitivity *(5)*, but usually at the expense of efficiency. In addition, many important biological substances do not possess a chromophore, thus requiring derivatization to detect them. In an effort to over-

From: *Clinical and Forensic Applications of Capillary Electrophoresis*
Edited by: J. R. Petersen and A. A. Mohammad © Humana Press Inc., Totowa, NJ

come this problem, indirect UV detection was developed *(6)*. This technique, however, has serious sensitivity limitations. Electrochemical detection (EC) has also been investigated but has found only limited applications since it depends on the electrochemical characteristics of the specific analyte *(7)*. In addition, interfacing EC with CE presents two unique problems: electrical decoupling of CE and EC electronics, and physical alignment of the electrode with the end of the capillary. In order to enhance sensitivity efforts have recently focused on the use of fluorescence, especially laser-induced fluorescence *(5,8–10)*, however, this detection mode is limited to compounds that are fluorescent. As with some of the other detection methods most of the compounds of interest have to be tagged, e.g., with a fluorophore. Such procedures require additional expertise, are tedious and generally compromise the advantages of CE. Another problem with spectroscopic detectors is that peak identity is generally confirmed using migration times. This information, however, is often insufficient to unequivocally identify compounds of interest since real world samples often contain unknown interferences and the parameters influencing migration time are not easily controlled in CE *(11)*.

Mass spectrometry, on the other hand, is rapidly becoming one of the detectors of choice in micro-separation techniques, including μ-LC and CE. This selective and highly sensitive detector opens up additional possibilities in analytical techniques by allowing high analysis speed in addition to providing information about the mass and, potentially, the structure of the separated compounds. This information is highly desirable to unequivocally identify components in complex mixtures. However, as a result of the small loading capacity and high separation efficiency, coupling of CE to MS is not without problems.

This chapter will not attempt to review the numerous methods that researchers have used to overcome the problem in interfacing (hyphenation) CE to MS since excellent reviews (on the interfacing of CE to MS) have been published during the last few years *(12–24)*. Instead, this chapter will focus on practical considerations for successful CE-MS coupling using electrospray ionization interface with special emphasis on the sheath flow or coaxial design which is currently applied in most CE-MS combinations. Practical aspects including background electrolyte composition for effecient and selective CE preparation as well as optimal ESI-MS detection are developed. Additionally, representative CE modes, such as capillary zone electrophoresis, nonaqueous CE, chiral CE and micellar electrokinetic chromatography (MEKC) illustrating the potential of CE-ESI-MS in drug analysis are discussed. Further, collision-induced dissociation to differentiate positional isomers which cannot be separated by CZE is also presented. Finally, a survey of CE-MS analytical applications dealing with small molecules, such as drugs and metabolites, is included.

2. COMBINING CE WITH ESI-MS

2.1. Electrospray Ionization

Since the first report developed by Olivares and coworkers *(25)*, several ionization methods have been applied for CE-MS coupling. Matrix-assisted laser desorption ionization (MALDI), inductively coupled plasma (ICP) ionization, as well as soft ionization techniques, such as continuous flow fast atom bombardment (FAB) and electrospray ionization (ESI), have been described for the coupling of CE to MS. However, as indicated by literature, electrospray ionization *(26)* is still the most widely used ionization technique. It has been applied to a large variety of compounds interfacing with many types of MS, including quadrupoles *(25,27,28)*, magnetic sector *(29)*, fourier transform ion cyclotron resonance *(30)*, time-of-flight *(31,32)*, and trapping devices *(33)*.

Electrospray (ES), first introduced by Yamashita and Fenn *(34,35)*, is a method by which ions present in a solution can be transferred to the gas phase. Today, it is generally agreed that the ES process involves three steps prior to mass analysis *(36–38)*:

1. Generation and charging of the electrospray droplets at the ESI capillary tip;
2. Shrinkage of the charged droplets by solvent evaporation and repeated droplet disintegration, ultimately leading to very small highly charged droplets capable of producing gas-phase ions; and
3. The actual mechanism by which gas-phase ions are produced from the very small and highly charged droplets.

The benefits of ESI include the ability to produce extensively multiply charged ions and direct mass information on virtually all types of mass spectrometers *(39)*, small sample requirement, and compatibility with high resolution techniques, such as CE. The ESI technique is especially suited for the analysis of moderately polar and thermo labile compounds possessing a mass range from 10^2 to 10^5 Daltons.

2.2. CE-MS Interface

The interface between CE and ESI-MS is one of the keys to the success of CE-ESI-MS technique. Unlike UV-VIS or fluorescence detection, which can be performed on-column, the effluent from CE must be physically transported to the mass spectrometer without sacrificing separation efficiency. Three main interfaces have been described, including liquid–liquid junction interfaces *(27,40)*, sheath–liquid interfaces *(25,41,42)*, and sheathless interfaces *(43,44)*. However, because of its instrumental simplicity and versatility, along with the possibility of enhancing the ionization process by chemical reaction, the coaxial sheath-flow interface is by far the most popular interface for CE-ESI-MS *(45)*. A concise description of the interfaces used and their working principle are described in considerably more detail elsewhere *(15,19,22)*.

However, to successfully interface CE to ESI-MS, a number of points have to be considered and specific problems overcome, as outline below:

- In conventional CE the capillary ends (at the anode and cathode) are placed in separation buffer reservoirs and an electric field is applied to achieve electrophoretic separation. Thus, the first purpose of the CE-MS interface is to establish an electrical connection at the capillary terminus, which serves to define the electric field along the CE capillary. The electrical connection at the capillary terminus also serves to establish an electrospray source voltage difference (3–5 kV) between the terminus and sample aperture of the mass spectrometer.

- The electrospray process is optimal for an effluent flow rate on the order of 1–10 µL/min. In order for the interface to function properly it is necessary to closely match the CE flow rate, typically between 0 and 100 nL/min, with the flow rates generally required by ESI techniques. To overcome this difference in flow rate, an additional fluid (make-up flow) is added coaxially to the CE capillary outlet supplementing the CE flow to that required for ESI. The addition of an external sheath liquid may, however, induce dilution of the separated analytes. In this context, the use of micro- or nanospray sources are interesting alternatives to produce a stable electrospray at the very low flow rates typical of CE while still providing a highly sensitive and efficient interface.

- CE-ESI-MS coupling induces some limitations concerning the type and concentration of the background electrolyte solution *(46)*. As such, nonvolatile buffers commonly used in capillary zone electrophoresis (CZE), such as phosphate, borate, and citrate, are not compatible with CE-MS. The use of a make-up flow containing 50–80% organic solvent, however, may overcome this problem *(47)*. Nonvolatile buffers also adversely affect the performance of the MS by enhancing the risk of contamination of the ionization chamber and suppressing the analyte signal. In addition, other additives, such as surfactants, cyclodextrins, as well as ion-pairing agents, commonly used to improve selectivity in CZE, are not suitable for ESI-MS. Because of these problems, volatile buffers *(48,49)*, such as formic acid, acetic acid, ammonium acetate, ammonium formate, and ammonium carbonate, are often recommended for CE-ESI-MS (Table 1). The use of capillary electrochromatography *(50)*, partial-filling technique *(51)*, or nonaqueous media *(52)* are interesting alternatives to extend the application range of CE-MS and will be discussed in more detail in the following section. It is also well documented that efficiency of CZE is best in

Table 1
Suitable CE-MS Buffers

	CE-UV	CE-MS
Buffers	Citrate	Formic acid
	Phosphate	Ammonium formate
	Borate	Ammonium acetate
		Ammonium carbonate
Additives	Micelles (e.g., SDS)	Partial-filling technique
	Chiral selectors (e.g., CDs)	Electrochromatography
		MeOH/MeCN mixture containing
		volatile electrolytes

the presence of high ionic strength buffers, the opposite required for optimum ESI-MS to produce gas phase ions.

- The scan rate of MS may not be adequate to reflect the high separation efficiency (peak width of a few seconds) and resolution of CE. However, by using selected ion monitoring mode (SIM) on single quadrupole instruments, significant enhancement of detection limits compared to those obtained with scanning MS operation is possible. This is because of the greater dwell time for signal acquisition at each selected m/z value. Thus, if the MW is known prior to separation, SIM can be used to further improve separation resolution and reduce detection limits. Another alternative in dealing with the speed of CE is to use ion trap and time-of-flight analyzers, which can record a full-scan spectra over a large mass range within 100–200 ms *(33,53)*. In addition, using a reduced flow rate method, Goodlett and coworkers *(54)* were able to both improve sensitivity and alleviate scan speed limitations for CE-MS. In this technique just prior to elution of the first analyte of interest into the ESI source, the electrophoretic voltage is decreased, slowing solute elution, and thus allowing more scans to be recorded without significant loss in ion intensity. This has been found to be particularly useful for polypeptides and proteins where broad m/z range spectra can be important in determination of the molecular weight.

Once each of these issues has been identified and resolved CE can then be interfaced to MS. A typical coaxial interface consisting of three concentric capillaries is illustrated in Fig. 1 *(55)*. The fused silica capillary is located in the center of the sprayer and performs the electrophoretic separation. The middle capillary (usually stainless steel) provides a coaxial sheath liquid make-up flow to ensure stable electrospray as well as electrical contact at the capillary outlet. The outer capillary, also in stainless steel, supplies a nebulizing gas flow to assist in droplet generation and shrinkage during the

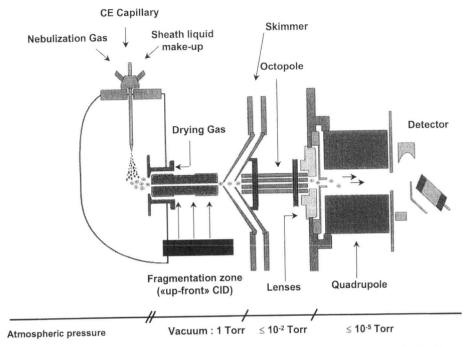

Fig. 1. Schematic drawing of Hewlett-Packard mass spectrometer including orthogonal flow sprayer for CE-MS and fragmentation zone in front of the single quadrupole *(55)*.

electrospray. In contrast to the API sources described so far, the sprayer is positioned orthogonally to the sampling orifice.

The addition of a nebulizing gas, in combination with a high voltage, is generally used to assist solvent evaporation, a prerequisite for successful electrospray ionization. This co-flow reduces the likelihood of ions penetrating from the sheath liquid into the CE capillary. However, the aspirating (siphoning) effect of a high flow rate of the coaxial sheath gas has been reported to affect separation quality resulting from a pressure-induced flow *(17,56,57)*. Moreover, to avoid siphoning effects, CE and MS instruments must be positioned close together and the outlet end of the CE capillary maintained at the same height as the inlet end.

Several investigations directed toward optimization of CE-MS performance have demonstrated *(58,59)* that small inner diameter capillaries (5–10 μm) provided a 25–50-fold gain in sensitivity as compared to 50–100 μm id capillaries. This sensitivity enhancement was attributed to an increase in ionization efficiency resulting from a decreased mass flow rate of the background electrolyte for smaller id capillaries. In addition to reducing the size of the capillaries, Tomlinson et al. *(60)* described methods for conditioning the CE capillary as well as configuring the CE-ESI-MS interface to further optimize CE-MS performance. Dimensions of the capillaries used to construct a typical coaxial CE-ESI-MS interface have also been shown to affect the sensitivity and stability *(61)*. These studies demonstrated that thick-walled capillaries can further enhance the system performance. Additionally, appropriate selection of the sheath liquid may improve significantly electrospray characteristics and ionization efficiency *(62)*. Finally, the positioning of the CE capillary with regard to the spray needle tip was found to significantly affect CE separation efficiency and resolution *(43,63,64)*. To achieve the best performance, the CE capillary must barely protrude from the ESI needle. If the capillary protrudes too much, stability of the Taylor cone is compromised and electrical contact with the CE capillary may be lost. If the CE capillary is withdrawn inside the ESI needle, separation efficiency can be dramatically affected, to an extent that the signal may be lost. Because of this problem commercial CE-ESI-MS interfaces have been designed to adjust capillary protrusion using a screw.

3. APPLICATIONS

Since CE-MS applications have already been presented and reviewed for analysis of large macromolecules like peptides (*see* Chapter 16), proteins, nucleotides, and oligosaccharides *(18,20,23)*, the present application review will be restricted to small molecules like drugs, byproducts, and metabolites. This section will concentrate on four major modes:

1. Capillary zone electrophoresis (CZE);
2. Nonaqueous CE (NACE);
3. Micellar electrokinetic chromatography (MEKC); and
4. Chiral CE.

The use of in-source collision induced dissociation is also addressed.

3.1. Capillary Zone Electrophoresis

CZE, which is strictly based on the electrophoretic properties of the analyte and buffer solution (*see* Chapter 2), is powerful and frequently used for CE-MS coupling. Two specific applications, amphetamines and carnitines, will be used to highlight the potential of CZE-MS coupling as well as the quantitative performance of the technique.

Because of their increasing illicit popularity, amphetamines and related derivatives are receiving more attention in clinical, pharmacological, and toxicological science, and monitoring their levels in biological fluids is of

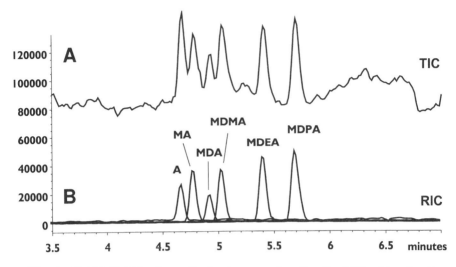

Fig. 2. CZE-ESI-MS of a spiked urine sample after liquid/liquid extraction procedure *(66)*. Peak identification: A, amphetamine; MA, methamphetamine; MDA, 3,4-methylenedioxyamphetamine; MDMA, 3,4-methylenedioxymethyl-amphetamine; MDEA, 3,4-methylenedioxyethylamphetamine; MDPA, 3,4-methyl-enedioxypropylamphetamine.

paramount importance. In our laboratory, a validated CZE method was reported for the determination of amphetamines and related derivatives sold on the black market in the form of tablets of various compositions *(65)*. However, because of the relatively low sensitivity afforded by the short optical path-length of the capillary, UV detection (UV) of these drugs in biological matrices (e.g., urine or serum) was a challenge. To overcome the limitation of sensitivity, CZE was interfaced with ESI-MS for the analysis of ecstasy and its derivatives. Considering the large number of parameters involved in CE-ESI-MS coupling, a chemometric approach was carried out to optimize such factors as nebulization pressure, drying gas temperature and flow rate, electrospray voltage, skimmer voltage, sheath liquid composition, and its flow rate *(66)*. After optimization of the CE-ESI-MS parameters and using a liquid–liquid extraction procedure, SIM was used to monitor only $(M+H)^+$ signals, which allowed a sensitive and unambiguous determination of these drugs in urine samples (Fig. 2).

The other CE-MS application was used to separate free carnitine and acylcarnitines (carnitine esters), which play an important role in the metabolism of fatty acids. Many genetic disorders are also characterized by abnormal production of these compounds in biological fluids. Henion et al.

(75) reported a CE-MS method for the determination of carnitine and several of its esters in human blood, plasma, and urine using preconcentration via sample preparation techniques. They tested a variety of MS detection modes, including scan, SIM, and selected-reaction monitoring (SRM) modes. For their application the latter (SRM) was preferred because of better selectivity and sensitivity. They also developed an abbreviated validation method to demonstrate the robustness of the SRM CE-MS method. Good quantitative data were achieved in terms of linearity, precision (0.8–14%), accuracy (85–111%), and limit of quantitation (0.1–1 nmol/mL). This application clearly indicates that CE-MS can meet the acceptance criteria for bioanalytical determinations and makes it an alternative for acylcarnitine determination in clinical samples.

The detection of several other classes of substances, e.g., designer drugs, nonopiod analgesics, nonsteroidal anti-inflammatory drugs (NSAIDs), benzodiazepines, β-adrenergic agents, plant metabolites, pesticides, and so forth have also been investigated (Table 2). Depending on the nature of the compounds, both positive and negative ionization modes have been applied. Most applications are performed in the presence of volatile buffers to preserve ESI-MS sensitivity and minimize ion source fouling problems. In addition, organic solvents are often used in the BGE to increase analyte solubility, improve resolution, and lower surface tension, thus enhancing the electrospray process. Low concentration nonvolatile buffers can be used, although at the expense of some loss of ionization efficiency resulting from competition with analytes in ESI.

3.2. MEKC-MS

In addition to CZE, micellar electrokinetic chromatography (MEKC) is one of the most widely used CE modes. Electrokinetic chromatography separation involving micelles was first described by Terabe et al. *(145)* to extend application of CE to electrically neutral substances. Today, MEKC is an accepted method for the simultaneous separation of both neutral and ionic solutes. The method requires addition of a surfactant, such as sodium dodecyl sulfate (SDS), to the BGE at a concentration above its critical micelle concentration. Selectivity is based on the differential partitioning of solutes between micellar and aqueous phases and differential electrokinetic migration, including electro-osmotic and electrophoretic mobilities. Recently, Watari developed microemulsion electrokinetic chromatography (MEEKC) as an extension of MEKC *(146)*. However, hyphenation of MEKC with MS is severely hampered by the presence of nonvolatile ionic surfactants, which often leads to a significant loss of electrospray efficiency and ion source contamination. The signal suppression mechanism can best

Table 2
Small Molecules Analyzed by CE-MS

Compounds	CE mode	Reference
Drugs of abuse	CZE-ESI-MS	*66–70*
(amphetamine and derivatives,	CZE-ESI-MS-MS	*71–73*
LSD, heroin, cocaine)	NACE-ESI-MS	*57,74*
Carnitine, acylcarnitines	CZE-ESI-MS-MS	*75*
Tricyclic antidepressant drugs	EKC-ESI-MS	*76*
	NACE-ESI-MS	*56*
β-Adrenergic blocker drugs	EKC-ESI-MS	*76*
(propranolol, alprenolol)		
β-Agonists (clenbuterol and analogs)	ITP-CZE-ESI-MS	*77*
	CZE-ESI-MS-MS	*78*
Venlafaxine and metabolites	NACE-ESI-MS	*79*
	Chiral CE-ESI-MS	*80*
Tramadol and metabolites	Chiral CE-ESI-MS	*80,81*
Methadone and EDDP	Chiral CE-ESI-MS	*80*
	CZE-ESI-MS-MS	*82*
Haloperidol and metabolites	CZE-ESI-MS	*52,83–86*
Pyrazolacridines	NACE-ESI-MS	*86,87*
Paracetamol, phenacetine, metabolites	CZE-ESI-MS	*88*
Pseudoephedrine, dextrometorphan	CZE-ESI-MS-MS	*89*
phenylpropanolamine, pyrilamine		
guaiafenesin, acetaminophen		
Benzodiazepines and metabolites	CZE-ESI-MS	*90,92*
	CZE-ESI-MS-MS	*91,93,144*
Nonsteroidal anti-inflammatory drugs	CZE-ESI-MS	*95*
	NACE-ESI-MS	*94*
	Chiral CE-ESI-MS	*96*
Morphine	CZE-ESI-MS-MS	*143*
Sulfonamides	CZE-API-MS	*90*
	CZE-ESI-MS-MS	*45,97*
Terbutaline, ketamine, propranolol	Chiral CE-ESI-MS	*98,99*
Ephedrine	Chiral CE-ESI-MS	*99*
Caffeine and metabolites	MEKC-ESI-MS	*150,155*
Local anesthetics	Chiral CE-ESI-MS	*100*
	Chiral CE-ESI-MS-MS	*101*
	CZE-ESI-MS	*70*
Camphoresulfonic acid, tropic acid,	Chiral CE-ESI-MS	*102*
arylpropionic acid, warfarin		
Mifentidine and metabolites	NACE-ESI-MS	*52,86,103–105*
Paracetamol and metabolites	CZE-ESI-MS	*106*
Nonopioid analgesics and metabolites	CZE-ESI-MS	*107*

Compounds	CE mode	Reference
Diagnostic metabolites	CE-ESI-MS-MS	*108*
Etilefrine, mianserine, tropic acid	Chiral CE-ESI-MS	*109*
3-Phenylamino-1,2-propanediol	CZE-ESI-MS	*110*
Tamoxifen and metabolites	NACE-ESI-MS	*111*
Macrolides antibiotics	CE-ESI-MS	*112*
Anthracyclines	ITP-CE-ESI-MS	*113*
Antibiotics	CZE-ESI-MS-MS	*45*
Prostaglandins	CZE-ESI-MS	*114*
Opium powder (morphine, codeine, thebaine, papaverine, noscapine)	CZE-TOF-MS	*115*
Antibacterial alkaloids	CZE-IS-MS	*116*
Berberine, coptisine, palmatine	CZE-ESI-MS-MS	*117*
Monoterpenoid indole alkaloids	CZE-ESI-MS	*118*
Photoberberines, β-carboline alkaloids	CZE-ESI-MS	*118*
Rauwolfia alkaloids	CZE-ESI-MS	*119*
Opium alkaloids	CZE-ESI-MS	*120*
Quebracho alkaloids alkaloids	CZE-ESI-MS	*120*
Tropane alkaloids	CZE-ESI-MS	*121,122*
Isoquinolines	CZE-ESI-MS	*123,124*
Isoflavones	CZE-ESI-MS	*125,126*
Sulfonylurea	CZE-ISP-MS	*92*
Alkyl sulfonates	CZE-ESI-MS-MS	*89*
Inositoles phosphates	CZE-ESI-MS	*127*
Phenoxy acid herbicides	ITP-CZE-ESI-MS	*17*
	Chiral CE-ESI-MS	*128*
Triazines	CZE-ESI-MS	*129*
	MEKC-ESI-MS	*130*
Tetramine	CZE-ESI-MS-MS	*131*
Paraquat and diquat herbicides	CZE-ESI-MS	*132*
Quaternary ammonium herbicides	CZE-ESI-MS-MS	*133*
Chlorinated acid herbicides	CZE-ESI-MS	*134*
Marine toxins	CZE-ESI-MS-MS	*45*
Sulfonated azo dyes	CZE-ESI-MS	*135*
Dyestuff degradation products	CZE-ESI-MS	*136*
Food dyes	CZE-ESI-MS-MS	*89*
Laser dyes	CZE-ESI-MS	*137*
Carboxylic acids	CZE-ESI-MS	*138*
Fatty acids	CZE-ESI-MS	*114*
Haloacetic acids	NACE-ESI-MS	*139*
Phospholipids	NACE-ESI-MS-MS	*140*
Chemical warfare agents	CZE-IS-MS	*141*
	CZE-ESI-MS-MS	*142*

be explained by two factors *(147)*: the reduction in the amount of solution that can be sprayed by ESI interface at elevated SDS concentrations, and interference of the transfer of cationic analytes from the droplet to the gas phase, because of coulombic interactions between analytes and negatively charged surfactant (SDS) ions. Various approaches have been reported for the on-line coupling of MEKC with MS and a recent review was given by Yang and Lee *(148)*. MEKC-ESI-MS using high-molecular-mass surfactants (e.g., 40,000) to reduce the level of background ions in the low m/z region has been described *(76,149,150)*. This method was applied to the separation and detection of a standard mixture of sulfamides. MEKC-MS hyphenation using a chemical ionization interface was also described for the analysis of aromatic amines *(151)*. These authors pointed out that although ion intensity was not appreciably affected by the high concentration of nonvolatile salts and surfactants, the signal was completely quenched in the ESI mode.

In analogy to the phase-switching approach in liquid chromatography, a coupled capillary set-up allowing the possibility of voltage switching and buffer renewal has also been described *(152)*. This system allows the transfer of zones of interest in the MEKC capillary to a second capillary and then to the MS. Foley and Masucci have also demonstrated that a semipermeable membrane can selectively allow small analyte molecules to pass through to a MS while retaining large buffer additives, such as surfactants *(153)*. Anodically migrating micelles moving away from the ESI-MS have also been used to prevent micelles from entering the MS interface *(154)*. This was done by adjusting the buffer pH and was applied to the analysis of chlortriazine herbicides and barbiturates. Alternatively, the partial-filling (PF) technique was found to be very useful for MEKC-MS applications *(130,155,156)*. This technique involves filling the capillary with a BGE minus SDS, followed by a short period of introduction of enough solution containing SDS to achieve separation, and finally by a sample injection. Mechanistic studies of PF-MEKC have been discussed by Nelson and Lee *(156)*. On-line PF-MEKC-MS applying an APCI interface was demonstrated for some pharmaceuticals as well as for industrial surfactants.

3.3. NACE-ESI-MS

Recently, the use of nonaqueous NA buffers in CE has been an area of increasing interest *(74,157,158)*. When compared to water, the different chemical and physical properties of organic solvents (viscosity, dielectric constant, polarity, auto-protolysis-constant, electrical conductivity, and so forth) can improve selectivity considerably (a challenging task in the separation science) and reduce Joule heating. Moreover, organic solvents have

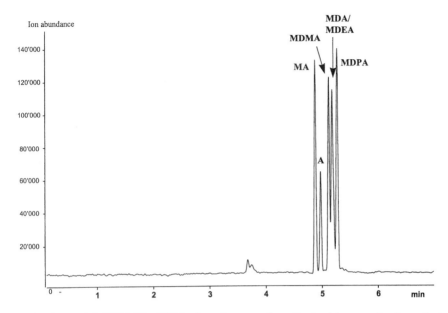

Fig. 3. NACE-ESI-MS of RIC of a urine sample spiked with a standard amphetamine mixture *(57)*. Peak assignment as in Fig. 2.

proved to be useful in analyzing hydrophobic compounds as well as drugs and metabolites, which are difficult to separate in aqueous buffers. Very high efficiency and resolution, short analysis times, and the ability to selectively increase analyte solubility are the main reasons for this success. The selectivity differences observed between aqueous and nonaqueous media have been attributed to changes in solvation of the analytes, dissociation of both analytes and silanol groups from the capillary surface, as well as possible ion-pairing effects. Finally, using an organic solvent with a volatile electrolyte affords MS compatibility because it improves the evaporation of the electrospray droplets *(52,159)*.

When we were investigating the potential of electrophoretic techniques for the analysis of amphetamines, NACE was interfaced with ESI-MS and UV detection at 200 nm *(57)*. This method was optimized and applied to the analysis of amphetamine derivatives in urine samples (Fig. 3). The quantitative performances of the method were also evaluated and showed high sensitivity as well as good reproducibility in terms of migration time and peak area ratio. In comparison to aqueous CE-ESI-MS methods previously described, NACE had different selectivities and resulted in an efficiency improvement. In addition, the electric current was very low in presence of the methanol-acetonitrile mixture and allowed good CE-MS compatibility.

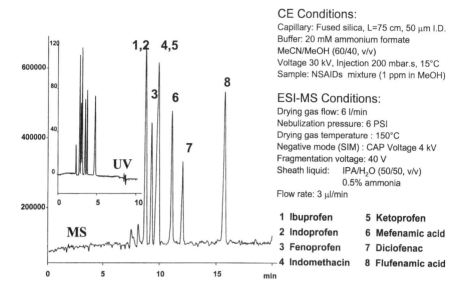

CE Conditions:
Capillary: Fused silica, L=75 cm, 50 µm I.D.
Buffer: 20 mM ammonium formate
MeCN/MeOH (60/40, v/v)
Voltage 30 kV, Injection 200 mbar.s, 15°C
Sample: NSAIDs mixture (1 ppm in MeOH)

ESI-MS Conditions:
Drying gas flow: 6 l/min
Nebulization pressure: 6 PSI
Drying gas temperature : 150°C
Negative mode (SIM) : CAP Voltage 4 kV
Fragmentation voltage: 40 V
Sheath liquid: IPA/H$_2$O (50/50, v/v)
                  0.5% ammonia
Flow rate: 3 µl/min

1 Ibuprofen	5 Ketoprofen
2 Indoprofen	6 Mefenamic acid
3 Fenoprofen	7 Diclofenac
4 Indomethacin	8 Flufenamic acid

Fig. 4. NACE-ESI-MS of nonsteroidal anti-inflamatory drugs. (**A**) UV signal; (**B**) reconstructed ion current *(94)*.

A NACE-ESI-MS method was also developed and successfully applied to the analysis of several NSAIDs *(94)*. UV detection was performed at 200 nm, 20 cm from the inlet end, whereas ESI-MS detection occurred at the capillary outlet, which accounts for the apparently greater migration times for the ESI-MS separation (Fig. 4). Both MS and UV signals from the DAD were acquired in the same run, allowing peak assignment with a very high confidence. Moreover, with volatile organic solvents a lower electrospray voltage can be applied, considerably reducing the electric discharge that can be observed in the negative polarity mode. NACE has been successfully applied to a large number of clinically relevant compounds (Table 2), including phospholipids *(140)*, organic acids *(139)*, venlafaxine and metabolites *(79)*, tamoxifen *(111)*, and tricyclic antidepressants *(56)*. NACE-ESI-MS was also useful in determining the mechanism of the in vitro microsomal metabolism of pyrazoloacridine, an antitumor drug *(86,87)*, as well as the in vitro metabolism of H2-antagonist mifentidine *(103–105)*.

3.4. Chiral CE-MS

Enantiomeric separation of chiral molecules is an area of utmost importance in separation science since enantiomer may have different pharmacological and toxicological properties. Thus, rapid, efficient, and sensitive analytical methods must be developed for the chiral purity control of drugs as well as pharmacokinetic and/or clinical studies. Recently, CE has become an interesting alternative to classical chromatographic techniques, such as GC and HPLC, for the stereoselective analysis of chiral drugs *(161)*. Enantioseparations are generally performed by adding a chiral selector to the running buffer. Various additives acting as chiral selectors, such as cyclodextrins (CDs), crown ethers, proteins, antibiotics, bile salts, and chiral micelles, have been reported in the literature. Nevertheless, CDs are by far the most widely used selectors in chiral CE. Neutral CD derivatives, presenting various functional groups, have been developed to induce different stereoselective interactions and enhance enantiomeric resolution. Recently, anionic substituted CDs, such as sulfated, sulfobutylether, phosphated, and carboxymethylated CDs, as well as cationic CDs, such as quaternary ammonium β-CD, have become commercially available and have been applied as chiral selectors. Just like MEKC-MS, coupling chiral CE with ESI-MS can be difficult because of the negative effect of nonvolatile chiral selectors on MS performance.

Using MEKC-MS as a guide, Lamoree et al. described the on-line coupling of CE with MS for the enantioseparation of ropivacaine *(100)*. Chiral purity determination by CE-MS was also demonstrated for pharmaceuticals, including terbutaline, ephedrine, ketamine, and propranolol. Under these conditions *(98,99)*, the suppression effect of CD on the analyte signal was reported. However, by using the partial filling technique introduction of chiral selector into the MS was avoided *(80,81,96,101,109)*. Similar to PF-MEKC, this involves filling a discrete portion of the capillary with a background electrolyte containing a chiral selector to achieve enantiomeric separation. Generally, a coated capillary is recommended to avoid any electroosmotic flow. In the case of basic compounds, negatively charged CDs are chosen since the application of the electric field results in a countercurrent process in which the chiral selector and the enantiomers migrate in opposite directions. This approach was applied in our laboratory for the enantioseparation of various pharmaceutical drugs and metabolites, including methadone *(80)*, venlafaxine *(80)*, and tramadol *(80,81)*. The stereoselective analysis of tramadol and its metabolites is illustrated in Fig. 5. In addition, negatively charged CDs add to the already high selectivity of MS to distinguish between metabolites with the same molecular mass, such as M1 and M2 as well as M3 and M5. CE-ESI-MS employing partial-filling technique was also reported in the literature for the separation of acidic and basic drugs in the presence of CDs *(101,109)*, vancomycin *(96,102)*, or avidin *(102)*.

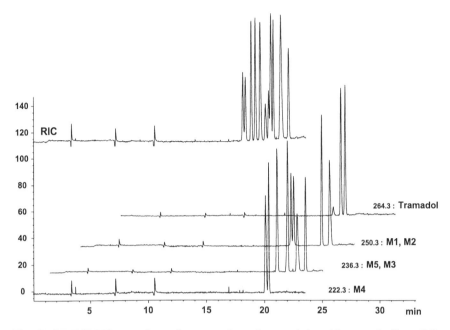

Fig. 5. CE-ESI-MS enantiomeric separation of tramadol and its metabolites *(81)*.

3.5. Collision-Induced Dissociation

Although electrospray is a soft ionization source, ions can be fragmented and structural information about a particular ion is sometimes available. Fragmentation can also be performed by means of tandem mass spectrometry (MS-MS), which requires a triple quadrupole or ion trap schemes for collision-induced dissociation (CID) of specified parent ions. It is, however, possible to perform fragmentation with a single quadrupole instrument by increasing the potential between the entrance capillary and the first skimmer (referred to as fragmentation voltage) within the ion-focusing region. (Insource CID is often used to provide information for structural elucidation of unknown compounds and confirmation of target analytes by using the abundance ratios of several diagnostic fragment ions.) CID with a single quadrupole system was successfully applied in our laboratory to separate and identify structural isomers, 3,4-methylenedioxyethylamphetamine (MDEA), and *N*-methyl-1-(3,4-methylenedioxyphenyl)-2-butamine (MBDB) *(66,67)*, as well as plant secondary metabolites, hyocsyamine, and its positional isomer littorine *(121,122)*. As shown in Fig. 6, in addition to the protonated molecular ion m/z 290, both MS spectra showed a peak at m/z 124, which corresponds to the loss of tropic acid and phenyllactic acid

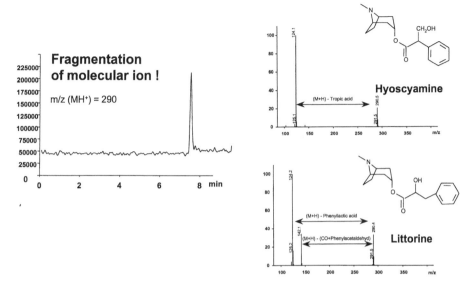

Fig. 6. MS spectra of hyoscyamine and littorine after CID (skimmer at 200 V). The daughter ion at m/z 124 corresponds to the loss of tropic acid and phenyllactic acid for hyoscyamine and littorine, respectively. In the case of littorine, the m/z 142 signal is caused by the loss of phenylacetaldehyde and carbon monoxide *(121)*.

for hyoscyamine and littorine, respectively. However, at high fragmenting voltage, the intermediate complex of littorine is less stable and results in the formation of tropine with a mass of 142. Therefore, at 200 V, this additional mass at m/z 142 indicates, without ambiguity, the presence of littorine in a plant extract. These results were assessed by tandem mass spectrometry (ESI/MS/MS) instrumentation. Thus, up-front CID can either afford structural information or generate confirmation ions in quantitative analysis with single MS, which increases result reliability.

4. CONCLUSIONS AND PERSPECTIVES

The coupling of CE (with its high separation efficiency) and electrospray ionization MS (with its high selectivity and low concentration detection limits) can provide rapid, sensitive, and unequivocal quantification and identification of drugs and metabolites in body fluids and complex mixtures. Various laboratories are awaiting this potential for purity testing, quantitation, elucidation, and confirmation of drug metabolism as well as pharmacological and toxicological studies.

Combining CE with MS allows efficient separation and identification of important biological compounds, such as pharmaceuticals, carbohydrates, peptides, proteins, and glycoforms. As more instruments interfacing CE with MS become more available, the number of applications will continue to grow. However, since most of the published applications have used model compounds, future work should focus on real-life samples. Moreover, additional studies will be necessary to evaluate whether this technique fulfills the validation criteria recommended by official guidelines required for the quantification of drugs and metabolites. Widespread acceptance of CE-MS within the electrophoretic and chromatographic community, as well as clinical and forensic laboratories, can only be realized by achieving such objectives.

Future CE-MS development will depend on increased sensitivity improvements. To overcome the insufficient concentration detection limit of CE caused by low injection volumes (approx 1–10 nL), several approaches are under investigation. These include sample stacking, isotachophoresis, and other sample concentration techniques commonly used in liquid chromatography, such as liquid–liquid and solid phase extraction, and more recently nanoelectrospray sources operating at low nanoliter per minute flow rates. With the advent of nonconventional MS instrumentation, such as ion-trap and TOF-MS, further sensitivity enhancements can be expected. Finally, considerable effort is directed toward the miniaturization of these techniques. Along these lines, direct coupling of compact and versatile micromachined chip devices to nanoelectrospray mass spectrometry systems is under development in different laboratories to achieve fast, selective, and sensitive analyses.

REFERENCES

1. Jorgenson, J. W. and Lukacs, K. D. (1981) Zone electrophoresis in open tubular glass capillaries. Anal. Chem. 53, 1298–1302.
2. Jorgenson, J. W. and Lukacs, K. D. (1983) Capillary zone electrophoresis. Science 222, 266–272.
3. Grossman, P. D. and Colburn, J. C. (1992) Capillary Electrophoresis: Theory and Practice, Academic Press, San Diego, CA.
4. Kunkel, A., Degenhardt, M., Schrim, B. and Wätzig, H. (1997) Performance of instruments and aspects of methodology and validation in quantitative CE. An update. J. Chromatogr. A 768, 17–27.
5. Pentoney, S. L., and Sweedler, J. V. (1993) Optical detection techniques for capillary electrophoresis, in Handbook of Capillary Electrophoresis (Landers, J. P., ed.), Marcel Dekker, New York, pp. 147–183.
6. Bruins, G. J. M., Van Asten, A. C., Xu, X., and Poppe, H. (1992) Theoretical and experimental aspects of indirect detection in capillary electrophoresis. J. Chromatogr. 608, 97–107.

7. Voegel, P. D. and Baldwin, R. P. (1997) Electrochemical detection in capillary electrophoresis. Electrophoresis 18, 2267–2278.

8. Timpermann, A. and Sweedler, J. V. (1996) Capillary electrophoresis with wavelength-resolved fluorescence detection. Analyst 121, 45R–52R.

9. Hernandez, L., Joshi, N., Verdeguer, P., and Guzman, N. A. (1993) Laser-induced fluorescence detection for capillary electrophoresis: a powerful analytical tool for the separation and detection of trace amounts of analytes, in Capillary Electrophoresis Technology (Guzman, N. A., ed.), Marcel Dekker, New York, pp. 605–614.

10. Schwartz, H. E., Ulfelder, K. J., Chen, F-T. A., and Pentoney, S. L. (1994) The utility of laser-induced fluorescence detection in applications of CE. J. Cap. Elec. 1, 36–54.

11. Chang, H. T. and Yeung, E. S. (1995) Dynamic control to improve the separation performance in capillary electrophoresis. Electrophoresis 16, 2069–2073.

12. Niessen, W. M. A., Tjaden, U. R., and Vandergreef, J. (1993) Capillary electrophoresis-mass spectrometry. J. Chromatogr. 636, 3–19.

13. Tomer, K. B. (1993) CZE-MS: continuous flow FAB and ESI, in Capillary Electrophoresis Technology (Guzman, N. A., ed.), Marcel Dekker, New York, pp. 569–586.

14. Smith, R. D. and Udseth, H. R. (1993) Mass spectrometric detection for capillary electrophoresis, in Capillary Electrophoresis Technology (Guzman, N. A., ed.), Marcel Dekker, New York, pp. 525–567.

15. Smith, R. D., Wahl, J. H., Goodlett, D. R., and Hofstadler, S. A. (1993) Capillary electrophoresis-mass spectrometry. Anal. Chem. 65, 574A–584A.

16. Cai, J. Y. and Henion, J. (1995) Capillary electrophoresis-mass spectrometry. J. Chromatogr. A 703, 667–692.

17. Nielen, M. W. F. (1995) Industrial applications of capillary zone electrophoresis-mass spectrometry. J. Chromatogr. A 712, 269–284.

18. Figeys, D. and Aebersold, R. (1989) High sensitivity analysis of proteins and peptides by capillary electrophoresis-tandem mass spectrometry: recent developments in technology and applications, Electrophoresis 19, 885–892.

19. Tomlinson, A. J., Guzman, N. A., and Naylor, S. (1995) Enhancement of concentration limit of detection in CE and CE-MS: A review of on-line sample extraction, clean-up, analyte pre-concentration, and micro-reactor technology, J. Cap. Elec. 2, 247–266.

20. Tomer, K. B., Parker, C. E., and Deterding, L. J. (1996) Capillary electrophoresis interfaced with mass spectrometry: electrospray ionization and continuous flow fast atom bombardment, in Capillary Electrophoresis in Analytical Biotechnology (Righetti, P. G., ed.), CRC series in Analytical Biotechnology, CRC Press, Boca Raton, FL, pp. 123–154.

21. Smith, R. D., Goodlet, D. R., and Wahl, J. H. (1993) Capillary electrophoresis mass spectrometry, in Handbook of Capillary Electrophoresis (Landers, J. P., ed.), Marcel Dekker, New York, pp. 185–206.

22. Banks, J. F. (1997) Recent advances in capillary electrophoresis-electrospray-mass spectrometry. Electrophoresis 18, 2255–2266.

23. Severs, J. C. and Smith, R. D. (1997) Capillary electrophoresis-electrospray ionization mass spectrometry, in Electrospray Ionization Mass Spectrometry;

Fundamentals, Instrumentation and Applications (Cole, R. B., ed.), John Wiley and Sons Inc., New York, pp. 343–382.

24. Kok, S. J., Velthorst, N. H., Gooijer, C., and Brimkman, U. A. T. (1998) Analyte identification in capillary electrophoresis separation. Electrophoresis 19, 2753–2776.

25. Olivares, J. A., Nguyen, N. T., Yonker, C. R., and Smith, R. D. (1987) On-line mass spectrometric detection for capillary zone electrophoresis. Anal. Chem. 59, 1230–1232.

26. Fenn, J. B., Mann, M., Meng, C. K., and Wong, S. F. (1990) Electrospray ionization: principle and practice. Mass Spectrom. Rev. 9, 37–70.

27. Lee, E. D., Muck, W., Henion, J. D., and Covey, T. R. (1988) On-line capillary zone electrophoresis-ion spray tandem mass spectrometry. J. Chromatogr. 458, 313–321.

28. Thibault, P., Pleasance, S., and Layocock, M. V. (1991) Analysis of paralytic shellfish poisons in capillary electrophoresis. J. Chromatogr. 542, 483–501.

29. Perkins, J. R. and Tomer, K. B. (1994) Capillary electrophoresis-electrospray mass spectrometry using a high performance magnetic sector mass spectrometer. Anal. Chem. 66, 2835–2840.

30. Hofstadler, S. A., Wahl, J. H., Bakhtair, R., Anderson, G. A., Bruce, J. E., and Smith, R. (1994) Capillary electrophoresis-Fourier transform ion cyclotron resonance mass spectrometry with sustained off-resonance irradiation for the characterization of protein and peptide mixtures. J. Am. Soc. Mass Spectrom. 5, 894–899.

31. Fang, L., Zhang, R., Williams, E. R., and Zare, R. N. (1994) On-line TOF-MS analysis of peptides separated by CE. Anal. Chem. 66, 3696–3701.

32. Banks, J. F. and Dresch, T. (1996) Detection of fast capillary electrophoresis peptide and proteins separations using electrospray ionization with a time of flight mass spectrometer. Anal. Chem. 68, 1480–1485.

33. Lee, E. D., Muck, W., Henion, J. D., and Covey, T. R. (1989) Liquid junction coupling for capillary zone electrophoresis/ion spray mass spectrometry. Biomed. Environ. Mass Spectrom. 18, 253–260.

34. Yamashita, M. and Fenn, J. B. (1984) Electrospray ion source: another variation of the free jet theme. J. Phys. Chem. 88, 4451–4459.

35. Yamashita, M. and Fenn, J. B. (1984) Negative ion production with electrospray ion source. J. Phys. Chem. 88, 4671–7674.

36. Kebarle, P. and Tang, L. (1993) From ions in solution to ions in the gas phase—the mechanism of electrospray mass spectrometry. Anal. Chem. 65, 972A–986A.

37. Kebarle, P. and Yeunghaw, H. (1997) On the mechanism of electrospray mass spectrometry, in Electrospray Ionization Mass Spectrometry; Fundamentals, Instrumentation and Applications (Cole, R. B., ed.), John Wiley and Sons Inc., New York, pp. 3–63.

38. Bruins, A. P. (1998) Mechanistic aspects of electrospray ionization. J. Chromatogr. A 794, 345–357.

39. Chowdhury, S. K. and Chait, B. T. (1991) Method of electrospray ionization of highly conductive solutions. Anal. Chem. 63, 1660–1664.

40. Johanson, I. M., Huang, E. C., Henion, J. D., and Zweigenbaum, J. (1991) Capillary electrophoresis-atmospheric pressure ionization-mass spectrometry for the characterization of peptides: instrumental considerations for MS detection. J. Chromatogr. 554, 311–327.

41. Ramsey, R. S. and McLuckey, S. A. (1995) Capillary electrophoresis/electrospray ionization ion trap mass spectrometry using a sheathless interface. J. Microcolumn Sep. 7, 461–469.

42. Wahl, J. H., Gale, D. C., and Smith, R. D. (1994) Sheathless capillary electrophoresis-electrospray ionization mass spectrometry using 10 µm i.d. capillaries: analyses of tryptic digests of cytochrome C. J. Chromatogr. 659, 217–222.

43. Smith, R. D., Barinaga, C. J., and Udseth, H. R. (1988) Improved electrospray ionization interface for capillary zone electrophoresis-mass spectrometry. Anal. Chem. 60, 1948–1952.

44. Smith, R. D., Loo, J. A., Barinaga, C. J., Edmonds, C. J., and Udseth, H. R. (1989) CZE and ITP-MS of polypeptides and proteins based upon ESI interface. J. Chromatogr. 480, 211–232.

45. Pleasance, S., Thibault, P., and Kelly, J. (1992) Comparison of liquid junction and coaxial interfaces for capillary electrophoresis-mass spectrometry with application to compounds of concern to the aquaculture industry. J. Chromatogr. 591, 325–339.

46. Thomson, B. A. and Iribarne, J. V. (1979) Field induced ion evaporation from liquid surfaces at atmospheric pressure. J. Chem. Phys. 71, 4451–4463.

47. Bruins, A. P., Covey, T. R., and Henion, J. D. (1987) Ion spray interface for combined LC/API-MS. Anal. Chem. 59, 2642–2646.

48. Tanaka, Y., Kishimoto, Y., Otsuka, K., and Terabe, S. (1998) Strategy for selecting separation solutions in CE-MS. J. Chromatogr. A. 817, 49–57.

49. Banks, F. J. (1995) Optimization of conditions for the analysis of a peptide mixture and a tryptic digest of a cytochrome C by CE-ESI-MS with an improved liquid sheath probe. J. Chromatogr. A 712, 245–252.

50. Hugener, M., Tinke, A. P., Niessen, W. M. A., Tjaden, U. R., and Van der Greef, J. (1993) Pseudo-electrochromatography-negative ion electrospray-mass spectrometry of aromatic glucoronides and food colors. J. Chromatogr5, . A. 647, 375–385.

51. Valtcheva, L., Mohammad, J., Petersson, G., and Hjerten, S. (1993) Chiral separation of β-blockers by HPCE based on non-immobilized cellulase as – enantioselective proteins. J. Chromatogr. 638, 263–267.

52. Tomlinson, A. J., Benson, L. M., and Naylor, S. (1995) Advantages of non-aqueous solvents in the analysis of drug metabolites using CE and on-line CE-MS. LC-GC Int. 8, 210–216.

53. Hopfgartner, G., Zell, M., Husser, C., Maschka-Selig, A., and Lausecker, B. (1999) The application of liquid chromatography and capillary zone electrophoresis combined with atmospheric pressure ionisation mass spectrometry for the analysis of pharmaceutical compounds in biological fluids. Chimia 53, 469–477.

54. Goodlet, D. R., Wahl, J. H., Udseth, H. R., and Smith, R. D. (1993) Reduced elution speed detection for capillary electrophoresis-mass spectrometry. J. Microcolumn Sep. 5, 57–62.

55. Agilent Technologies Technical Note. "CE-ESI-MS: An Integrated Solution". Publication Number 5968-1328E.
56. Liu, C. S., Li, X. F., Pinto, D., Hansen, E. B., Cerniglia, C. E., and Dovichi, N. J. (1998) On-line nonaqueous capillary electrophoresis and electrospray mass spectrometry of tricyclic antidepressants and metabolic profiling of amitriptyline by cunninghamella. Electrophoresis 19, 3183–3189.
57. Geiser, L., Cherkaoui, S., and Veuthey, J. L. (2000) Simultaneous analysis of some amphetamine derivatives in urine by nonaqueous capillary electrophoresis coupled to electrospray ionization mass spectrometry. J. Chromatogr. A, 895, 111–121.
58. Wahl, J. H., Goodlet, D. R., Udseth, H. R., and Smith, R. D. (1992) Attomole level capillary electrophoresis-mass spectrometric protein analysis using 5 μm i. d. capillaries. Anal. Chem. 64, 3194–3196.
59. Wahl, J. H., Goodlet, D. R., Udseth, H. R., and Smith, R. D. (1993) Use of small diameter capillaries for increasing peptide and protein detection sensitivity in capillary electrophoresis-mass spectrometry. Electrophoresis 14, 448–457,
60. Johnson, K. L., Tomlinson, A. J., and Naylor, S. (1996) Capillary conditioning and electrospray ionization configuration for optimal CE-MS performance. Rapid Commun. Mass Spectrom. 10, 1159, 1160.
61. Foret, F., Thompson, T. J., Vouros, P., Karger, B. L., Gebauer, P., and Bocek, P. (1994) Liquid sheath effects on the separation of proteins in capillary electrophoresis/electrospray mass spectrometry. Anal. Chem. 66, 4450–4458.
62. Tetler, L. W., Copper, P. A., and Powel, B. (1995) Influence of capillary dimensions on the performance of a coaxial capillary electrophoresis-electrospray mass spectrometry interface. J. Chromatogr. 700, 21–26.
63. Kirby, D. P., Thorne, J. M., Gotzinger, W. K., and Karger, B. L. (1996) A CE-ESI-MS interface for stable low flow operation. Anal. Chem. 68, 4451–4457.
64. Lazar, I. M., Lee, E. D., Rockwood, A. L., and Lee, M. L. (1997) Evaluation of an electrospray interface for CE-TOF-MS. J. Chromatogr. A 791, 269–278.
65. Sadeghipour, F., Varesio, E., Giroud, C., Rivier, L., and Veuthey, J. L. (1997) Analysis of amphetamines by capillary electrophoresis and liquid chromatography: application to drug seizures and cross-validation. Forens. Sci. Int. 86, 1–13.
66. Varesio, E., Cherkaoui, S., and Veuthey, J. L. (1998) Optimization of CE-ESI-MS parameters for the analysis of ecstasy and derivatives in urine. J. High Resol. Chromatogr. 21(12), 653–657.
67. Cherkaoui, S., Rudaz, S., Varesio, E., and Veuthey, J. L. (1999) On-line capillary electrophoresis-electrospray mass spectrometry for the analysis of pharmaceuticals. Chimia 53, 501–505.
68. Gaus, H. J., Gögüs, Z. Z., Schmeer, K., Behnke, B., Kovar, K. A., and Bayer, E. (1996) Separation and identification of designer drugs with capillary electrophoresis and on-line connection with ionspray mass spectrometry. J. Chromatogr. A 735, 221–226.
69. Lazar, I. M., Naisbitt, G., and Lee, M. L. (1998) Capillary electrophoresis-time-of-flight mass spectrometry of drugs of abuse. Analyst 123, 1449–1454.

70. Curcuruto, O., Zaramella, A., Hamdan, M., Turrina, S., and Tagliaro, F. (1995) CZE-ESI-MS for the characterization of drugs of forensic interest, Rapid Comm. Mass Spectrom. 9, 1487–1491.

71. Ramseier, A., Siethoff, C., Caslavska, J., and Thormann, W. (2000) Confirmation of amphetamines and designer drugs in human urine by capillary electrophoresis-ion trap mass spectrometry. Electrophoresis 21, 380–387.

72. Siethoff, C., Wagner-Redeker, W., Schäfer, M., and Linscheid, M. (1999) HPLC-MS with an ion trap mass spectrometer. Chimia 53, 484–491.

73. Cai, J. and Henion, J. (1996) Elucidation of LSD in vitro metabolism by liquid chromatography and capillary electrophoresis with tandem mass spectrometry. J. Anal. Toxicol. 20, 27–37.

74. Bjornsdottir, I., Tjornelund, J., and Hansen, S. H. (1998) Nonaqueous capillary electrophoresis—its applicability in the analysis of food, pharmaceuticals and biological fluids. Electrophoresis 19, 2179–2186.

75. Heinig, K. and Henion, J. (1999) Determination of carnitine and acylcarnitines in biological samples by capillary electrophoresis-mass spectrometry. J. Chromatogr. B 735, 171–188.

76. Lu, W., Shamsi, S., McCarley, T. D., and Warner, I. M. (1998) On-line capillary electrophoresis-electrospray ionization mass spectrometry using a polymerized anionic surfactant. Electrophoresis 19, 2193–2199.

77. Lamoree, M. H., Reinhoud, N. J., Tjaden, U. R., and Niessen, W. M. A., and Van der Greef, J. (1994) On-capillary isotachophoresis for loadability enhancement in capillary zone electrophoresis-mass spectrometry of β-agonists. Biol. Mass. Spectrom. 23, 339–345.

78. Wachs, T., Sheppard, R. L., and Henion, J. (1996) Design and applications of self-aligning liquid junction-electrospray interface for capillary electrophoresis-mass spectrometry. J. Chromatogr. B 685, 335–342.

79. Cherkaoui, S., Rudaz, S., and Veuthey, J. L. (2000) Nonaqueous capillary electrophoresis—mass spectrometry for separation of venlafaxine and its phase I metabolites. Electrophoresis (Submitted).

80. Rudaz, S., Cherkaoui, S., and Veuthey, J. L. (2000) Enantiomeric separation of pharmaceuticals using on-line capillary electrophoresis-electrospray ionization mass spectrometry. 13th International Symposium on High Performance Capillary Electrophoresis and Related Microscale Techniques, Saarbrücken, Germany, 20–24 February 2000.

81. Rudaz, S., Cherkaoui, S., Dayer, P., Fanali, S., and Veuthey, J. L. (2000) Simultaneous stereoselective analysis of tramadol and its main phase I metabolites by on-line capillary zone electrophoresis-electrospray ionization mass spectrometry. J. Chromatogr. A 868, 295–303.

82. Thormann, W., Lanz, M., Caslavska, J., Siegenthaler, P., and Portmann, R. (1998) Screening for urinary methadone by capillary electrophoretic immunoassays and confirmation by capillary electrophoresis-mass spectrometry. Electrophoresis 19, 57–65.

83. Tomlinson, A. J., Benson, L. M., Johnson, K. L., and Naylor, S. (1993) Investigation of the metabolic fate of the neuroleptic drug haloperidol by capillary

electrophoresis-electrospray ionization mass spectrometry. J. Chromatogr. Biomed. Appl. 621, 239–248.

84. Tomlinson, A. J., Benson, L. M., Oda, R. P., Braddock, W. D., Riggs, B. L., Katzmann, J. A., and Naylor, S. (1995) Novel modifications and clinical applications of preconcentration-capillary electrophoresis-mass spectrometry. J. Cap. Elec. 2, 97–104.

85. Tomlinson, A. J., Benson, L. M., Jameson, S., Johnson, D. H., and Naylor, S. (1997) Utility of membrane preconcentration CE-MS in overcoming limited sample loading for analysis of biologically derived drug metabolites, peptides and proteins. J. Am. Soc. Mass Spectrom. 8, 15–24.

86. Tomlinson, A. J., Benson, L. M., and Naylor, S. (1994) On-line CE-MS for the analysis of drug metabolites mixture: practical considerations. J. Cap. Elec. 1, 127–135.

87. Benson, L. M., Tomlinson, A. J., Reid, J. M., Walker, D. L., Ames, M. M., and Naylor S. (1993) Study of in vivo pyrazolacridine metabolism by capillary electrophoresis using isotachophoresis preconcentration in non-aqueous separation buffer. J. High Resol. Chromatogr. 16, 324–326.

88. Aschcroft, A. E., Major, H. J., Wilson, I. D., Nicholls, A., and Nicholson, J. K. (1997) Application of capillary electrophoresis-mass spectrometry to the analysis of urine samples from animals and man containing paracetamol and phenacetin and their metabolites. Anal. Commun. 34, 41–43.

89. Wheat, T. E., Lilley, K. A., and Banks, J. F. (1997) Capillary electrophoresis with electrospray mass spectrometry detection of low-molecular mass compounds. J. Chromatogr. A 781, 99–105.

90. Johansson, I. M., Pavelka, R., and Henion, J. D. (1991) Determination of small drug molecules by capillary electrophoresis-atmospheric pressure ionization mass spectrometry. J. Chromatogr. 559, 515–528.

91. Lausecker, B., Hopfgartner, G., and Hesse, M. (1998) Capillary electrophoresis-mass spectrometry versus micro-high-performance liquid chromatography-mass spectrometry coupling: a case study. J. Chromatogr. B, 718, 1–13.

92. Garcia, F. and Henion, J. (1992) Fast capillary electrophoresis-ion spray mass spectrometric determination. J. Chromatogr. 606, 237–247.

93. McClean, S., O'Kane, E., Hillis, J., and Smyth, W. F. (1999) Determination of 1,4-benzodiazepines and their metabolites by capillary electrophoresis and high-performance liquid chromatography using ultraviolet and electrospray ionisation mass spectrometry. J. Chromatogr. A 838, 273–291.

94. Cherkaoui, S. and Veuthey, J. L. On-line capillary electrophoresis-electrospray mass spectrometry for the analysis of pharmaceuticals. Presented: Thirteenth International Symposium of High Performance Capillary Electrophoresis and Related Microscale Techniques, Saarbouvcken, Germany Feb. 20–24, 2000.

95. Aschcroft, A. E., Major, H. J., Lowes, S., and Wilson, I. D. (1995) Identification of non-steroidal anti-inflamatory drugs and their metabolites in solid phase extracts of human urine using capillary electrophoresis-mass spectrometry. Anal. Proc. Incl. Anal. Commun. 32, 459–462.

96. Fanali, S., Desiderio, C., Schulte, G., Heitmeier, S., Strickmann, D., Chankvetadze, B., and Blaschke, G. (1998) Chiral capillary electrophoresis-

electrospray mass spectrometry coupling using vancomycin as chiral selector. J. Chromatogr. A 800, 69–76.

97. Perkins, J. R. (1992) Nanoscale separations combined with ESI-MS: sulfonamide determination. J. Am. Soc. Mass Spectrom. 3, 139–149.

98. Lu, W. and Cole, R. B. (1998) Determination of chiral pharmaceutical compounds, terbutaline, ketamine and propranolol, by on-line capillary electrophoresis-electrospray ionization mass spectrometry. J. Chromatogr. B 714, 69–75.

99. Sheppard, R. L., Tong, X., Cai, J., and Henion, J. D. (1995) Chiral separation and detection of terbutaline and ephedrine by capillary electrophoresis coupled with ion spray mass spectrometry. Anal. Chem. 67, 2054–2058.

100. Lamoree, M. H., Sprang, A. F. H., Tjaden, U. R., and Van der Greef, J. (1996) Use of heptakis (2,6-di-O-methyl)-β-cyclodextrin in on-line capillary zone electrophoresis-mass spectrometry for the chiral separation of ropivacaine. J. Chromatogr. A 742, 235–242.

101. Jäverfalk, E. M., Amini, A., Westerlund, D., and Andren, P. E. (1998) Chiral separation of local anesthetics by a capillary electrophoresis/partial filling technique coupled on-line to micro-electrospray mass spectrometry. J. Mass Spectrom. 33, 183–186.

102. Tanaka, Y., Kishimoto, Y., and Terabe, S. (1998) Separation of acidic enantiomers by capillary electrophoresis-mass spectrometry employing a partial filling technique. J. Chromatogr. A 802, 83–88.

103. Tomlinson, A. J., Benson, L. M., and Naylor S. (1994) Effects of organic solvent in the capillary electrophoresis and on-line capillary electrophoresis-mass spectrometry analysis of drug metabolite mixtures. Am. Lab. 26(9), 29–36.

104. Tomlinson, A. J., Benson, L. M., Gorrod, J. W., and Naylor S. (1994) Investigation of the in vitro metabolism of the H2-antagonist mifentidine by on-line CE-MS using nonaqueous separation conditions. J. Chromatogr. 657, 373–381.

105. Tomlinson, A. J., Benson, L. M., and Naylor, S. (1994) Nonaqueous solvents in the on-line capillary electrophoresis-mass spectrometry analysis of drug metabolites. J. High Resol. Chromatogr. 17, 175–177.

106. Heitmeier, S. and Blaschke, G. (1999) Direct assay of nonopioid analgesics and their metabolites in human urine by capillary electrophoresis and capillary electrophoresis mass spectrometry. J. Chromatogr. B 721, 109–125.

107. Heitmeier, S. and Blaschke, G. (1999) Direct determination of paracetamol and its metabolites in urine and serum by capillary electrophoresis with ultraviolet and mass spectrometric detection. J. Chromatogr. B 721, 93–108.

108. He, T., Quinn, D., Fu, E., and Wang, Y. K. (1999) Analysis of diagnostic metabolites by capillary electrophoresis-mass spectrometry. J. Chromatogr. B 727, 43–52.

109. Schulte, G., Heitmeier, S., Chankvetadze, B., and Blaschke, G. (1998) Chiral capillary electrophoresis-electrospray mass spectrometry coupling with charged cyclodextrin derivatives as chiral selectors. J. Chromatogr. A 800, 77–82.

110. Benson, L. M., Tomlinson, A. J., Mayeno, A. N., Gleich, G. J., Wells, D., and Naylor, S. (1996) Membrane preconcentration-capillary electrophoresis-mass

spectrometry (mPC-CE-MS) analysis of 3-phenylamino-1,2-Propanediol (PAP) metabolites. J. High Resol. Chromatogr. 19, 291–294.

111. Lu, W., Poon, G. K., Garmichael, P. L., and Cole, R. B. (1996) Analysis of tamoxifen and its metabolites by on-line capillary electrophoresis-electrospray ionization mass spectrometry employing nonaqueous media containing surfactants. Anal. Chem. 68, 668–674.

112. Parker, J. R. (1992) Application of nanoscale packed capillaries LC (75 μm i.d.) and CZE-ESI-MS for the analysis of macrolides antibiotics. J. Am. Soc. Mass. Spectrom. 3, 563–574.

113. Reinhoud, N. J., Tinke, A. P., Tjaden, U. R., Niessen, W. M. A., and Van der Greef, J. (1992) Capillary isotachophoretic analyte focusing for capillary electrophoresis with mass spectrometric detection using electrospray ionization. J. Chromatogr. 838, 273–291.

114. Petersson, A. P., Hulthe, G., and Fogelqvist, E. (1999) New sheathless interface for coupling capillary electrophoresis to electrospray mass spectrometry evaluated by the analysis of fatty acids and prostaglandins. J. Chromatogr. A 854, 141–154.

115. Lazar, I. M., Naisbitt, G., and Lee, M. L. (1999) Capillary electrophoresis time-of-flight mass spectrometry of an opium powder. Chromatographia 50, 188–194.

116. Hsieh, F. Y. L., Cai, J., and Henion, J. (1994) Determination of trace impurities of peptides and alkaloids by capillary electrophoresis-ion spray mass spectrometry. J. Chromatogr. A 679, 206–211.

117. Chen, Y. R., Wen, K. C., and Her, G. R. (2000) Analysis of coptisine, berberine and palmatine in adulterated chinese medicine by capillary electrophoresis-electrospray ion trap mass spectrometry. J. Chromatogr. A 866, 273–280.

118. Unger, M., Stöckigt, D., Belder, D., and Stöckigt, J. (1997) General approach for the analysis of various alkaloid classes using capillary electrophoresis and capillary electrophoresis-mass spectrometry. J. Chromatogr. A 767, 263–276.

119. Stöckigt, D., Unger, M., Belder, D., and Stöckigt, J. (1997) Analysis of rauwolfia alkaloids employing capillary electrophoresis-mass spectrometry. Nat. Prod. Letts. 9, 265–272.

120. Unger, M, Stöckigt, D., Belder, D., and Stöckigt, J. (1997) Alkaloid determination in crude extracts from cortex quebracho and opium applying capillary electrophoresis and capillary electrophoresis-mass spectrometry coupling. Pharmazie 52, 691–695.

121. Mateus, L., Cherkaoui, S., Christen, P., and Veuthey, J. L. (1999) Capillary electrophoresis-diode array detection-electrospray mass spectrometry for the analysis of selected tropane alkaloids in plant extracts. Electrophoresis 20, 3402–3409.

122. Mateus, L., Cherkaoui, S., Christen, P., and Oksman-Caldentey, K. M. (2000) Simultaneous determination of scopolamine, hyoscyamine and littorine in plants and different root clones of hyoscyamus muticus by micellar electrokinetic chromatography. Phytochemistry, 54, 517–523.

123. Sturm, S. and Stuppner, H. (1998) Analysis of isoquinoline alkaloids in medicinal plants by capillary electrophoresis-mass spectrometry. Electrophoresis 19, 3026–3032.

124. Henion, J. D., Mordehal, A. V., and Cai, J. (1994) Quantitative capillary electrophoresis-ion spray mass spectrometry on a benchtop ion trap for the determination of isoquinoline alkaloids. Anal. Chem. 66, 2103–2109.

125. Aramendia, M. A., Borau, V., Garcia, I., Jimenez, C., Lafont, F., Marinas, J. M., Porras, A., and Urbano, F. J. (1995) Determination of isoflavones by capillary electrophoresis-electrospray ionization mass spectrometry. J. Mass Spectrom. Rapid Commun. Mass Spectrom. 153–157.

126. Aramendia, M. A., Garcia, I., Lafont, F., and Marinas, J. M. (1995) Determination of isoflavones using capillary electrophoresis in combination with electrospray mass spectrometry. J. Chromatogr. A 707, 327–333.

127. Buscher, B. A. P., Hofte, A. J. P., Tjaden, U. R., and Van der Greef, J. (1997) On-line electrodialysis-capillary zone electrophoresis-mass spectrometry of inositol phosphates in complex matrices. J. Chromatogr. A 777, 51–60.

128. Otsuka, K., Smith, C. J., Grainger, J., Barr, J. R., Patterson, D. G., Tanaka, J. N., and Terabe, S. (1998) Stereoselective separation and detection of phenoxy acid herbicide enantiomers by cyclodextrin-modified capillary zone electrophoresis-electrospray ionization mass spectrometry. J. Chromatogr. A 718, 75–81.

129. Tsai, C. Y., Chen, Y. R., and Her, G. R. (1998) Analysis of triazines by reversed electroosmotic flow capillary electrophoresis-electrospray mass spectrometry. J. Chromatogr. A 813, 379–386.

130. Nelson, W. M., Tang, Q., Harrata, A. K., and Lee, C. S. (1996) On-line partial filling micellar electrokinetic chromatography-electrospray ionization mass spectrometry. J. Chromatogr. A 749, 219–226.

131. Zhao, J. Y., Thibault, P., Tazawa, T., and Quilliam, M. A. (1997) Analysis of tetramine in sea snails by capillary electrophoresis-tandem mass spectrometry. J. Chromatogr. 781, 555–564.

132. Lazar, I. M. and Lee, M. L. (1999) Capillary electrophoresis time of flight mass spectrometry of paraquat and diquat herbicides. J. Microcolumn Sep. 11(2), 117–123.

133. Moyano, E., Games, D. E., and Galceran, M. T. (1996) Determination of quaternary ammonium herbicides by capillary electrophoresis/mass spectrometry. Rapid Commun. Mass Spectrom. 10, 1379–1385.

134. Song, X. and Budde, W. L. (1998) Determination of chlorinated acid herbicides and related compounds in water by capillary electrophoresis-electrospray negative ion mass spectrometry. J. Chromatogr. A 829, 327–340.

135. Riu, J., Schönsee, I., and Barcelo, D. (1998) Determination of sulfonated azo dyes in groundwater and industrial effluents by automated solid-phase extraction followed by capillary electrophoresis-mass spectrometry. J. Mass. Spectrom. 33, 653–663.

136. Takeda, S., Tanaka, Y., Nishimura, Y., Yamane, M., Siroma, Z., and Wakida, S. I. (1999) Analysis of dyestuff degradation products by capillary electrophoresis. J. Chromatogr. A 853, 503–509.

137. Varghese, J. and Cole, R. B. (1993) Optimization of capillary zone electrophoresis-electrospray mass spectrometry for cationic and anionic laser dye analysis employing opposite polarities at the injector and interface. J. Chromatogr. 639, 303–316.
138. Johnson, S. K., Houk, L. L., Johnson, D. C., and Houk, R. S. (1999) Determination of small carboxylic acids by capillary electrophoresis with electrospray-mass spectrometry. Anal. Chim. Acta 389, 1–8.
139. Ahrer, W. and Buchberger, W. (1999) Determination of haloacetic acids by the combination of non-aqueous capillary electrophoresis and mass spectrometry. Fres. J. Anal. Chem. 365, 604–609.
140. Raith, K., Wolf, R., Wagner, J., and Neubert, R. H. H. (1998) Separation of phospholipids by nonaqueous capillary electrophoresis with electrospray ionisation mass spectrometry. J. Chromatogr. A 802, 185–188.
141. Kostiainen, R. and Bruins, A. P. (1993) Identification of degradation products of some chemical warfare agents by capillary electrophoresis-ionspray mass spectrometry. J. Chromatogr. 634, 113–118.
142. Mercier, J. P., Chaimbault, P., Morin, Ph., Dreux, M., and Tambuté, A. (1998) Identification of phosphonic acids by capillary electrophoresis-ionspray mass spectrometry. J. Chromatogr. A 825, 71–80.
143. Tsai, J. L., Wu, W. S., and Lee, H. H. (2000) Qualitative determination of urinary morphine by CZE and ion trap mass spectrometry. Electrophoresis 21, 1580–1586.
144. McClean, S., O'Kane, E. J., and Smyth, W. F. (2000) The identification and determination of selected 1,4-benzodiazepines by an optimised capillary electrophoresis-electrospray mass spectrometry method. Electrophoresis 7, 1381–1389.
145. Terabe, S., Otsuka, K., Ichikawa, K., Tsuchiya, A., and Ando, T. (1984) Electrokinetic separations with micellar solutions and open-tubular capillaries. Anal. Chem. 56, 111–113.
146. Watari, H. (1991) Microemulsion capillary electrophoresis. Chem. Lett. 391–394.
147. Rundlett, K. L. and Armstrong, D. W. (1996) Mechanism of signal suppression by anionic surfactants in capillary electrophoresis-electrospray ionization mass spectrometry. Anal. Chem. 68, 3493–3497.
148. Yang, L. and Lee, C. S. (1997) Micellar electrokinetic chromatography-mass spectrometry. J. Chromatogr. A 780, 207–218.
149. Ozaki, H., Itou, N., Terabe, S., Takada, Y., Sakairi, M., and Koizumi, H. (1995) Micellar electrokinetic chromatography-mass spectrometry using a high-molecular mass surfactant. On line coupling with an electrospray ionization interface. J. Chromatogr. A 716, 69–79.
150. Ozaki, H. and Terabe, S. (1998) On-line micellar electrokinetic chromatography-mass spectrometry with a high-molecular mass surfactant. J. Chromatogr. A 794, 317–325.
151. Takada, Y., Sakairi, M., and Koizumi, H. (1995) Atmospheric pressure chemical ionization interface for capillary electrophoresis mass spectrometry. Anal. Chem. 67, 1474–1476.

152. Lamoree, M. H., Tjaden, U. R., and Van der Greef, J. (1995) On-line coupling of micellar electrokinetic chromatography to electrospray mass spectrometry using anodically migrating micelles. J. Chromatogr. A 712, 219–225.

153. Foley, J. P. and Masucci, J. A. (1995) Proceedings of the Seventeenthth International Symposium on Capillary Chromatography and Electrophoresis, p. 278.

154. Yang, L., Harrata, K., and Lee, C. S. (1997) On-line micellar electrokinetic chromatography-electrospray ionization mass spectrometry using anodically migrating micelles. Anal. Chem. 69, 1820–1826.

155. Muijselaar, P. G., Otsuka, L., and Terabe, S. (1998) On-line coupling of partial-filling micellar electrokinetic chromatography with mass spectrometry. J. Chromatogr. A, 802, 3–15.

156. Nelson, W. M. and Lee, C. S. (1996) Mechanistic studies of partial-filling micellar electrokinetic chromatography. Anal. Chem. 68, 3265–3269.

157. Valko, I. E., Siren, H., and Riekkola, M. L. (1997) Capillary electrophoresis in nonaqueous media: An overview. LC-GC Int. 3, 190–196.

158. Hansen, S. H., Tjornelund, J., and Bjornsdottir, I. (1996) Selectivity enhancement in capillary electrophoresis using nonaqueous media. Trends Anal. Chem. 15, 175–180.

159. Yang, Q., Benson, L. M., Johnson, K. L., and Naylor S. (1999) Analysis of lipophilic peptides and therapeutic drugs: on-line-nonaqueous capillary electrophoresis-mass spectrometry. J. Biochem. Biophys. Methods 38, 103–121.

160. Chankvetadze, B. (1997) Capillary Electrophoresis in Chiral Analysis. John Wiley and Sons, New York.

VI

Mass Spectrometry, Therapeutic Drug Monitoring, and Toxicology

16

Capillary Electrophoresis-Mass Spectrometry of Biologically Active Peptides and Proteins

Stephen Naylor and Andy J. Tomlinson

1. INTRODUCTION

Capillary electrophoresis (CE) is characterized by rapid analysis times and ultra-high resolution capabilities. Indeed, these characteristics, in conjunction with low sample consumption and improved analyte recovery, were expected to revolutionize the analysis of complex biological mixtures of peptides and proteins (1–3). Furthermore, the family of CE separation techniques affords numerous other separation mechanisms that differ from high-performance liquid chromatography (HPLC) separation of peptides and proteins. In addition to free solution separations such as capillary zone electrophoresis (CZE) (4), analyte separation of peptides and proteins can also be effected by isoelectric focusing (IEF) (5–8), isotachophoresis (9), molecular weight sieving (10), and micellar electrokinetic chromatography (MEKC) (11).

The use of mass spectrometry (MS) in conjunction with CE for the analyses of peptides and proteins has experienced explosive growth in recent years (12–17). In large part this can be attributed to the development of electrospray ionization (ESI) and its miniaturization, microspray ionization (µESI) and nanospray ionization (nano-ESI) (18–20). These techniques enable rapid analysis of thermally labile, hydrophilic biopolymers, such as peptides and protein, in addition to being compatible with CE (18–21). The development of µESI and nano-ESI enabled the use of very low flow infusion rates (nanoliter/min) of analyte mixtures using only small amounts of precious peptide and protein sample mixutes (22,23).

As discussed in the previous chapter, CE-MS was pioneered independently by Smith using a coaxial sheath liquid approach (24,25) and by

From: *Clinical and Forensic Applications of Capillary Electrophoresis*
Edited by: J. R. Petersen and A. A. Mohammad © Humana Press Inc., Totowa, NJ

Henion who developed the liquid-junction interface *(26,27)*. Since the first report of on-line CE-MS, it has undergone considerable developments in both instrumentation and applications, and has been the subject of a number of reviews *(28–32)*. However, the development of on-line CE-MS has not been without significant challenges. First, optimal analyte resolution on CE and CE-MS is only achieved when the sample injection volume is <2% of the total capillary volume *(33)*. Hence, sample injection volumes are usually in the range of tens of nanoliters for commonly used capillaries (e.g., 50 μm i.d.) to low picoliters for small internal diameter capillaries (<10 μm i.d.) *(34,35)*. The concentration sensitivity of CE and CE-MS is, therefore, significantly inferior to HPLC, which can accommodate anywhere from 100 μL to >1 mL sample injection volumes. Thus, a high sample concentration is critical for CE and CE-MS analysis, which is not ideal for peptides or protein mixtures present in sample vials. At high analyte concentrations, these biopolymers often aggregate and then precipitate. In addition, at such high concentrations, peptides and proteins also readily adhere to pipet tips and sample vial surfaces, leading to significant sample losses. A variety of approaches have been developed to overcome this limitation for peptides and proteins and include analyte stacking *(36–38)*, focusing *(39,40)*, capillary isotachophoresis *(41–43)*, and on-line analyte concentrators that include solid phase (*see* refs. *34* and *44* for review), and membrane preconcentration cartridges (*see* refs. *34* and *44* for review, *see also* refs. *45–51*). These approaches will be discussed later.

Another problem associated with CE and CE-MS analysis of peptides and proteins is that the bare silica of the capillary is not chemically inert. When filled with an aqueous solution, the silica surface takes on a charge that is pH-dependent *(52)*. Although this is a primary factor in the development of electro-osmotic flow (EOF), it also provides an active surface for adsorption of peptides and proteins. Hence, the CE and CE-MS analysis of peptides and proteins often results in significant analyte loss and compromised resolution *(53–55)*. Various approaches have been utilized, including pH extremes *(56)*; the use of coated capillaries *(57)*, and these approaches will be reviewed later.

This chapter will focus on the use of CE-MS in the analysis of biologically active peptides and proteins. In particular, emphasis is placed on the robustness and sensitivity of the technology needed to analyze complex mixtures where the constituents are present at very low concentrations. Furthermore, strategies that facilitate on-line manipulation of samples to effect isolation, concentration, and analysis of compounds will also be described.

2. ANALYTICAL CONSIDERATIONS

Typically, the analysis of biologically active peptides and proteins requires minimal sample handling and maximum resolution and detection sensitivity of individual analytes. In this regard CE-MS appears to afford the "best of all worlds." However, it is important to realize that often times the biologically active or significant component in the complex mixture is present at very low concentrations and/or low absolute amounts. It is important to consider carefully the sample-handling strategy, as well as the intricacies of the method to be used in analysis of such compounds.

2.1. Method Preparation

Analysis of biologically active peptide and protein mixtures by CE and CE-MS requires attainment of reproducible migration times. In order to achieve this, it is necessary to prepare the CE capillary. The simplest approach is to use a hydroxide (or methoxide) solution to etch and clean the silica surface, followed by washing first with H_2O and, finally, with background electrolyte solution *(58)*. For peptide analysis, it is usual to condition the capillary prior to CE separation. Typically, 2–5 analyses of a standard solution containing a peptide mixture is sufficient. In cases where a more rigorous cleaning regime is required, we have subsequently shown that a solution of 70% formic acid/30% n-propanol, followed by conditioning, will ensure migration time reproducibility *(59)*.

It has been demonstrated that in free solution, peptide migration is proportional to $m^{2/3}/z$ (where m is mass and z is the charge of the peptide) *(60)*. A number of predictive programs now exist to correlate the pI of a peptide with the charge on the molecule at a specified pH. Thus, if the peptide composition of a mixture is known, the free solution conditions to effect CE separation can be predicted. In this instance the most important parameter to consider is the pH of the background electrolyte (BGE). Obviously, other important parameters to consider are the ionic strength of BGE, capillary dimensions, temperature and applied voltages. However, for peptides the most direct route to optimal separation conditions is to change the pH of the BGE. It is important that only volatile salts are used in the BGE for CE-MS *(see* Chapter 15). Hence, acidic BGEs are usually prepared with mixtures of NH_4OAc and CH_3COOH solutions. Basic pH conditions are usually achieved using mixtures of NH_4OAc, NH_4HCO_3, and NH_4OH. It is also important to note that these solutions do not have high buffering capacity and this can lead to irreproducible migration times as ions are depleted from the BGE. In order to overcome this limitation, frequent replenishment of BGE with fresh solution is necessary *(58)*. We have found that in the analysis of peptides, a solution of 2 m*M* ammonium acetate in 1% acetic acid provides an excellent BGE for analysis by CE-MS *(45–47)*. In addition, increasing the acetic acid to 5% (v/v) enhances peptide separation, which is attributed to increased BGE viscosity *(18)*.

As noted earlier, the use of bare fused silica capillaries can lead to significant losses in peptide during analysis by CE and CE-MS. Thus, the use of polybrene-coated capillaries has found significant use in the CE-MS analysis of peptides *(18,61)*. The polybrene coating reverses the charge on the capillary wall and under acidic BGE conditions prevents peptide adsorption to the wall. Typically, coating and conditioning the capillary allows optimal separation performance for 15–20 analyses. The capillary is then completely stripped and recoated to carry out further analyses. It should be noted that it is not possible to coat dynamically the CE capillary in the CE-MS analysis of peptides because this would adversely affect ESI-MS performance.

The development of CE-MS conditions for the separation of proteins is considerably more complex than for optimization of peptide separations. Protein denaturation, aggregation, precipitation, and solubility as well as severe adsorption to the capillary wall can all degrade CE and CE-MS performance *(62,63)*. Therefore, for almost all CE and CE-MS protein analyses, a coated capillary is necessary. We recently evaluated the performance of a number of coated capillaries in the analysis of proteins derived from aqueous humor *(64)*. We found that the salt matrix of this physiologically derived fluid interferred with the separation of the proteins that are present in this fluid. In most cases, only a single peak was detected. However, use of a polybrene capillary enabled good resolution of the components of this important physiological fluid. We have also found that a BGE composed of ammonium acetate and acetic acid to be very suitable for protein analysis by CE-MS, with increased acetic acid concentration often improving analyte resolution *(63)*.

2.2. Sample Preparation

As noted above, extreme caution is required during preparation of dilute solutions of peptides and proteins. These analytes readily adhere to every surface that they contact. Therefore, manipulations need to be minimized. However, biologically relevant peptides and proteins are often most soluble in solutions of high ionic strength. Such solutions are usually not optimal for separation by CE. Typically, these solutions will reduce the effect of stacking mechanisms, or compress the pH gradient in cIEF separations *(7,65)*. Clearly, the salt concentrations need to be reduced. This, however, should not be at the expense of analyte concentration. In this regard, use of an on-line sample preparation (e.g., solid-phase extraction (SPE)-CE-MS or membrane preconcentration (mPC)-CE-MS) appears to be most appropriate *(34,44)*. As described in detail later, these techniques enable analyte preconcentration and sample cleanup with minimal intervention by the operator with resulting improved analyte recovery. Furthermore, as we have found in our studies, the salt in the sample matrix may aid protein recovery from the solid phase or impregnated membrane *(62,63)*. Also, traces of salt that remain after on-line cleanup may improve analyte stacking, provided a positively charged capillary is used for analyte separation. For peptides, the combination of reversed-phase HPLC (RP-HPLC) off-line with mPC-CE-MS has been proven to be a sensitive method of analysis, since subsequent sample preparation involves merely removing the organic solvent from fractions and diluting the residue in a suitable aqueous solvent *(46,47)*. This method could be further improved by on-line coupling of these techniques, as has been demonstrated by Jorgenson's group *(66)*. However, this tandem technique requires that the mass spectrometer be capable of high sensitivity at fast scan rates, since the CE separation is usually complete in just a few seconds. As such, the development of fast-scanning, highly-sensitive electrospray-time of flight mass spectrometers (ESI-TOF-MS) will make this technology more viable *(67)*.

An area that has received only scant attention is that of on-line digestion CE-MS *(68)*. Such methodology, demonstrated by Kuhr and his group, appears to be a useful way of generating peptide maps of small amounts of biologically relevant proteins *(68,69)*. In conjunction with on-line SPE-CE-MS or mPC-CE-MS, digestion in an open tubular enzyme capillary, or an enzyme-modified solid support, would appear to be a powerful methodology for proteomic research. In addition, up-front separation by an appropriate chromatographic step (either HPLC or CE) could provide an attractive method for characterizing the protein composition of a biological system, that once optimized would need little operator intervention. Hence, analyte losses and sample contamination should be minimized. On-line, automated peptide/protein sequencing using tandem MS could also be achieved by this integrated approach.

2.3. Sample Injection

Typically three modes of sample injection into the CE capillary are used for analyte analysis with on-line MS detection. These include electrokinetic injecton, during which high voltage is applied to the sample solution. Analytes migrate into the capillary according to their electrophoretic mobility or may be transported by the migration of solvated ions *(65)*. This mode of injection is affected by the salt concentration of the sample matrix. Thus the amount of analyte injected into the capillary can vary from sample to sample unless care is taken to ensure that each sample is isotonic. In addition, analytes of differing charge will migrate into the capillary at different rates introducings selectivity into the analysis. For these reasons, electrokinetic injection is not particularly useful for the analysis of biologically derived mixtures of peptides and proteins.

The two other sample injection modes for CE-MS are based on hydrodynamic flow. In one mode, the inlet of CE capillary is immersed in the sample vial and raised for a specific period to a predefined height above its outlet *(65)*. The volume of sample injected is dependent on the back pressure of the capillary, the height differential between the capillary inlet and outlet, and the time of the injection. This technique is often used when a homemade CE system is connected to the mass spectrometer. For commercially available units, the CE capillary is inserted into a sealed sample vial to which a nitrogen head pressure is applied for a specific length of time. Sample is forced from the vial into the capillary. Since both of these techniques are based upon hydrodynamic flow, all components of a complex mixture are injected into the CE capillary, minimizing the selectivity observed with electrokinetic injections. However, salt from the matrix of biologically derived samples will be introduced along with analytes of interest into the capillary. This will significantly affect the performance characteristics of the separation, and this subject will be addressed in the sections that follow.

2.4. On-Line Sample Concentration

A significant problem in the CE and CE-MS analysis of biologically active peptides and proteins is that the analytes are often present at very low concentration levels. In addition, the low internal volume of CE capillaries leads to a requirement of high analyte concentration for all CE and CE-MS studies. Analyte preconcentration can be achieved by off-line sample preparation, using lyophilization, or adsorption onto a solid phase to enable both sample cleanup and analyte concentration. However, manipulations of dilute solutions of peptides and proteins should be minimized since sample losses can be significant. Therefore, many investigators have attempted to improve the sample loading capacity of the CE capillary while maintaining optimal analyte resolution and separation efficiency.

Initially, a variety of electrophoretic concentration methods, including analyte stacking, *(36–38)* field amplification *(39,40)*, and transient isotachophoresis (tITP) *(41–43)* were developed to preconcentrate analytes following injection of the sample into the capillary. All of these techniques occur as voltage is applied across the CE capillary causing analyte zones to concentrate due to different field strengths or chemical microenvironments that form within the CE capillary *(65)*. Consequently, larger volumes can be analyzed with minimal loss of resolution and separation efficiency. In the most favorable cases, the sample can constitute up to approx 90% of the total CE capillary volume with minimal loss of CE performance. However, since the total capillary volume is small, maximum sample loading is usually limited to <1 μL. Also, as mentioned earlier, salts in the sample matrix can disrupt such analyte stacking and focusing processes. Such matrix components introduce zones of low electric field within the capillary upon application of high voltage *(34,44,65)*. Analyte migration velocities are slower, and this can prevent the analytes from focusing into discrete zones. Therefore, preprocessing of biologically derived mixtures may be required to reduce their salt concentration prior to use of these stacking and focusing techniques. Nevertheless, use of CE-tITP-MS has provided a means for analyte preconcentration to a level sufficient to allow its use for the analysis of peptide and protein mixtures *(43)*.

A technique that emerged from single-column tITP was the use of CE-cITP-MS *(70,71)*. For this approach, cITP separations are performed in wide-bore (100–200 μm i.d.), larger volume capillaries. Following the cITP step, analytes are transferred into the CE capillary for further separation, and subsequent MS detection. This technique permits the analysis of sample volumes as large as 20 μL, and as such, it provides a practical means of enhancing the concentration sensitivity of CE-MS. However, this technique is significantly more complex than other strategies for concentration sensitivity enhancement, and is not well-suited to routine operation.

In another approach, capillary isoelectric focusing-mass spectrometry (cIEF-MS) enables the analysis of a full capillary volume of sample *(5–7,72,75)*. This technique has proved to be particularly useful for the analysis of complex mixtures of proteins. Separations are usually performed in a coated capillary that exhibits negligible EOF. In a focusing step, ampholites, which are premixed with the sample, migrate through the capillary to form a pH gradient. Simultaneously, proteins migrate until they reach the pH zone that corresponds to their isoelectric point (pI), where they become neutral, hence no longer migrate. The proteins are focused into discrete zones and preconcentrated. Ultimately, a stationary state is achieved when all proteins have migrated into the pH zones that correspond to their pI. Mobilization of the proteins into the mass spectrometer is achieved using an electrophoretic approach, hydrodynamic flow or a combination of these techniques. While cIEF-MS has been shown to be useful for the analysis of proteins, the process of pH gradient formation and analyte focusing are severely compromised by the presence of salts. High salt concentrations lead to excessive currents during the focusing phase of the experiment, causing ampholyte zone broadening and a less well-defined pH gradient.

Recently, we have found that use of a 5–10 min gradient application of voltage facilitates on-line removal of salts *(7,75)*. The current profiles observed in these experiments led us to conclude that the relatively slow application of the focusing voltage enables the ejection of highly mobile salts as the pH gradient is developed and proteins migrate to zones that correspond to their pl. Two protein solutions were analyzed using the same polyvinyl alcohol coated capillary. First, a solution containing lysozyme, cytochrome C, myoglobin, carbonic anhydrase, and trypsin inhibitor in water was analyzed using a standard cIEF approach. All five proteins were baseline resolved. Subsequently, the same proteins were dissolved in 200 mM sodium chloride. In this case analysis by a standard cIEF approach failed. As a voltage of 20 kV was applied to the capillary (over 30 s) to affect analyte focusing, the current rose to 45 μA and became unstable. It was impossible to obtain satisfactory results from this system without first removing the sodium chloride by means of a slow voltage ramp. This technique worked well and has been reproducible in our hands. As expected, a small shrinkage of the pH gradient was observed. This occurred during the desalting process when cations and anions are mobilized from the capillary and are replaced by counterions of the background electrolyte. While a UV detector was used to acquire the data described here, we subsequently demonstrated the efficacy of this approach for analysis of physiologically derived protein mixtures by cIEF-MS. It the latter study we demonstrated the detection of glycated hemoglobin chains in diabetic blood and the direct analysis of cerebral spinal fluid by cIEF-MS *(75,76)*.

Analyte concentrators and membrane preconcentration devices have also been developed to overcome the relatively poor concentration limits of detection of CE and CE-MS. This technology was recently the subject of three extensive reviews *(34,44,77)*. Briefly, such technology is based on the insertion of a small bed of adsorptive phase or impregnated membrane at the inlet of the capillary coupled to the MS (*see* Fig. 1). Analytes are adsorbed onto the absorptive phase to concentrate them. Injection volumes in excess of 200 μL are routine with this technology, which corresponds to an increase in concentration sensitivity of 100–1000 times that of a conventional CE injection method. In addition, since analytes are adsorbed onto a solid phase or impregnated membrane, on-line sample cleanup can be effected by washing with a suitable solvent *(46,47)*. For biologically derived peptide and pro-

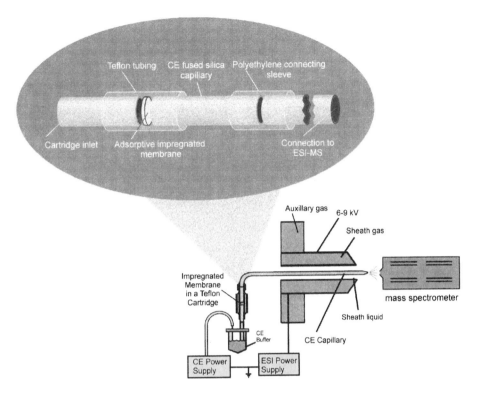

Fig. 1. Schematic of on-line membrane preconcentration-capillary electrophoresis-mass spectrometry (mPC-CE-MS), using electrospray ionization with a coaxial sheath liquid configuration.

tein samples, this process enables the removal of salt and other hydrophilic contaminants that interfere with the electrophoretic separation. This eliminates the need for excessive off-line pretreatment, improving analyte recovery, which ultimately enhances concentration sensitivity.

Some of these techniques (e.g., membrane preconcentration) have also been shown to be compatible with contemporary CE stacking and focusing chemistries. Indeed, mPC-tITP-CE-MS has been shown to be an optimal technique for the separation and sequencing of low concentrations of peptides *(45–47)*. A major consideration for optimal mPC-CE-MS performance is the use of a sufficient volume of an elution solvent (e.g., 80% methanol or acetonitrile in water) to ensure maximized peptide recovery. However, the use of an excessive volume of elution solvent severely degrades the performance of the analysis. Use of a tITP focusing strategy in conjunction with membrane preconcentration can overcome this problem, since analytes are

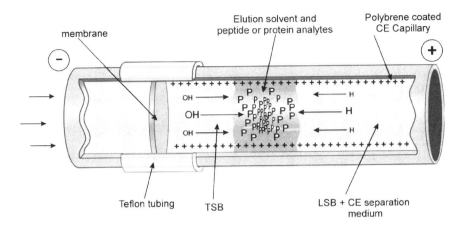

Fig. 2. Schematic of moving boundary ITP after peptide or protein analytes have been eluted from the adsorptive membrane. CE voltage applied after analytes have been eluted in aqueous/organic solvent.

focused into discrete zones as voltage is applied across the capillary. The tITP condition that we developed for use in conjunction with mPC-CE-MS is shown schematically in Fig. 2. In a systematic study we have shown that this stacking/focusing regime is a complex combination of transient cIEF-tITP and analyte stacking, that needs to be fully optimized for each mPC-CE capillary used *(46–48)*. However, once optimized, this system works extremely well.

Although peptide analysis by mPC-tITP-CE-MS can be achieved using an uncoated fused silica capillary and an acidic BGE, it is our experience that peptides and proteins are more optimally analyzed using a coated capillary *(18,63)*. In our studies of MHC class I peptides, tear proteins, and the composition of aqueous humor, we have found a polybrene-coated capillary is most suitable *(18,62–64)*. Again, the use of tITP in conjunction with mPC-CE-MS ensures that a larger volume of an elution solvent can be used with little degradation of performance. Indeed, unless a relatively large volume of elution solvent is used, proteins are not efficiently recovered from currently available impregnated membrane. In a systematic study, we found that the composition of the elution solvent was critical for elution of proteins from a C_2 impregnated membrane *(62)*. Increasing acetonitrile concentration from 40 to 80% in water significantly improved protein recovery from the membrane, and overcame a selectivity problem at the lower acetonitrile concentrations. Furthermore, we demonstrated that there was no requirement for the addition of an acid to this elution solvent. Addition of

0.1% trifluoroacetic acid to the 80% acetonitrile elution solvent adversely affected protein separation. We attributed this result to localized interaction of the TFA, an efficient ion-pair reagent, with the positively charged polybrene-coated capillary. In addition, we found that use of a less efficient ion-pair reagent (such as acetic acid) did not influence protein recovery. We attributed this result to the fact that gaps are deliberately introduced in mPC cartridges as they are prepared. This prevents perturbation of EOF by the cartridge. However, turbulent mixing of injected solvent will occur. Thus, when using an elution solvent of 80% acetonitrile in water proteins will be eluted from the membrane by the formation of a solvent gradient. As acetic acid is a constituent of a typical BGE for this application, the front edge of the elution solvent will be modified with this reagent. We postulated that this would be beneficial for the recovery of analytes from the membrane.

From our studies it is clear that mPC-CE-MS analysis of protein mixtures is still in its infancy, being limited by the choice of impregnated membranes. This approach will undoubtedly be improved in the future as new impregnated membranes with more appropriate physico-chemical properties (e.g., wide-pore polymeric phases, such as PLRP-S 4000 Å) become available. In addition, further development of affinity capture analyte concentrators will prove to be very valuable for the isolation and analysis of target proteins.

2.5. Capillary Surface Technology

As noted earlier, CE was initially thought to be a new approach that would revolutionize the analysis of peptides and proteins. For some applications (e.g., the sequencing of MHC class I peptides) CE has been proved to be extremely valuable. However, capillary-surface technology has proved to be a major challenge for the analysis of these important biopolymers. The manufacture of fused silica capillaries that exhibit constant surface properties has been the subject of much industrial research by companies that supply this consumable to the users of CE. In our own hands, we have found that although a single CE capillary that is prepared from a bulk supply may provide high performance, the next length of fused silica may not condition at all. In addition, there is no way of predicting in advance which piece of fused silica will work. This can be both frustrating and time consuming. For peptides and proteins, capillary preparation is further complicated by potential analyte-wall interactions. As noted earlier, the internal surface of a fused silica capillary is ionized when filled with an aqueous BGE. While the degree of ionization is dependent upon the pH of the BGE, the ionized silanol groups of the CE capillary provide an active anionic surface to which peptides and proteins can adsorb (53–55). This problem is particularly evident for proteins. These analytes are amphiphilic, having a structure that allows the chemical environment to determine their characteristics (e.g., charge, polarity, and hydrophobicity).

The interactions of proteins at the liquid-solid boundary of fused silica CE capillaries have been thoroughly investigated *(53–55)*. Forces that are invoked during these interactions include electrostatic, ion pairing, hydrophobic, and the formation of hydrogen bonds. In CE separations, adsorption equilibrium between proteins and the capillary wall cause severe zone broadening. Peaks also become asymmetric, which leads to decreased analyte resolution and separation efficiency. Furthermore, a changing capillary surface also affects the magnitude of the EOF causing analyte separations to become irreproducible.

To negate analyte-wall interactions, major efforts have been directed toward shielding or inverting the negative charge on the capillary wall. Various capillary coatings have been described (for a recent review of this subject, *see* ref. *57*). These include polymers, such as polyacrylamide (PAA), polyethylene glycol (PEG), polyethylene imine (PEI), polyvinyl alcohol (PVA), aminopropyltrimethoxysilane (APS), and C8 or C18 phases that contain siloxane bound anchor groups for covalent attachment to the capillary surface. Alternatively, static coatings, such as PEI and polybrene, have been adsorbed onto the capillary surface prior to the analysis of peptides or proteins. Similarly, dynamic coatings, such as PVA, can be added to the background electrolyte in an attempt to eliminate the interaction of analytes with the capillary wall. There have also been some investigations on the use of polymeric capillaries *(78–80)*. However, these were difficult to make with a consistent small internal diameter and did not readily overcome the issue of protein interaction with the capillary wall since even polymers can take on a charge during electrophoresis.

By design, all capillary coatings change the chemistry of the silica surface. Characteristics of the polymer or chemical coating determine the nature of the capillary surface. For example, hydrophilic neutral coatings (such as PVA, PEG, and PAA) impart no charge to the capillary wall and effectively eliminate EOF *(57)*. In these capillaries, analyte resolution is based solely on the differences of electrophoretic mobility of each analyte. Other coatings, such as PEI, APS, polybrene, or surfactants (such as cetyltrimethylammonium bromide), reverse the charge on the capillary wall, and EOF flows from cathode to anode. CE capillaries coated with such positively charge materials have been shown to be especially advantageous for the analysis of basic proteins. More recently, we have reported that a polybrene-coated capillary is very useful for the analysis of the protein composition of physiologically derived fluids (such as aqueous humor) *(62,63)*. Indeed, separations in a polybrene-coated capillary were found to be less affected by the salty matrix of this fluid than other capillary coatings tested. In fact, in capillaries that were coated with a neutral polymer, we found that the high salt concentration of these samples prevented the separation of the proteins that were present in physiologically derived fluids. Often, only one peak was observed during separations under these conditions.

For CE-MS experiments, the use of a coated capillary further complicates this methodology. If the coating is not sufficiently anchored to the capillary wall, it can bleed into the MS. Here it may be ionized, thereby generating a large chemical background, or interfering with the electrospray processes to impair stability or reduce analyte sensitivity. Hence, in addition to preventing analyte adsorption, the coating has to be stable and remain in the capillary. Most of those described above, with the exception of the dynamic coating strategy, have been successfully used for protein analysis by CE-MS. In general, coatings that invert the charge on the capillary wall have been preferred for CE-MS analysis of proteins (16,63,81–87). This can be attributed to the stability of such coating in acidic background electrolytes, which is a regime that also promotes the formation of positively charged analytes, thereby enabling the use of positive ion MS conditions.

2.6. CE-MS Compatible Buffers

As mentioned earlier, the use of nonvolatile BGE in the CE capillary to separate analytes can be detrimental to electrospray MS performance (88,89). Buffers of relatively high ionic strength are often used for CE separations, since these help to prevent analyte–analyte and analyte–wall interactions. Involatile salts are also a favorite choice for CE separations when used in conjunction with detection devices other than MS. In contrast, volatile buffers (e.g., ammonium salts) of low concentration, ionic strength, and conductivity are typically used for most CE-MS experiments. This is to ensure stable electrospray conditions and help prevent MS contamination by salts and ultimately instrument breakdown. For peptides and proteins, Moseley et al. found that acidic buffers of low ionic strength provided best CE-MS sensitivity when using a sheath-liquid interface (88). Wahl and Smith compared the effect of BGE composition on CE-MS using both sheath-liquid and sheathless electrospray interfaces (89). The results of this study were in good agreement with theory and showed that CE-MS sensitivity was reduced with increasing buffer concentration and ionic strength. In addition, comparison of ammonium acetate/acetic acid and sodium phosphate buffer systems indicated that at a 1 mM concentration the latter buffer provided sevenfold less signal to background than the volatile acetate system. This was attributed to the difference in ionic strength and volatility of the BGEs examined. Other results of these studies demonstrated that the sheathless interface often provided better analyte detectability than a sheath-liquid interface for most buffer systems. Likewise, a smaller-bore capillary enabled improved tolerance of the buffer system, and this was attribute to the lower BGE flow rate. BGE flow rate in a 10 μm i.d. capillary is approx 0.8 nL/min for a 10 m*M* ammonium acetate/acetic acid BGE *(89)*.

In other studies, organic modifiers have been added to the BGE to aid analyte solubility *(90,91)*. Use of organic modifiers also changes the physical properties of the separation solution, which can lead to a reduced EOF. The organic solvent can alter the thickness of the electrical double-layer at the capillary wall, and/or change the viscosity of the BGE. As demonstrated in Fig. 3, a nonaqueous BGE can also offer advantages for CE-MS analyses of hydrophobic peptides. Here, an ammonium acetate/formic acid BGE system dissolved in a mixture containing only acetonitrile and methanol (75:25 [v/v]) was used to separate two hydrophobic peptides, namely, Gramicidine S and Bacitracin. Both of these analytes are only sparingly soluble in aqueous solution, and poor analyte sensitivity was demonstrated using a conventional aqueous CE-MS BGE (data not shown). However, a nonaqueous BGE enabled efficient analysis of these analytes by CE-MS when using a sheath-liquid interface (consisting of 5 m*M* ammonium acetate in 80:20 [v/v] isopropanol:water). Indeed, we were able to detect a number of minor contaminants in the samples of both peptides by CE-MS using the nonaqueous BGE system *(94)*.

3. CE-MS INTERFACES FOR PEPTIDE AND PROTEIN ANALYSIS

A number of elegant but different approaches have been reported in coupling off-line and interfacing on-line CE with MS. This subject area has been reviewed extensively *(16,17,28–32,92)* and is also discussed in some detail in Chapter 15. In this section we will briefly discuss coupling and interfacing strategies as they pertain to analysis of peptides and proteins. In

---

Fig. 3. *(opposite page)* Nonaqueous-CE-MS (NACE-MS) analysis of gramicidin S and bacitracin. The separation buffer is 20 m*M* ammonium acetate and 114 m*M* formic acid in acetonitrile and methanol (75:25 [v/v]); 25 kV applied voltage and 7.5 μA CE current. Capillary 50 μm i.d. × 70 cm; 10-s low pressure injection of 200 ng/μL mixed standards. Liquid sheath, 5 m*M* ammonium acetate in 80% 2-propanol and 20% water (2 μL/min flow rate). ESI spray voltage 3.45 kV and current 3.3 μA. (**A**) NACE-MS ion electropherogram. (**B**) NACE-MS spectra of gramicidin S and minor impurities. (**C**) NACE-MS spectra of bacitracin and minor impurities.

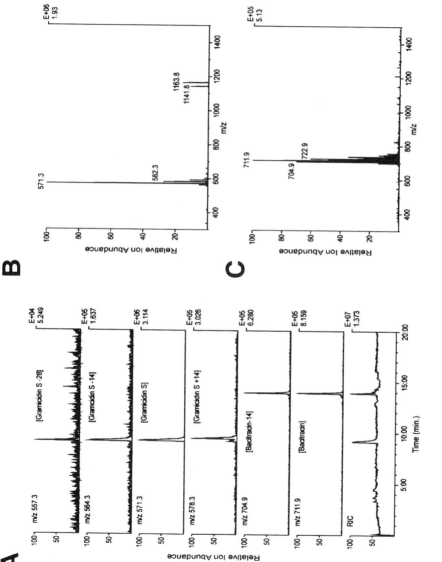

Fig. 3

particular the sheath-liquid interface has been one of the most widely used methods for connecting the CE capillary to the MS. Briefly, the CE capillary is extended through the ion source and is surrounded by a coaxial delivered sheath liquid used as a make-up flow and analyte entrainment process, as well as providing the electrical contact point for the ESI voltage *(25)*. In their studies on protein mixtures, Karger et al. investigated ionic mobility in CE-MS using a sheath-liquid interface *(93)*. Since ions migrate towards both anode and cathode, ionic components of the sheath liquid can migrate into the separation capillary. Both sharp and diffuse ionic boundaries were detected and resulted in migration delays, inversion of migration order, and often loss of analyte resolution. Here, while the BGE was the same in the two experiments, substitution of a sheath liquid containing 1% acetic acid in 50% methanol/water by 20 mM TFA in 50% methanol/water had a dramatic effect on the analysis of a mixture of these proteins. The time of the separation was compressed, and protein resolution was significantly different. Hence, the sheath liquid is a further parameter that requires close attention. In addition to avoiding the possible detrimental effects on analyte separation (described earlier), careful selection of the sheath liquid can also lead to the use of background electrolytes that contain involatile buffers. Ions present in the sheath liquid can penetrate the CE capillary to prevent such involatile salts from entering the interface. Furthermore, this process can effectively remove adducts (e.g., phosphates) from proteins prior to entering the mass spectrometer. We have also noted on occasion that proteins may not be detected at the mass spectrometer (even though they have been seen to migrate past a UV window that is close to the inlet of the CE capillary) when using a mostly organic sheath-liquid interface. In addition to the previous explanation, we have postulated that the mostly organic sheath liquid causes the proteins to precipitate as they elute from the CE capillary. As a result, proteins are neither ionized nor detected.

An alternative approach for coupling CE to MS is with the use of a liquid-junction reservoir. This approach was pioneered by Henion *(26,27)* and consists of CE capillary placed in a buffer reservoir and analytes are transported into the MS via a transfer capillary that acts as an outlet from the buffer reservoir. One of the advantages of the liquid-junction interface in the analyses of peptides and proteins is its tolerance to involatile buffer agents. Such buffers are preferentially favored for optimal peptide and protein solubility *(28)*.

More recently the development of the sheathless interface has significantly reduced chemical background noise and enhanced MS sensitivity of analyte detection *(18–23,94,95)*. A number of different designs have been described and have recently been compared and evaluated *(95)*. Clearly, such miniaturized CE-MS interfaces will dominate the way analysis of peptides and proteins occurs in the future *(17)*.

4. CE-MS AND TANDEM MS: BIOLOGICAL SAMPLES

It is very clear that CE-MS and CE-tandem mass spectrometry (CE-MS/MS) can play a significant role in the analysis of biologically active peptides and proteins. However, to date, these techniques have been underutilized and underexploited. In particular it is interesting to note that in three very recent general reviews of pharmaceuticals and drugs *(96)*, clinical chemistry *(97)* and forensic science *(98)*, no citation of CE-MS usage was noted in any of the reviews. We and others have utilized CE-MS and CE-MS/MS in the analysis of complex peptide and protein mixtures derived from physiological fluids and tissues, and some of these examples are described in this section of the chapter. Although not all examples are specific to clinical chemistry, toxicology, or forensic science, it is hoped that the applications described highlight the usefulness and power of such an approach and will encourage greater use in the future.

4.1. Biologically Active Peptides

A significant and noteworthy use of CE-MS in the analysis of a complex peptide mixture from snake venom was carried out by Perkins and Tomer *(99)*. They took lower molecular mass fractions (<8500 Daltons) from snake venom of the Jameson's Mamba (*Dendroaspis jamesoni kaimosae*) and the Eastern Coral Snake (*Mierurus fulvius*) and subjected them to CE-MS with single ion monitoring to enhance sensitivity detection limits. Using this approach, they were able to detect the presence of 83 peptides in the venom of the Jameson Mamba and 49 peptides from the coral snake, all in the molecular mass range of 6000–8500 Daltons. Their approaches readily demonstrate the excellent resolving capability of CE, coupled with the superb detection capability of on-line MS. Subsequently, Afifiyan et al. *(101)* used a combination of RP-HPLC (and CE in conjunction with MS to isolate and identify four short chain neurotoxic peptides from the Malayan spitting cobra (*Naja naja sputatrix*). In this case, however, cDNA from the cobra were cloned and expressed in *Escherichia coli* and the peptides purified and identified using CE and MS.

More recently CE-MS has been utilized in the analysis of degradation products from neuropeptide Y (101). Optimal CE conditions were obtained with high formic acid concentrations (250 mM, pH 2.75) in conjunction with 25–50 mM triethylamine. The degradation products could be readily separated from the parent peptide. In addition, CE-MS analysis allowed the determination of which amino acids had been lost from the parent peptide.

Finally, Hennebicq et al. *(102,103)* have used CE-MS in the analysis of different microsomal preparations obtained from gastric and colonic mucosa obtained from normal and tumor tissue. They analyzed the *O*-glycosylated products obtained from the selected-acceptor substrate peptide (TTSAPTTS) in the presence of *N*-acetylgalactosaminyltransferases (GalNAc). Their analytical data was consistent with the existence of more than one form of GalnAc transferase, which were expressed differentially in the gastrointestinal tract (stomach or colon). They also showed that levels of enzyme activity were tissue-specific. Furthermore, they demonstrated using CE-MS that high dipeptidylaminotransferase activity was present in tumor gastric, as well as normal colonic tissue. This work indicates the strong potential of CE-MS in the detection and identification of new markers of disease, as well as affording a rapid screen for known markers of diseased tissue.

The use of CE-MS/MS in the analysis of biologically active peptides requires that an on-line preconcentration step of analytes occurs prior to sequence analysis. Almost all the work in this area has used mPC-CE-MS/MS and is described in more detail later (*see* Section 4.3.).

4.2. Biologically Active Proteins

Most approaches for the analysis of proteins have utilized some type of on-line concentration step prior to CE separation and detection. One successful approach has been to use cIEF-MS. This has been demonstrated as a useful approach for the analysis of proteins by a number of groups including Lee *(73,104)*, Smith *(14,105)*, and Naylor *(7,75)*. It has been useful in rapidly screening protein mixtures derived from whole blood *(75)*, cerebrospinal fluid *(75)*, and *E. coli* lysate from cultures *(105)*. We have utilized this approach in the direct one-step analysis of human cerebrospinal fluid and this is shown in Fig. 4. By determining molecular weight of protein responses and interrogating the protein database, it is possible to readily identify proteins present in such a complex mixture. Obviously such an approach affords a very powerful tool in the clinical diagnosis of disease using protein markers. The other concentration analysis utilizes on-line preconcentration-CE-MS and is discussed in more detail in the next section (*see* Section 4.3.).

4.3. On-Line Preconcentration-CE-MS of Peptides and Proteins

As noted earlier, most analyses of biologically active peptides and proteins have been carried out using on-line preconcentration-CE-MS (*see* Section 2.4. for details). In particular, the group at Mayo has used on-line membrane preconcentration CE-MS (mPC-CE-MS) and CE-MS/MS (mPC-CE-MS/MS) *(106)*. Furthermore, in addition to analyte preconcentration,

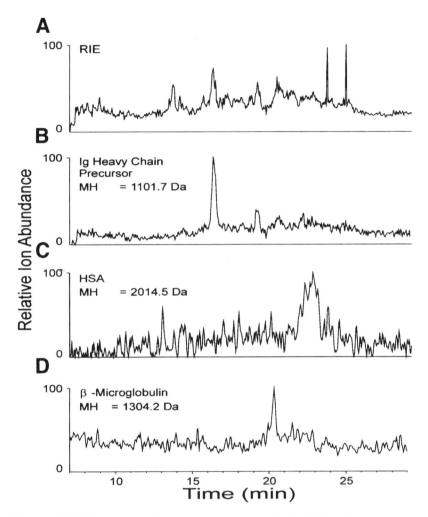

Fig. 4. cIEF-MS analysis of human cerebrospinal fluid (CSF). (**A**) Reconstructed ion electropherogram demonstrating the complexity of this physiological sample. Many analytes have been clearly resolved from this sample. (**B**) Tentative identification of β_2-microglobulin within the CSF. These analytes appear as some of the most intense within the data. All analytes were identified by molecular weight data. (**C**) Identification of human serum albumin (HSA). (**D**) Identification of β_2-microglobulin within the CSF. These analytes appear as some of the most intense within the data. All analytes were identified by molecular weight data.

mPC-CE can also be used for efficient sample cleanup. Obviously, sample cleanup is particularly important for biologically active peptides and proteins derived from physiological fluids, such as blood, bile, and urine. The presence of high salt concentrations in such fluids can dramatically affect analyte separation efficiency in CE. Also, these biological matrix components can complicate and even degrade electrophoretic stacking and focusing procedures (35,45). The mPC-CE-MS approach is relatively unaffected by such contaminants and the process actually removes them prior to CE electrophoretic separation.

4.3.1. Biologically Active Peptides

A number of studies have been undertaken in the use of mPC-CE-MS and tandem MS for the separation, detection, and sequencing of peptides (34,44,106). However, the ultimate goal was to develop a microanalytical technique for the analysis of peptides present in complex mixtures at low concentration levels (nM–pM), typically found in biological fluids, tissue, and cell cultures. In this regard, we have investigated the most suitable preconcentration membrane for use in such analyses (106,107), optimal peptide elution conditions (46,47), moving boundary tITP conditions (45,47), capillary coatings (18,62,63), and capillary internal diameter (47). Furthermore, we have demonstrated the use of an integrated approach of mPC-tITP-CE with microspray MS (18), as well as improved tandem MS sensitivity in conjunction with mPC-CE-MS (47). This is summarized in Table 1.

Membrane PC-CE-MS has been used in the detection of growth factors IgF-I and IgF-II derived from cell media (107). However, the primary impetus for the development and optimization of mPC-CE-MS and tandem MS was in the analysis of MHC class I peptides. These 8–10 amino-acid peptides are important signals in mammalian immune systems. However, characterization and sequence determination of individual peptides presents a formidable analytical challenge. This because ~10,000–15,000 such peptides, each of unique sequence, can be presented at the cell surface. Also, many of these peptides are found at very low concentrations (10^{-12}–10^{-18} M).

The strategy we have developed for sequencing MHC class I peptides has been described in detail (50,108–110), but, briefly, HPLC fractions (~100 μL) containing MHC class I peptides are collected. The organic solvent (CH_3OH or CH_3CN) is removed under vacuum and each fraction is diluted with CE separation buffer to a total volume of ~150 μL. Approximately 50 μL is loaded off-line via the pressurized bomb (108) and subjected to mPC-CE-MS for molecular mass determination. Subsequently, precursor ions (MH^+) of antigenic peptides or peptides of interest are subjected to mPC-CE-MS/MS in order to obtain sequence information. These latter analyses are carried out using the remaining ~100 μL of sample.

Table 1
Examples of mPC-CE-MS and Tandem MS Analysis of Peptide and Protein Mixtures

Analytes (origin)	Conditions (detection, membrane, capillary i.d., coating, focusing)	References
Peptides		
Peptides (standards)	mPC-CE-UV; SDB, 50 μm, bfs[b], tITP	(45)
	mPC-CE-MS; SDB, 50 μm, bfs, tITP	(46)
	mPC-CE-MS;SDB, 25 μm, bfs, tITP	(47)
	mPC-CE-MS/MS;SDB, 50 μm, bfs, tITP	(47)
	mPC-CE-MS/MS;SDB, 25 μm, bfs, tITP	(47)
	mPC-CE-MS(MS)[c];SDB, 25 μm, polybrene, tITP	(18)
Trypsin digest of α-casein	mPC-CE-MS;SDB, n.g.[d]; polybrene	(111)
IgF-I and IgF-II (cell media)	mPC-CE-MS;SDB, 50 μm, polybrene	(107)
MHC class I (K[b] EL-4)	mPC-CE-MS(MS)[c,e];SDB, 25 μm, bfs, tITP	(108,109)
MHC class I (K[b] EG-7)	mPC-CE-MS[e];SDB, 25 μm, bfs, tITP	(50)
MHC class I (K[b] EG-7)	mPC-CE-MS(MS)[c,e];SDB, 25 μm, polybrene, tITP-microspray	(18)
MHC class I (PVG R1 rat spleens)	mPC-CE-MS(MS)[c,e];SDB, 25 μm, bfs, tITP	(44)
Proteins		
Proteins (standards)	mPC-CE-UV, C-2, 50 μm, polybrene, tITP	(62)
Proteins (aqueous humor)	mPC-CE-UV, C-2, 50 μm, polybrene, tITP	(62)
Proteins-Bence Jones (urine)	mPC-CE-MS, SDB, 50 μm, polybrene	(50,107)
Proteins (blood dialysate)	mPC-CE-MS, SDB, 50 μm, polybrene	(44)
Proteins (brain dialysate)	mPC-CE-MS, SDB, 50 μm, polybrene	(44)
Proteins (CSF)	mPC-CE-MS, SDB, 50 μm, polybrene	(44)
Proteins (aqueous humor)	mPC-CE-MS, C-8, 50 μm, polybrene	(50)
Proteins (aqueous humor)	mPC-CE-MS, c-2, 50 μm, polybrene, tITP	(63)
Proteins (tears)	mPC-CE-MS, SDB, 50 μm, polybrene, tITP	(44)
Proteins (renal dialysate)	mPC-CE-MS(MS)[d], SDB, 50 μm, polybrene, tITP	(112)

[a] see refs. 34, 44, for review. [b] bfs, bare fused silica. [c] both MS and tandem MS analysis. [d] Details not given. [e] Off-line sample loading.

337

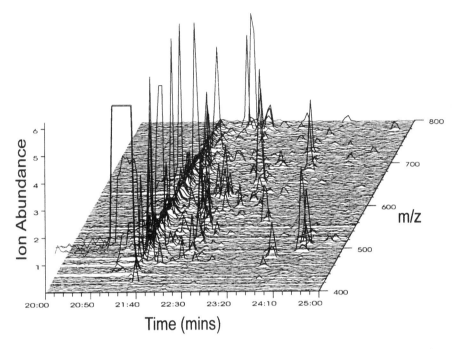

Fig. 5. Three dimensional plot of mPC-CE-MS analysis of an HPLC fraction from ~10^9 EG-7 mouse tumor cells containing peptide(s) that induced a positive T-cell stimulation response. Twenty-five microliters of the diluted HPLC fraction pressure injected and adsorbed onto an SDB membrane. Analyte elution was with ~80 nL 80:20 MeOH:H_2O sandwiched between an LSB of 0.1% NH_4OH and a TSB of 1% AcOH followed by separation buffer (2 mM NH_4OAc:1% AcOH). Separation was carried out in bare fused silica capillary (25 µm i.d. × 75 cm in length) at a voltage of 25 kV. MS was performed on a MAT 900 over a mass range 300–1300 amu at 3 s/decade, accelerating voltage 4.8 kV and an ESI spray voltage of 3.4 kV. ESI capillary was 200°C.

In a specific instance, naturally processed MHC class I peptides were isolated from ~10^9 EG-7 mouse tumor cells. This cell line had been transvected with the ovalbumin gene, along with the actin promoter. The cells were harvested, lysed, and MHC class I peptides obtained as described previously *(108,110)*. Subsequently, all HPLC fractions were subjected to a T-cell stimulation immunoassay *(110)*. Once such fraction exhibited a positive T-cell stimulation response. This fraction (~50 µL) was then subjected to mPC-CE-MS analysis to ascertain the number and molecular weights of peptides present, and this is shown in Fig. 5. A myriad of peptide responses were detected, indicating that in most cases such analyses should be carried out in conjunction with a targeted immunoassay or other bioassay approach

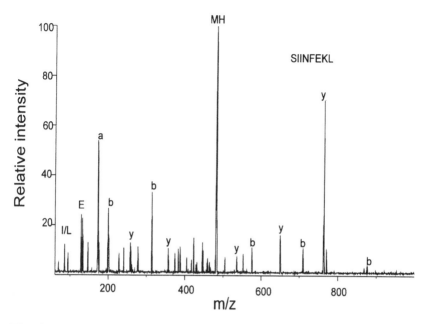

Fig. 6. Membrane PC-tITP-CE-microspray-MS/MS analysis of $MH_2^{2+} = 482.3$. Sample obtained from another preparation of ~10^9 EG-7 tumor cells. Approximately 10 μL was pressure injected onto an SDB membrane. Peptides were eluted with ~110 nL of 80% MeOH/H_2O followed by a TSB of ~115 nL 0.1% NH_4OH. Separation was carried out in a polybrene coated capillary (75 μm i.d. × 80 cm) at 15 kV with reversed polarity. It was connected via a liquid junction to a capillary emitter (25 μm i.d. × 15 mm), which was positioned ~15 mm away from the heated capillary. Separation solvent was 0.05% AcOH in 10% MeOH. Collision induced dissociation of $MH_2^{2+} = 582.3$ was carried out using argon as collision gas at 1 × 10^{-5} mbar pressure and a collision energy of 28 eV.

(50). However, in this particular case, a peptide with migration time ~23 min afforded an ion $MH_2^{2+} = 482.3$. This corresponds to the molecular weight of an ovalbumin peptide, OVA, a known antigen of this particular mouse model system. Another EG-7 tumor cell preparation was ultimately subjected to mPC-CE-MS/MS using a polybrene-coated capillary in conjunction with microspray-MS, in order to achieve maximum sensitivity and sequence data on the peptide. The ion at m/z 482.3 was subjected to collision induced dissociation conditions previously shown to afford significant fragmentation of the precursor ion *(13)*, and the resulting product ion spectrum is shown in Fig. 6. Based on both the clear 'y' and 'b' series of ions, as well as the returned SEAQUEST search, the sequence was determined to be SIINFEKL, confirming the presence of the OVA peptide in this fraction. This overall

strategy has been used to successfully analyze and obtain other peptides sequence data from K[b] EG-7, K[b] EL-4, and PVG R1 rat spleen cell lines, and this is all summarized along with mPC-CE-MS conditions in Table 1.

4.3.2. Proteins from Physiological Fluids

One-step, on-line analysis of physiological fluids (e.g., urine, bile, plasma, tears) by mPC-CE-MS has substantial potential in the development of suitable biomarkers for diagnosis of disease states. We have previously reported the utilization of this approach for the detection of Bence-Jones protein(s) in urine *(107)*. This protein(s) is a known biomarker for patients suffering from multiple myeloma. Typically, a 24-h urine sample is collected followed by numerous sample handling and separation steps in order to detect the presence of the protein. This is in stark contrast to the ~30-min analysis time of the urine sample by mPC-CE-MS. Approximately 1.5 µL of urine obtained from a patient suffering from acute multiple myeloma was subjected to mPC-CE-MS analysis. The mass spectrum revealed a number of glycoforms of the protein at 23,680, (Parent), 23,941, and 24,144 Daltons *(12,20)*. It is possible that the ratio of these previously undetected glycoforms may give further insight into onset and development of the disease, and this is currently under investigation.

Other demonstrations of the direct analysis of physiological fluids by mPC-CE-MS have been reported. They include blood and brain dialysate *(44)*, cerebrospinal fluid *(44)*, aqueous humor *(50,63)*, tears *(44)*, and kidney dialysate *(112)*, and is summarized in Table 1. An analysis of physiologically of such derived fluids affords a myriad of responses, many of which are unidentified proteins. For example, aqueous humor is the extracellular fluid that fills the anterior chamber of the eye and bathes the lens, cornea, and trabecular regions. It is composed of inorganic ions, small organic molecular, and numerous peptides and proteins. It has been proposed that levels of endogenous proteins, as well as the presence of exogenous proteins may be of some diagnostic significance. In that regard we compared the mPC-CE-MS profile of aqueous humor from patients with cataracts ("normal") to patients suffering from glaucoma. This is shown in Fig. 7A and B for the base peak ion chromatogram of normal (Fig. 7A) versus glaucoma (Fig. 7B) aqueous humor. It is clear that the 'normal' aqueous humor contains many more protein responses than that of the glaucoma aqueous humor, and we are in the process of attempting to identify individual protein constituents in order to understand the comparative differences. This may give more insight into the basic mechanisms involved in the onset of glaucoma.

A

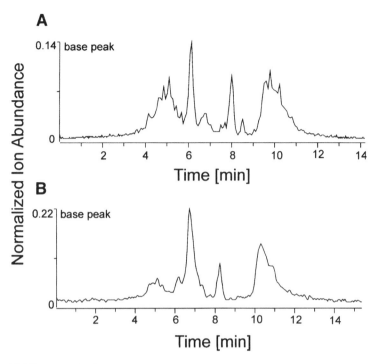

Fig. 7. Direct analysis by mPC-CE-MS of aqueous humor from a patient under-going surgery for (**A**) cataracts, (**B**) glaucoma by mPC-CE-MS. One microliter of aqueous humor was pressure-injected onto a C-2 reversed phase membrane. The membrane was washed with 2 (L of 2 mM NH$_4$OAc in 5% AcOH, and analytes were subsequently eluted with 60 nL of 80% CH$_3$CN in H$_2$O, followed by a TSB of 60 nL 0.5% NH$_4$OH. Separation was carried out in a polybrene coated capillary (50 µm i.d. × 80 cm in length) at a voltage of 15 kV. MS was performed on a MAT 900 over a mass range of 650–2200 amu at 3 s/decade. Accelerating voltage 4.7 kV and an ESI spray voltage of 3.4 kV. Instrument resolution ~500, analyte detection with PATRIC detector.

It is clear from the mPC-CE-MS analysis of aqueous humor, described earlier, that ultimately rapid identification of proteins derived from physi-ological fluids is necessary. This has recently been described for the identi-fication of a renal dialysate protein *(112)*. A number of patients at Mayo had a rare renal tumor that was shown to inhibit renal epithelial phosphate trans-port. Approximately 200 L of renal dialysate was collected from these patients and ultimately reduced to ~6 mL. This was achieved through a series of dialysis and size-exclusion chromatography concentration steps. The active component(s) was tracked at each stage using an opossum kidney-cell phosphate (^{32}P-labeled) uptake assay. Approximately 100 µL of the dialysate active fraction was assigned for mPC-CE-MS and tandem MS analyses. Initially, 20 μL was subjected to mPC-CE-MS and one major ion response was detected at M_r = 11,729 Daltons (Fig. 8A). The remaining ~80 μL was then digested with lysine-C proteolytic enzyme and the resulting digest subjected to mPC-CE-MS and tandem MS analysis. A series of peptides were detected including an ion at m/z 574.5, corresponding to the MH_2^{2+} = 574.5 shown in Fig. 8B. This spectrum was searched without prior interpretation using the SEAQUEST database. The resulting peptide sequence, VEHSDLSFSK was consistent with the peptide being derived from the protein $β_2$-microglobulin.

Surprisingly, this is a common protein found in human dialysate. At present it is not clear if the elevated levels of $β_2$-microglobulin interfere with phosphate uptake in renal epithelial cells or perhaps another minor component co-migrates with it. This problem is still under active investigation. Nevertheless, it is clear that mPC-CE-MS and tandem MS can play a significant role in rapidly and unequivocally identifying proteins.

5. FUTURE DIRECTIONS

The analysis of biologically derived peptides and proteins will continue to be dominated by the need for rapid analyses of complex mixtures at increasingly lower levels of analytes. This is particularly true for analytes in arenas such as clinical chemistry, toxicology, and forensics. Furthermore, developing practices in the area of proteomics will inevitably be more demanding of the sensitivity of analytical methods. Current practices demand that the sensitivity of protein sequencing methods is comparable to that of slab gel silver-staining techniques. While these approaches are yielding results, it is likely that many biologically significant proteins will not be detected or characterized. However, at the sensitivity levels that will be required in this area of research, sample manipulations become a major challenge. Both analyte losses and sample contamination by ubiquitous human proteins (such as keratin) become significant issues at picomolar concentrations. Automated preparation and analysis of low volume, low concentration samples of high complexity will be required to overcome these issues. Clean-room technology is also likely to become a major requirement of these investigations. Figeys and Abersold *(17)* recently proposed a solution to these issues. These investigators have suggested the use of coupled microfabricated, integrated analytical modules with mass spectrometry for this application, and they have recently proposed MFD-MS as the acronym for this technology. While research of these devices is in its infancy, such miniaturized approaches coupled with a sensitive mass spectrometer could

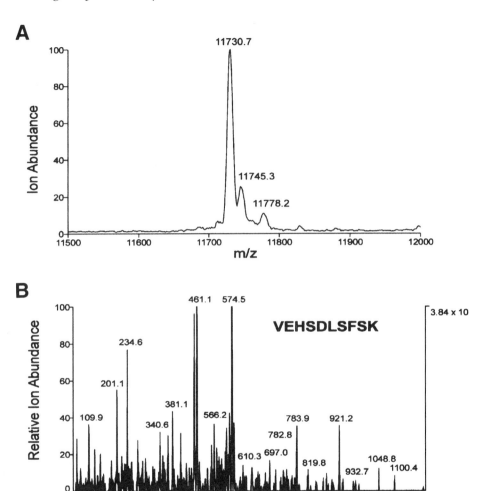

Fig. 8. Identification of human renal dialysate protein obtained from 200 L of dialysate by mPC-CE-MS and tandem MS. (**A**) mPC-CE-MS analysis of active fraction shown to inhibit phosphate uptake in renal epithelial cells. 20 μL of active fraction pressure injected onto an SDB membrane. Protein was eluted with 80:20 MeOH:H$_2$O. Separation was carried out on a bare fused silica capillary (50 μm × 78 cm) at a voltage of 15 kV. MS was performed on MAT 900 under similar conditions to those described in Fig. 7. (**B**) mPC-CE-MS/MS of precursor ion MH$_2^{2+}$ = 574.5 derived from lysine-C proteolytic digestion of protein (M$_r$ = 11,729 Daltons). 60 μL of lysine-C digest of protein was loaded onto an SDB membrane. Peptides were eluted with 60 nL 80:20 MeOH:H$_2$O between a LSB of 60 nL of 1% NH$_4$OH and TSB of 90 nL 2 mM NH$_4$OAc. All other conditions of CE capillary and MS/MS as described in Figs. 5 and 6, respectively.

provide the detection limits required in the next generation of proteomic studies. Furthermore, with careful design of the array, on-chip protein isolation, digestion, and analysis could be accommodated in this nano-environment. However, the use of nano-technologies will provide new challenges. First, creative coupling of the macro world of biochemistry to the nano-analytical environment will be required. In this regard, the lessons learned from the development of mPC-CE-MS and SPC-CE technologies should aid these studies. Particularly in the area of reducing potentially long sample injection times, caused by slow liquid flow rates in these nano-devices. The sensitivity of protein sequencing will also require further creative input. In this area, interfacing the microfabricated array to the mass spectrometer will need particular attention.

A further technology that is expected to improve MS sensitivity is the development of the highly sensitive electrospray time of flight (ESI-TOF-MS), electrospray quadrupole time of flight mass spectrometers (ESI-QTOF-MS), and quadrupole ion trap coupled with a reflecting time-of-flight instrument. The development of such instruments is well underway. In addition to high sensitivity, these instruments have a short duty cycle, which enables very fast data acquisition, with no loss of sensitivity. These instruments also provide a constant medium resolution (>5000 full width half maximum [fwhm] definition), and good mass accuracy. The use of isotopic labeling (as achieved when enzymatic protein digests are carried out in ^{18}O water) can aid peptide identification since MS/MS instruments allows ^{18}O enriched ions to be readily identified in spectra, facilitating peptide sequence identification.

In summary, it is clear that there will need to be a significant pursuit of more sensitivity for CE-MS. In this regard, MFD-MS may, with further development and possible coupling to a highly sensitive mass spectrometer (such as an ESI-TOF-MS), provide the technology that is needed for future generations of proteomic research. However, lessons learned in the macro world of CE-MS will need to be heeded as new MFDs and MS interfacing techniques are developed. In particular, input by material scientists may provide improved surfaces to prevent interaction and loss of peptides and proteins within the channels of MFDs. Assuming that these challenges will be overcome, technology for isolation, manipulation, digestion, and sequencing extremely low levels of biologically active peptides and proteins will become a reality within the next few years.

ACKNOWLEDGMENTS

We thank Mrs. Diana Ayerhart for her invaluable help in preparing this manuscript and the figures. We also thank Dr. David Wells (3M, St. Paul,

MN) for his assistance in providing us with the impregnated membranes. We also greatly acknowledge the contributions of our collaborators on the various projects described in this work, and they include Dr. Jerry Gleich (Department of Immunology, Mayo Clinic), Dr. Steve Jameson (University of Minnesota), Dr. Doug Johnson (Department of Ophthalmology, Mayo Clinic), and Dr. Raj Kumar (Department of Internal Medicine, Mayo Clinic). We also acknowledge funding from Finnigan MAT #1, Beckman Instruments, Vistakon, Blandin Foundation, and Mayo Foundation in order to carry out this work.

REFERENCES

1. Van de Goor, T., Apffel, A., Chakel, J., and Hancock, W. (1997) Capillary electrophoresis of peptides, in Handbook of Capillary Electrophoresis, 2nd ed. (Landers, J. P., ed.), John Wiley and Sons, New York, NY, pp. 214–258.
2. Pritchett, T. and Robey, F. A. (1997) Capillary electrophoresis of proteins, in Handbook of Capillary Electrophoresis, 2nd ed. (Landers, J. P., ed.), John Wiley and Sons, New York, NY, pp. 259–295.
3. Lloyd, D. K., Aubry, A. F., and De Lorenzi, E. (1997) Selectivity in capillary electrophoresis: the use of proteins (review). J. Chromatogr. A. 792, 349–369.
4. Baker, D. R. (1995) Capillary Electrophoresis. John Wiley and Sons, New York, NY, p. 244.
5. Wu, J. and Pawliszyn, J. (1994) Application of capillary isoelectric focusing with absorption imaging detection to the analysis of proteins. J. Chromatogr. B. 657, 327–332.
6. Liu, X., Sosic, Z., and Krull, I. S. (1996) Capillary isoelectric focusing as a tool in the examination of antibodies, peptides, and proteins of pharmaceutical interest. J. Chromatogr. A. 735, 165–190.
7. Clarke, N. J., Tomlinson, A. J., Schomberg, G., and Naylor, S. (1997) Capillary isoelectric focusing of physiologically derived proteins with on-line desalting of isotonic salt concentrations. Anal. Chem. 69, 2786–2792.
8. Pritchett, T. J. (1996) Capillary isoelectric focusing of proteins. Electrophoresis 17, 1195–1201.
9. Krivankova, L. and Bocek, P. (1998) Capillary isotachophoresis, in High Performance Capillary Electrophoresis: Theory, Techniques, and Applications, (Khaledi, M. G., ed.), John Wiley and Sons, New York, ACS Monograph Series, 146, pp. 251–275.
10. Shieh, P., Cooke, N., and Guttman, A. (1998) Capillary gel electrophoresis, in High Performance Capillary Electrophoresis: Theory, Techniques, and Applications (Khaledi, M. G., ed.), John Wiley and Sons, New York, ACS Monograph Series, 146, pp. 185–221.
11. Khaledi, M. G. (1998) Micellar electrokinetic chromatography, in High Performance Capillary Electrophoresis: Theory, Techniques, and Applications (Khaledi, M. G., ed.), John Wiley and Sons, New York, NY, ACS Monograph Series, 146, pp. 77–140.

12. Loo, J. A., Udseth, H. R., and Smith, R. D. (1989) Peptide and protein analysis by electrospray ionization-mass spectrometry and capillary electrophoresis-mass spectrometry. Anal. Biochem. 179, 404–412.

13. Rosnack, K. J., Stroh, J. G., Singleton, D. H., Guarino, B. C., and Andrews, G. C. (1994) Use of capillary electrophoresis-electrospray ionization mass spectrometry in the analysis of synthetic peptides. J. Chromatogr. A. 675, 219–225.

14. Severs, J. C, Hofstadler, S. A., Zhao, A., Senh, R. T., and Smith, R. D. (1996) The interface of capillary electrophoresis with high performance Fourier transform ion cyclotron resonance mass spectrometry for biomolecule characterization. Electrophoresis 17, 1808–1817.

15. Cole, R. B. (ed.) (1997) Electrospray Ionization Mass Spectrometry: Fundamentals Instrumentation and Applications. Wiley, New York, NY, p. 577.

16. Valaskovic, G. A., Kelleher, N. L., and McLafferty, F. W. (1996) Attomole protein characterization by capillary electrophoresis-mass spectrometry. Science 273, 1199–1202.

17. Figeys, D. and Aebersold, R. (1998) High sensitivity analysis of proteins and peptides by capillary electrophoresis-tandem mass spectrometry: recent developments in technology and applications. (Review) Electrophoresis 19, 885–892.

18. Naylor, S., Ji, Q., Johnson, K. L., Tomlinson, A. J., Kieper, W. C., and Jameson, S. C. (1998) Enhanced sensitivity for sequence determination of major histocompatibility complex class I peptides by membrane preconcentration-capillary electrophoresis-microspray-tandem mass spectrometry. Electrophoresis 19, 2207–2212.

19. Figeys, D., van Oostveen, I., Ducret, A., and Aebersold, R. (1996) Protein identification by capillary zone electrophoresis/microelectrospray ionization-tandem mass spectrometry at the subfemtomole level. Anal. Chem. 68, 1822–1828.

20. Hsieh, F., Baronas, E., Muir, C., and Martin, S. A. (1999) A novel nanospray capillary zone electrophoresis/mass spectrometry interface. Rapid Commun. Mass Spectrom. 13, 67–72.

21. Yates, J., III (1998) Mass spectrometry and the age of the proteome. J. Mass Spectrom. 33, 1–19.

22. Mann, M. and Wilm, M. (1994) Error-tolerant identification of peptides in sequence databases by peptide sequence tags. Anal. Chem. 66, 4390–4399.

23. Wilm, M. and Mann, M. (1996) Analytical properties of the nanoelectrospray ion source. Anal. Chem. 68, 1–8.

24. Smith, R. D., Olivares, J. A., Nguyen, N. T., and Udseth, H. R. (1988) Capillary zone electrophoresis-mass spectrometry using an electrospray ionization interface. Anal. Chem. 60, 436–441

25. Smith, R. D., Loo, J. A., Barinaga, C. J., Edmonds, C. G., and Udseth, H. R. (1989) Capillary zone electrophoresis and isotachophoresis-mass spectrometry of polypeptides and proteins based upon an electrospray ionization interface. J. Chromatogr. 480, 211–232.

26. Lee, E. D., Mueck, W., Henion, J. D., and Covey, T. R. (1988) On-line capillary zone electrophoresis in spray tandem mass spectrometry for the determination of dynorphins. J. Chromatogr. 458, 313–321.

27. Johannson, I. M., Huang, E. C., Henion, J. D., and Zweigenbaum, J. (1991) Capillary electrophoresis for the characterization of peptides. Instrumental considerations for mass spectrometeric detection. J. Chromatogr. 554, 311–327.

28. Cai, J. and Henion, J. D. (1995) Capillary electrophoresis-mass spectrometery. J. Chromatogr. 703, 667–692.

29. Smith, R. D., Udseth, H. R., Wahl, J. H., Goodlett, D. R., and Hofstadler, S. A. (1996) Capillary electrophoresis/mass spectrometry. Methods Enzymol. 271, 448–486.

30. Severs, C. J. and Smith R. D. (1997) Capillary electrophoresis–electrospray ionization–mass spectrometry, in Electrospray Ionization-Mass Spectrometry (Cole, R. B., ed.). Wiley, New York, NY, pp. 343–382.

31. Bank, J. F. (1997) Recent advances in capillary electrophoresis-electrospray-mass spectrometry. 18, 2255–2266.

32. Ding, J. and Vouros, P. (1999) Advances in CE/MS. Anal. Chem. 71, 378A–385A.

33. Cai, J. and El Rassi, Z. (1993) Selective on-line preconcentration of proteins by tandem metal chelate capillaries-capillary zone electrophoresis. J. Liq. Chromatogr. 16, 2007–2024.

34. Tomlinson, A. J., Guzman, N. A., and Naylor, S. (1995) Enhancement of concentration limits of detection in CE and CE-MS: a review of on-line sample extraction, cleanup, analyte preconcentration, and microreactor technology. J. Cap. Elect. 2, 247–266.

35. Wahl, J. H., Goodlett, D. R., Udseth, H. R., and Smith, R. D. (1992) Attomole level capillary electrophoresis-mass spectrometric protein analysis using 5-μm i.d. capillaries. Anal. Chem. 64, 3194–3196.

36. Moring, S. E., Colburn, J. C., Grossman, P. D., and Lauer, H. H. (1989) Analytical aspects of an autometed capillary electrophoresis system. LC-GC 8, 34–36.

37. Abersold, R. and Morrison, H. D. (1990) Analysis of dilute peptide samples by capillary zone electrophoresis. J. Chromatogr. 516, 79–88.

38. Schwer, C. and Lottspeich, F. (1992) Analytical and micropreparative separation of peptides by capillary zone electrophoresis using discontinuous buffer systems. J. Chromatogr. 623, 345–355.

39. Burgi, D. S. and Chien, R. (1991) Optimization in sample stacking for high performance capillary electrophoresis. Anal. Chem. 63, 2042–2047.

40. Chien, R. L. and Burgi, D. S. (1992) On-line sample concentration using field amplification in CZE. Anal. Chem. 64, 489A–496A.

41. Smith, R. D., Fields, S. M., Loo, J. A., Barinaga, C. J., Udseth, H. R., and Edmonds, C. G. (1990) Capillary isotachophoresis with UV and tandem mass spectrometry detection for peptides and proteins. Electrophoresis 11, 709–717.

42. Lamoree, M. H., Reinhoud, N. J., Tjaden, U. R., Niessen, W. M. A., and Van der Greef, J. (1994) On-capillary isotachophoresis for loadability enhancement in capillary zone electrophoresis/mass spectrometry of β-agonists, Biol. Mass Spectrom. 23, 339–345.

43. Thompson, T. J., Foret, F., Vouros, P., and Karger, B. L. (1993) Capillary electrophoresis/electrospray ionization mass spectrometry: improvement of protein detection limits using on-column transient isotachophoretic sample preconcentration. Anal. Chem. 65, 900–906.
44. Tomlinson, A. J., Benson, L. M., Guzman, N. A., and Naylor, S. (1996) Preconcentration and microreaction technology on-line with capillary electrophoresis. J. Chromatogr. 744, 3–15.
45. Tomlinson, A. J. and Naylor, S. (1995) Enhanced performance membrane preconcentration-capillary electrophoresis-mass spectrometry (mPC-CE-MS) in conjunction with transient isotachophoresis to analyze peptide mixtures. J. High Resol. Chromatogr. 18, 384–386.
46. Tomlinson, A. J. and Naylor S. (1995) Systematic development of on-line membrane preconcentration-capillary electrophoresis-mass spectrometry (mPC-CE-MS) for the analysis of peptide mixtures. J. Cap. Elec. 2, 225–233.
47. Tomlinson, A. J. and Naylor, S. (1995) A strategy for sequencing peptides from dilute mixtures at the low femtomole level using membrane preconcentration capillary electrophoresis tandem mass spectrometry. J. Liq. Chromatogr. 18, 3591–3615.
48. Naylor, S. and Tomlinson, A. J. (1996) Membrane preconcentration-capillary electrophoresis-mass spectrometry in the analysis of biologically derived metabolites and biopolymers. Biomed. Chromatogr. 10, 325–330.
49. Kurian, E., Prendergast, F. G., Tomlinson, A. J., Holmes, M. W., and Naylor, S. (1997) Identifying sites of protein modification by using matrix assisted laser desorption/ionization-time of flight-mass spectrometry and on-line membrane preconcentration-capillary electrophoresis-tandem mass spectrometry. J. Amer. Soc. Mass Spectrom. 8, 8–14.
50. Tomlinson, A. J., Benson, L. M., Jameson, S., Johnson, D. H., and Naylor, S. (1997) Utility of membrane preconcentration-capillary electrophoresis-mass spectrometry in overcoming limited sample loading for analysis of biologically derived drug metabolites, peptides, and proteins. J. Amer. Soc. Mass Spectrom. 8, 15–24.
51. Naylor, S. and Tomlinson, A. J. (1998) Membrane preconcentration-capillary electrophoresis-tandem mass spectrometry (mPC-CE-MS/MS) in the sequence analysis of biologically derived peptides. Talanta 45, 603–612.
52. Weinberger, R. (1993) Practical Capillary Electrophoresis. Academic, San Diego, CA, p. 312.
53. Kohr, J. and Engelhardt, H. (1993) Capillary electrophoresis with coated capillaries. Chromatogr. Sci. Ser. 64, 357.
54. Madgassi, S. and Kamyshni, A. (1996) Surface activity and functional properties of proteins, in Surface Activity of Proteins (Madgassi, S., ed.), Marcel Dekker, New York, p. 2.
55. Chiari, M., Nesi, M., and Righetti, P. G. (1996) Surface modifications of silica walls: a review of different methodologies, in Capillary Electrophoresis in Biotechnology (Righetti, P. G., ed.), CRC, Boca Raton, FL, pp. 1–36.

56. Thibault, P., Paris, C., and Pleasance, S. (1991) Analysis of peptides and proteins by capillary electrophoresis/mass spectrometry using acidic buffers and coated capillaries. Rapid Commun. Mass Spectrom. 5, 484–490.
57. Schomburg, G. (1998) Coated capillaries in high performance capillary electrophoresis, in High Performance Capillary Electrophoresis: Theory, Techniques, and Applications (Khaledi, M. G., ed.), John Wiley and Sons, New York, ACS Monograph Series, 146, pp. 481–523.
58. Naylor, S. Benson, L. M., and Tomlinson, A. J. (1994) Capillary zone electrophoresis for the analysis of small molecules: practical considerations. J. Cap. Elec. 3, 181–189.
59. Johnson, K. L., Tomlinson, A. J., and Naylor, S. (1996) Capillary conditioning and electrospray ionization for optimal capillary electrophoresis/mass spectrometry performance. Rapid Commun. Mass Spectrom. 10, 1159, 1160.
60. McCormick, R. M. (1994) Capillary zone electrophoresis of peptides, in Handbook of Capillary Electrophoresis: A Practical Approach, 1st ed. (Landers, J. P., ed.), CRC, Boca Raton, FL, pp. 287–323.
61. Kelly, J. F., Locke, S. J., Ramaley, L., and Thibault, P. (1996) Development of electrophoretic conditions for the characterization of protein glycoforms by capillary electrophoresis-electrospray mass spectrometry. J. Chromatogr. A 720, 409–427.
62. Rohde, E., Tomlinson, A. J., Johnson, D. H., and Naylor, S. (1998) Protein analysis by membrane preconcentration-capillary electrophoresis: systematic evaluation of parameters affecting preconcentration and separation. J. Chromatogr. B. 713, 301–311.
63. Rohde, E., Tomlinson, A. J., Johnson, D. H., and Naylor, S. (1998) Comparison of protein mixtures in aqueous humor by membrane preconcentration-capillary electrophoresis-mass spectrometry (mPC-CE-MS). Electrophoresis 19, 2361–2370.
64. Rohde, E., Tomlinson, A. J., Johnson, D. H., and Naylor, S. Evaluation of capillary coating for the capillary electrophoresis separation of proteins in aqueous humor. Biomed. Chromatogr. (Submitted)
65. Chien, R.-L. (1998) Sample introduction and stacking, in High Performance Capillary Electrophoresis: Theory, Techniques, and Applications (Khaledi, M. G., ed.), John Wiley and Sons, New York, ACS Monograph Series, 146, pp. 449–479.
66. Lewis, K. C., Opitack, G. J., Jorgenson, J. W., and Sheeley, D. M. (1997) Comprehensive on-line RPLC-CZE-MS of peptides. J. Amer. Soc. Mass Spectrom. 8, 495–500.
67. McComb, M. E., Krutchinsky, A. N., Ens, W., Standing, K. G., and Perreault, H. (1998) Sensitive high resolution analysis of biological molecules by capillary zone electrophoresis coupled with reflecting time-of-flight mass spectrometry. J. Chromatogr. 800, 1–11.
68. Licklider, L., Kuhr, W. G., Lacy, M. P., Keough, T., Purdon, M. P., and Takigiku, R. (1995) On-line microreactors/capillary electrophoresis/mass spectrometry for the analysis of proteins and peptides. Anal. Chem. 67, 4170–4177.

69. Amankwa, L. N. and Kuhr, W. G. (1993) On-line peptide mapping by capillary zone electrophoresis. Anal. Chem. 65, 2693–2697.
70. Stegehuis, D. S., Irth, H., Tjaden, U. R., and van der Greef, J. (1991) Isotachophoresis as an on-line concentration pretreatment technique in capillary electrophoresis. J. Chromatogr. 538, 393–402.
71. Tinke, A. P., Reinhoud, N. J., Niessen, W. M. A., Tjaden, U. R., and van der Greef, J. (1992) On-line isotachophoretic analyte focusing for improved detection limits in capillary electrophoresis/electrospray mass spectrometry. Rapid Commun. Mass Spectrom. 6, 560–563.
72. Kirby, D. P., Thorne, J. M., Gotzinger, W. K., and Karger, B. L. (1996) A CE/ESI-MS interface for stable, low-flow operation. Anal. Chem. 68, 4451–4457.
73. Tang, Q., Harrata, A. K., and Lee, C. (1995) Capillary isoelectric focusing-electrospray mass spectrometry for protein analysis. Anal. Chem. 67, 3515–3519.
74. Lamoree, M. H., Tjaden, U. R., and van der Greef, J. (1997) Use of microdialysis for the on-line choupling of capillary isoelectric focusing with electrospray mass spectrometry. J. Chromatogr. A. 777, 31–39.
75. Clarke, N. J., Tomlinson, A. J., and Naylor, S. (1997) On-line desalting of physiologically derived fluids in conjunction with capillary isoelectric focusing-mass spectrometry. J. Amer. Soc. Mass Spectrom. 8, 743–748.
76. Clarke, N. J., Croy, C. L., Tomlinson, A. J., and Naylor, S. Capillary isoelectric focusing (cIEF-MS) as an efficient method for the analysis of biologically derived protein mixtures, Anal. Biochem. (Submitted)
77. Guzman, N. A., Park, S. S., Schaufelberger, D., Hernandez, L., Paez, X., Rada, P., Tomlinson, A. J., and Naylor, S. (1997) New approaches in clinical chemistry: on-line analyte concentration and microreaction capillary electrophoresis for the determination of drugs, metabolic intermediates and biopolymers in biological fluids. J. Chromatogr. B 697, 37–66.
78. Ren, X. and Liu, P. Z. (1996) Cellulose modified polypropylene hollow fibers for capillary electrophoresis. J. Microcol. Sep. 8, 529–534.
79. Ren, X., Liu, P. Z., Malik, A., and Lee, M. L. (1996) Hydrophilic polymer-modified polypropylene hollow fibers with controllable electroosmotic flow for capillary electrophoresis. J. Microcol. Sep. 8, 535–540.
80. Fridstrom, A., Lundell, N., Ekstrom, B., and Markides, K. E. (1997) Dextran-modified polypropylene hollow fibers for use in capillary electrophoresis. J. Microcol. Sep. 9, 1–7.
81. Smith, R. D., Wahl, J. H., Goodlett, D. R., and Hofstadler, S. A. (1993) Capillary electrophoresis/mass spectrometry. Anal. Chem. 65, 574A–584A.
82. Hofstadler, S. A., Wahl, J. H., Bruce, J. E., and Smith, R. D. (1993) On-line capillary electrophoresis with Fourier transform ion cyclotron resonance mass spectrometry. J. Am. Chem. Soc. 115, 6983,6984.
83. Perkins, J. R., Parker, C. E., and Tomer, K. B. (1993) The characterization of snake venoms using capillary electrophoresis in conjunction with electrospray mass spectrometry: black mambas. Electrophoresis 14, 458–468.

84. Cole, R. B., Varghese, J., McCormick, R. M., and Kadlecek, D. (1994) Evaluation of a novel hydrophilic derivatized capillary for protein analysis of biological electrophoresis-electrospray mass spectrometry, J. Chromatogr. A 680, 363–373.

85. Hofstadler, S. A., Swanek, F. D., Gale, D. C., Ewing, A. G., and Smith, R. D. (1995) Capillary electrophoresis-electrospray ionization Fourier transform ion cyclotron resonance mass spectrometry for direct analysis of cellular proteins. Anal. Chem. 67, 1477–1480.

86. Kelly, J. F., Locke, S. J., Ramaley, L., and Tibault, P. (1996) Development of electrophoretic conditions for the characterization of protein glycoforms by capillary electrophoresis-electrospray mass spectrometry. J. Chromatogr. A 720, 409–427.

87. Figeys, D. and Aebersold, R. (1997) Capillary electrophoresis of peptides and proteins at neutral pH in capillaries covalently coated with polyethyleneimine. J. Chromatogr. B 695, 163–168.

88. Moseley, M. A., Jorgenson, J. W., Shabanowitz, J., Hunt, D. F., and Tomer, K. B. (1992) Optimization of capillary zone electrophoresis electrospray parameters for the mass spectrometry and tandem mass spectrometry of proteins. J. Am. Soc. Mass Spetrom. 3, 289–300.

89. Wahl, J. H. and Smith, R. D. (1994) Comparison of buffer systems and interface designs for capillary electrophoresis-mass spectrometry. J. Cap. Elec. 1, 62–71.

90. Yang, Q., Benson, L. M., Johnson, K. L., and Naylor, S. (1999) Analysis of lipophilic peptides and therapeutic drugs: on-line-nonaqueous capillary electrophoresis-mass spectrometry. J. Biochem. Biophys. Methods 38, 103–121.

91. Johnson, K. L., Tomlinson, A. J., Benson, L. M., and Naylor, S. (1997) Capillary electrophoresis using non-aqueous media interface with electrospray ionization mass spectrometer: analysis of hydrophobic peptide on uncoated CE capillaries. Finnigan MAT Application Note.

92. Tomer, K. B., Parker, C. E., and Deterding, L. J. (1998) High performance capillary electrophoresis-mass spectrometry, in High Performance Capillary Electrophoresis: Theory, Techniques, and Applications (Khaledi, M. G., ed.), Wiley, New York, NY, ACS Monograph Series, 146, 405–446.

93. Foret, F., Thompson, T. J., Vouros, P., and Karger, B. L. (1994) Liquid sheath effects on the separation of proteins in capillary electrophoresis/electrospray mass spectrometry. Anal. Chem. 66, 4450–4458.

94. Kriger, M. S., Cook, K. D., and Rasmey, R. S. (1995) Durable gold-coated fused silica capillaries for use in electrospray mass spectrometry. Anal. Chem. 67, 385–389.

95. Herring, C. J. and Qin, J. (1999) An on-line preconcentrator and the evaluation of electrospray interfaces for the capillary electrophoresis/mass spectrometry of peptides. Rapid. Commun. Mass Spectrom. 13, 1–7.

96. Gilpin, R. K. and Pachla, L. A. (1999) Pharmaceuticals and related drugs. Anal. Chem. 71, 217R–233R.

97. Anderson, D. J. (1999) Clinical chemistry. Anal. Chem. 71, 293R–372R.

98. Brettell, T. A., Inman, K., Rudin, N., and Saferstein, R. (1999) Forensic science. Anal. Chem. 71, 235R–255R.
99. Perkins, J. R. and Tomer, K. B. (1995) Characterization of the lower-molecular-mass fraction of venoms from *Dendroaspis jamesoni kaimosae* and *Micrurus fulvius* using capillary-electrophoresis electrospray mass spectrometry. Eur. J. Biochem. 233, 815–827.
100. Afifiyan, F., Armugam, A., Gopalakrishnakone, P., Tan, N. H., Tan, C. H., and Jeyaseelan, K. (1998) Four new postsynaptic neurotoxins from *Naja naja sputatrix* venom: cDNA cloning, protein expression, and phylogenetic analysis. Toxicon. 36, 1871–1885.
101. Ensing, K., de Boer, T., Schreuder, N., and de Zeeuw, R. A. (1999) Separation and identification of neuropeptide Y, two of its fragments and their degradation products using capillary electrophoresis mass spectrometry. J. Chromatogr. B. 727, 53–61.
102. Hennebicq, S., Tetaert, D., Soudan, B., Boersma, A., Briand, G., Richet, C., et al. (1998) Influence of the amino acid sequence on the MUC5ACmotif peptide O-glycosylation by human gastric UDP-GalNAc:polypeptide N-acetylgalactosaminyltransferase(s). Glycoconjugate J. 15, 275–282.
103. Hennebicq, S., Tetaert, D., Soudan, B., Briand, G., Richet, C., Demeyer, D., et al. (1998) Polypeptide: N-acetylgalactosaminyltransferase activities towards the mucin MUC5AC peptides motif using microsomal preparations of normal and tumoral digestive mucosa. Biochimie 80, 69–73.
104. Wei, J., Yang, L., Harrata, A. K., and Lee, C. S. (1998) High resolution analysis of protein phosphorylation using capillary isoelectric focusing-electrospray ionization-mass spectrometry. Electrophoresis 19, 2356–2360.
105. Jenson, P. K., Pasa-Tolic, L., Anderson, G. A., Horner, J. A., Lipton, M. S., Bruce, J. E., and Smith, R. D. (1999) Probing proteomes using capillary isoelectric focusing-electrospray ionization Fourier transform ion cyclotron resonance mass spectrometry. Anal. Chem. 71, 2076–2084.
106. Yang, Q., Tomlinson, A. J., and Naylor, S. (1999) Membrane preconcentration CE. Anal. Chem. 4, 183A–189A.
107. Tomlinson, A. J., Benson, L. M., Oda, R. P., Braddock, W. D., Riggs, B. L., Katzmann, J. A., and Naylor, S. (1995) Novel modifications and clinical applications of preconcentration-capillary electrophoresis-mass spectrometry. J. Cap. Elec. 2, 97–104.
108. Tomlinson, A. J., Benson, L. M., Jameson, S., and Naylor, S. (1996) Rapid loading of large sample volumes, analyte cleanup, and modified moving boundary transient isotachophoresis conditions for membrane preconcentration-capillary electrophoresis in small diameter capillaries. Electrophoresis 17, 1801–1807.
109. Tomlinson, A. J., Jameson, S., and Naylor, S. (1996) Strategy for isolating and sequencing biologically derived MHC class I peptides, J. Chromatogr. A. 744, 273–278.
110. Hogquist, K. A., Tomlinson, A. J., Kieper, W. C., McGargill, M. A., Hart, M. C., Naylor, S., and Jameson, S. C. (1997) Identification of a naturally occurring ligand for thymic positive selection. Immunity 6, 389–399.

111. Jonsher, K. R. and Yates, J. R. (1997) A novel and versatile liquid junction for microspray, CE, and membrane chromatography applications. Proceedings of the 45th ASMS Conference on MS and Allied Topics, Palm Springs, CA, June 1–5, 1997, p. 1192.

112. Naylor, S., Tomlinson, A. J., Londowski, J. M., and Kumar, R. (1996) Structural Characterization of Human Renal Dialysate Protein by mPC-CE-MS/MS. Proceedings of the 44th ASMS Conference on Mass Spectrometry and Allied Topics, Portland, OR, USA, May 12–16, 1996, p. 934.

17
Serum Drug Monitoring by Capillary Electrophoresis

Z. K. Shihabi

1. INTRODUCTION

Since it was found few decades ago that optimization of serum antiepileptic drug levels reduced the number of seizures and drug side effects, the field of therapeutic drug monitoring (TDM) has flourished. Historically TDM started with the spectrophotometric analysis of phenobarbital and phenytoin. However, due to the inability to use spectral data to differentiate closely related drugs, chromatographic techniques such as gas chromatography (GC) and high-performance liquid chromatography (HPLC) were introduced. These methods required skill, sample preparation, and a long turn-around time (TAT) from receipt of sample to reporting of results. Thus despite their high cost, immunoassays, which provided quicker TAT, have slowly replaced chromatographic methods. Although easier to perform and suited for automation, immunoassays are usually not available when a new drug is first released to use in the treatment of patients.

Capillary electrophoresis (CE) is a very versatile technique and can potentially be used to analyze not only the drug but also its metabolites. In fact, drug analysis represents one of the best potential applications of CE. However, as with any analytical method, CE has not only advantages but also drawbacks. The advantages and disadvantages of CE and the types of drugs suited for analysis by this technique are discussed in this chapter. In general, CE offers speed, ease of analysis, low cost of operation, and very high resolution. CE can also offer basic information on the physicochemical properties of the drug such as protein binding and ionization. However, it suffers from matrix effects (especially when using serum), poor detection limits, and less than desirable precision. To use CE successfully for the

From: *Clinical and Forensic Applications of Capillary Electrophoresis*
Edited by: J. R. Petersen and A. A. Mohammad © Humana Press Inc., Totowa, NJ

analysis of drugs, four areas require careful attention: 1) choice of the separation type (CZE, MEKC, Chiral); 2) sample preparation (especially critical for serum samples); 3) instrument setup (optimum voltage, maximum injection volume); and 4) precision (choice of capillary wash and internal standards). These points will be discussed in this chapter.

2. COMPARISON OF CE AND HPLC

In the past, small molecules, such as drugs, have not been analyzed by electrophoretic techniques due to the lack of sensitivity. Generally, drugs were analyzed by chromatographic techniques, such as HPLC, that are based on the interaction of the compound with the column packing (e.g., hydrophobicity). CE, on the other hand, utilizes charge (directly or indirectly) to separate and identify the drug of interest.

Several studies have shown that for TDM, CE is better than HPLC, being faster and easier to use (1–6). CE also has better resolution (7), especially for polar compounds (5), and costs less to operate (7). Wynia et al. (6) determined the precision, linearity, ruggedness, and detection limits for CE and HPLC using the antidepressant drug mirtazapine. They found that the relative standard deviation (RSD) for CE was higher than that for HPLC, 0.6 vs 0.2, respectively. The linearity for CE (10–1400 µg/mL) was also different than HPLC (4–800 µg/mL). Altria and Bestford (8) reviewed the analysis of a variety of pharmaceuticals and found that CE has many advantages over HPLC. Many researchers have also found that CE has advantages in terms of reduced sample pretreatment, consumable costs, and analysis time. Additionally, CE has the ability to separate a wide range of compounds using a single set of operating conditions. Most workers however, agree that in general HPLC tends to give better precision and better sensitivity.

Because CE and HPLC can analyze the same molecules, in many instances they can seem complementary to each other. CE is better suited for the analysis of polar or charged compounds with high molar absorbitivity or those that are present in a relatively high concentration. Nonpolar compounds or those with low molar absorbitivity may be better analyzed by HPLC. However, by using a combination of stacking methods and special flow cells with extended light path, CE can achieve sensitivity close to that found for HPLC.

3. CE PROBLEMS FOR TDM

The poor sensitivity and matrix effects are two major problems that may seem insurmountable to newcomers to the field of CE. This is especially true for TDM. In addition, CE also has less than desirable reproducibility. These problems and how to overcome them are discussed later.

3.1. Sensitivity

Owing to the narrow path length of the detection window in the capillary, the absorbance signal in CE is not very strong. Sometimes in order to improve the separation efficiency (theoretical plate number) or to speed up the analysis, the capillary diameter is decreased. This in turn causes a further decrease in the signal. To overcome this problem, capillaries with an extended light path, e.g., Z-cell, bubble cell, or the high sensitivity cell, have been developed for some CE instruments. Even with these new detection windows, many of the drugs routinely analyzed for TDM are present in serum at concentration of 0.01–1 mg/L, well below the detection limits. Thus, the majority of the drugs have to be concentrated before analysis by CE, either on or outside the capillary. Fortunately electrophoretic techniques offer a very simple means called stacking to concentrate the analyte directly on the capillary.

Initial studies with two commonly used drugs, theophylline and phenobarbital, have demonstrated that detection of therapeutic levels are attainable with simple stacking methods and little sample preparation. Some drugs, however, still require complex extraction and concentration steps.

3.2. Matrix Effects

In CE, unlike most other techniques, many basic parameters such as resolution, plate number, migration time, and precision are greatly affected by the sample matrix, especially when inorganic ions or proteins are present. As the sample size increases, matrix effects become more significant *(9)*. Generally CE easily analyzes pure standards. However, analysis of serum samples, the usual sample matrix for TDM is more difficult. The salts present in serum (~150 mmol/L) affect the field strength and consequently the velocity of the analyte causing band broadening. Proteins in the serum (~60 g/L), on the other hand, bind to the capillary walls *(9)*, producing secondary interactions, and affecting the reproducibility of the method.

4. FORMS OF CE USED TO SEPARATE DRUGS

In the analysis of drugs and other small molecules, three basic forms of CE, capillary zone electrophoresis (CZE), micellar electrokinetic capillary chromatography (MEKC), and chiral separation are often used.

4.1. Capillary Zone Electrophoresis (CZE)

In CZE, separation is based on charge of the analyte in a buffered solution. The method is used for analysis of drugs that either have a positive or negative charge.

4.2. Micellar Electrokinetic Capillary Chromatography (MEKC)

MEKC is where separation is based on the differential distribution of the drug of interest between the aqueous phase and micelles formed using a surfactant such as sodium dodecyl sulfate (SDS). Separation in this system is based on hydrophobicity. This method can be used for analysis of neutral as well as charged molecules. Serum can be injected directly, provided the migration of the serum proteins does not overlap with the drugs being analyzed. The correct amount of SDS, ionic strength of the buffer, and modifiers are manipulated to achieve this effect *(1,10,11)*.

4.3. Chiral Separation

Chiral separation is a form of CE where special additives, e.g., cyclodextrins (CD) or proteins, are incorporated into the separation buffer affecting the migration of one isomer more than the other isomer. Chiral separation by CE is much easier to perform than by HPLC. To date, it is most often used in the pharmaceutical industry and has yet to be used in TDM.

5. SERUM SAMPLE PREPARATION

One of the advantages of CE is the simplicity of the sample preparation. For example, sometimes the sample can be introduced directly without preparation. However, due to matrix effects, analysis of drugs in serum often requires special preparation such as dilution, protein precipitation, or extraction. Drugs such as the antifungal fluconazole have been analyzed after a variety of sample preparation methods *(7)* to illustrate the differences in speed, linearity, detection limits, and precision. For example, direct injection of plasma or supernatant after protein precipitation by acetonitrile has detected fluconazole levels of >5 µg/mL. Using liquid–liquid extraction (dichloromethane), the detection limit is about 1 µg/mL. However by using disposable solid-phase C18 cartridges and 1 mL of plasma to extract the drug, levels as low as 0.1 µg/mL can be detected.

For MEKC, if the drug concentration is high enough the serum can be simply diluted in buffer before injection onto the capillary (direct serum analysis), minimizing the matrix effects. This is because the small amounts of serum are solubilized by the micelles of the surfactant. Thormann and colleagues *(12,13)* have successfully applied this technique to the analysis of several drugs such as theophylline, caffeine, and barbiturates by directly injecting serum. Similarly, we applied this technique in the analysis of the new antiepileptic drug felbamate *(1)* (*see* Fig. 1). The simplicity, high resolving power, and the small sample size used for the assay render this method suitable for monitoring the levels of these drugs in pediatric patients (Fig. 1).

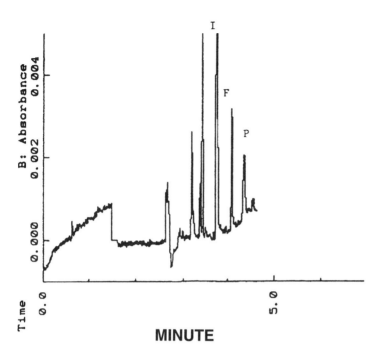

Fig. 1. Felbamate analysis by CE with direct serum injection after the addition of an internal standard. Patient receiving felbamate (53 mg/L, F) and phenobarbital (18 mg/L, P), (I, internal standard). CE Analysis (Beckman CE): equal volumes of serum and the internal standard (acetacetanilide 200 mg/L,I) were mixed and injected on the instrument. Capillary 50 cm × 50 μm. Wavelength 214 nm, fixed current at 38 uA, pressure injection 5 s. Buffer, boric acid 100 m*M*, pH 8.4, containing 55.4 m*M* SDS. (Adapted with permission from ref *[1]*).

In CZE, small amounts of proteins (<3 g/L) can be tolerated provided the ionic strength of the buffer is high enough and the capillary is washed thoroughly with sodium hydroxide after each injection. Ions in the sample also decrease the field strength and can cause band broadening. To minimize these effects, the sample is diluted in a low ionic strength buffer while the ionic strength of the electrophoresis buffer is increased (typically >100 m*M*) *(14,15)*. If the protein concentration is too high, they can bind to the capillaries, modifying the surface charge and affect the separation of subsequent samples. Proteins can be removed before injecting the sample by precipitation with acids, heavy metal ions, or alcohols. However, acids and heavy metals ions add salt to the sample that can degrade the separation.

To overcome the problem of sample matrix, several strategies have been developed by using membranes, protein precipitation, and extraction methods.

5.1. Use of Membranes

Membranes with a low molecular weight cut-off can be used to remove proteins and other large molecules. However, salts that can interfere in the separation remain in the filtrate. Membrane filters are also relatively expensive, and can require a long time to filter the serum. As an example, the membrane filters have been used in the analysis of serum nitrate by CE *(16)*. Membrane filtration to remove protein bound drugs can also be used to separate free drugs for further analysis by CE *(17)* (*see* Fig. 2).

5.2. Protein Precipitation

Precipitation of proteins by acetonitrile is an effective and simple method to pre-treat serum samples for analysis by CZE. In addition to removing proteins, acetonitrile, also permits injection of a large volume of sample (5–20% of the capillary volume) leading to 5–20-fold concentration by the capillary because of "stacking," as discussed later. The use of this simple method of concentration allows many drugs to be determined at concentrations of approaching 0.5 mg/L. Deproteinization also decreases the need for washing of the capillary between samples, thus speeding the analysis. This method, however, is limited to analysis of small molecules by the CZE and is not suitable for MEKC *(9,18)*.

5.3. Extraction

Use of an organic solvent or by a solid phase to extract drugs from serum also removes the proteins and salts present. In addition to sample clean-up, extraction methods can also be used to concentrate the drug. In routine analysis, solvent and solid-phase extractions followed by solvent evaporation are usually avoided as much as possible because of the time, labor, and skill required. However, drugs present in serum below 1 mg/L usually require extraction and concentration. Different strategies of sample pretreatment and methods for direct injection of bio-fluids for drug analysis by CE have been recently reviewed by Lloyd *(19)*.

6. CONCENTRATION BY CAPILLARY STACKING

As mentioned earlier in this chapter, electrophoretic techniques offer a relatively simple means to concentrate the sample directly on the capillary by injecting a large volume of sample. Under nonstacking conditions, the sample volume is kept below 1% of the capillary volume. However this volume can be increased to 10–30% of the capillary volume using stacking conditions. The drug "stacks" at the interface of the injection buffer and the run buffer (*see also* Chapter 2 for a more detailed discussion). This helps to

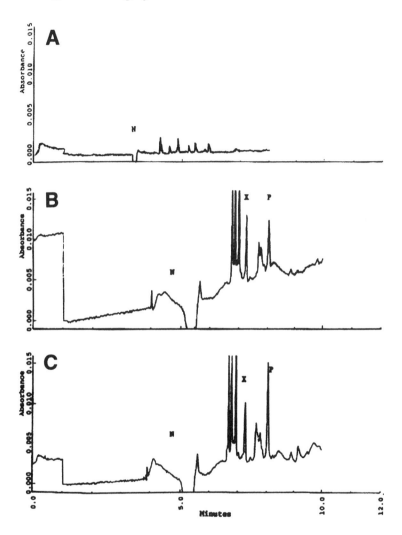

Fig. 2. Analysis of serum free phenytoin (P) from a patient (1.8 mg /L) using a Beckman CE Model 2000. Serum was filtered in a Centrifree filter (Amicon, Beverly, MA), 50 µL of the filtrate was removed, mixed with 100 µL acetonitrile containing 2 mg/L isobutyl methylxanthine (X) as an internal standard, and injected on a capillary: 50 µm × 40 cm at 9 kV (N, neutral molecules).The separation buffer, borate 300 m*M*, pH 8.7. **(A)** The patient at loading of 1%, 214 nm. **(B)** The patient at 10%. **(C)** The patient at 10% loading spike with 2.5 mg/L. (Note that injecting the traditional small volume of sample <1% of the capillary does not give enough sensitivity to detect the free phenytoin. Increasing the sample volume to 10% of the capillary gives good sensitivity provided acetonitrile is present in the sample. In the absence of acetonitrile *(18)* the peaks are short, distorted, and overlap, not shown.)

alleviate the poor detection limits of CE. Stacking, however, requires careful planning and an understanding of the method. For example, the field strength should be very high in the injected sample relative to the electrophoresis buffer so the drugs migrate rapidly to the solvent interface before the separation step takes place. Buffers, that do not generate much Joule heating, such as, e.g., borate, become important for this step *(20)*. Methods have been described for stacking by: low ionic strength buffer in the sample, stacking by inclusion of acetonitrile in the sample, and isotachophoresis. Stacking in MEKC is more difficult but a few methods have been described recently.

6.1. Low Ionic Strength Buffers

Dissolving the sample in the separation buffer, but at a 10 times lower ionic strength, or conversely, by injecting a small plug of water before the sample, increases the peak height 3–10 times by stacking *(9,21)* (*see* Fig. 3B). A similar stacking can be obtained in the electrokinetic injection (Field Amplified Injection), provided the sample matrix is free from salts. For example, Zhang et al. *(22)* used this technique to increase the sensitivity for amiodarone analysis by several orders of magnitude. This type of on-column stacking is best suited for analysis of compounds present in a clean matrix, e.g., extracted samples.

6.2. Acetonitrile-Salt

Addition of acetonitrile to the sample (not in the electrolyte) leads to stacking, especially when inorganic salts are present at concentration of ~1% *(9,18,20,23)*. Thus, acetonitrile stacking is useful for samples with physiological amounts of salts and proteins such as serum. The acetonitrile and salts (~50 mmol/L of NaCl in the final mixture) allow for increasing the sample size (using hydrodynamic injection) up to 50% of the capillary volume, yielding a 5–20-fold concentration.

Acetonitrile stacking depends on several factors, such as the pH and ions in the sample *(20)*, in addition to the ionic strength of the separation buffer *(18)*. Weakly anionic compounds are easier to stack using acetonitrile in borate buffer compared to cationic compounds. The latter group stacks better in buffers containing amines and zwitterions *(24)*. Stacking by acetonitrile, as illustrated in Fig. 3D, allows many drugs to be analyzed in serum at the low level of ~0.5 mg/L. In this figure, the relative width of the drug peak to that of the neutral molecules indicates visually the degree of stacking achieved by this method.

6.3. Field-Amplified Injection in Presence of Salts

Recently, we found that electrokinetic injection in presence of physiological amounts of salts (~1%) can give sharp peaks provided the sample con-

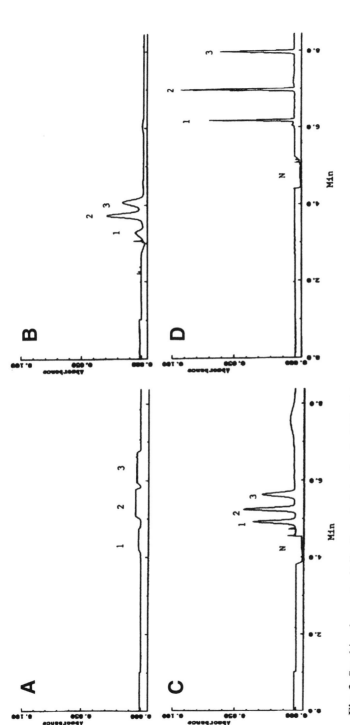

Fig. 3. Stacking by acetonitrile. Sample injection is 17% of the capillary volume. The compounds iohexol (1), theophylline (2), and phenobarbital (3) were dissolved in: (**A**) the separation buffer (borate 250 m*M*, pH 8.9, non-stacking), (**B**) the separation buffer at 25 m*M*, (**C**) acetonitrile-water (2:1 [v:v]), (**D**) acetonitrile-1% NaCl (2:1 [v:v]). Adapted with permission from ref. *(18)*. (Note that usually the sample size is kept <1% of the capillary volume to get sharp peaks. Here, the sample size is increased to 17%.)

tains 66% acetonitrile. The advantage of this type of injection over the previous hydrodynamic injection is a better theoretical plate number.

6.4. Transient Isotachophoresis

Isotachophoresis (*see* Chapter 2 for a detail description) is a powerful method for concentrating drugs on the capillary. It is well-suited for samples with a high salt content. However, coupling it to CE is difficult. A transient isotachophoretic step or self-stacking occurring in the early stages of the electrophoresis is more practical. Under these conditions a suitable, complementary ion is added to the sample to act as a leading/terminating ion *(25–27)* and a large volume is injected. The conditions for ITP can be fulfilled before the separation is changed to CZE. Knowledge of migration rate of the different ions and a clever choice of the buffers are important for the success of this technique.

6.5. Stacking in MEKC

Stacking in MEKC is more difficult than in CZE. However, several methods have been described recently by Terabe and others. They are based on solubilizing neutral molecules in micelles with accelerated micelle migration using a lower conductivity matrix. For example, Quirino and Terabe *(28)* described the use of low conductivity in the sample (dissolved in water) in the normal injection mode. Liu et al. *(29)* dissolved the sample in a solution containing SDS with a concentration lower than the separation buffer and injected at a negative polarity. After a brief period needed for analyte stacking and removal of the sample matrix, the polarity is switched to positive for separation and detection. Quirino and Terabe *(30)* have also described a similar stacking method, including the use of high molecular weight surfactants. They also described a simpler approach by using reversed-migration micelles for stacking *(31)*. In this technique, the pH of the separation buffer is acidic so the micelles have a higher electrophoretic velocity than the electroosmotic flow (EOF). A large sample, prepared in water or dilute buffer, is injected under reversed polarity allowing a concentration factor of ~100-fold.

7. PRECISION

The precision of both peak area (used for quantification) and migration time (used for identification) in CE is not as good as that in HPLC. However, studies aimed at understanding this problem will improve precision, as has been the case with other emerging techniques.

In many instances, imprecision in migration time is related to the interaction of the compound with the capillary wall and to changes in the EOF.

Fortunately, in CE the migration time is more predictable than the peak height (area). By employing one or more references points or internal standards, precision can be improved *(32)*. Dose and Guichon *(33)* reported that a RSD of 1% for migration time and peak area is possible by using two internal standards. Siren et al. *(34)* also showed that using multiple standards whose migration time closely brackets the compound being analyzed improves the reproducibility to <1%. Migration time can also be more reproducible when a constant current is used than a constant voltage *(35)*. In addition, calculations based on the effective mobility are more reproducible than migration time giving a RSD of mobility of 0.01–0.03% *(36)*.

Imprecision in peak height or area on the other hand is related to two factors: injection volume or time and capillary wall effects. It has been found that the RSD of peak height (area) is inversely related to the sample concentration *(37,38)*. Thus, as the sample concentration increases precision improves. This is especially true when peak area instead of peak height is used *(32,38,39)*. Stacking methods that concentrate the sample on the capillary improve the precision for peak area *(9)*. In general, peak area shows less variation than the peak height with a wider range of linearity *(32,38)*. In the absence of the sample extraction, internal standards will improve slightly the precision of peak height or area.

Several other factors can affect precision in CE. Controlling the temperature of the buffer inside the capillary has been found to be a critical factor in reproducibility *(40)*. Kunkel et al. *(41)* compared the RSD of several CE instruments. They pointed out that the technology for the detector has been improved and the main source of error for most of the instruments is sample injection, which can be decreased by using internal standards.

Changes in the capillary surface can also affect precision. A thorough wash with NaOH (0.1–1 *M*) *(42)*, phosphoric acid (100 m*M*), acetonitrile, or SDS *(43)* decreases the wall effects and improves greatly the reproducibility of the migration time and peak height (area). Kelly et al. *(44)* presented data on electrolysis of the buffer and its effect on the precision. They found that high ionic strength buffers at low current or zwitterionic buffers (which generate low current) improve precision. They also presented several suggestions to decrease the effect of electrolysis. Water injection (2–3 s) after the sample also improves precision.

8. DRUGS ANALYZED BY CE

A single drug can be analyzed for different purposes, e.g., TDM, metabolic, forensic, pharmaceutical, or pharmacological. In the pharmaceutical industry CE is used to determine drug purity or to study its metabolism. The same conditions used for these studies, buffer, pH, voltage, internal standards, and so on, can be extended or modified for use in separation of therapeutic drugs. However, unlike the pharmaceutical industry, the emphasis in TDM is on speed, precision, automation, and sample clean up. However, it turns out many of the methods developed for the different drugs are very similar to each other. For this reason, Altria et al. described a general CE method employing a high pH borate buffer, which was validated to allow analysis of a wide range of acidic pharmaceutical compounds using a variety of internal standards *(45)*. They also validated a similar procedure for the analysis of basic compounds *(46)*. Based on our experience for TDM, anionic drugs are separated best in borate buffer, 200 mmol/L, after sample deproteinization with 2 vol of acetonitrile. Sample loading can be from 1–10% of the capillary volume *(9)*. Cationic compounds, on the other hand, are better analyzed using triethanolamine buffers *(24)*. Neutral compounds can be analyzed in either borate or phosphate buffers containing SDS (MEKC). Standards are added to the serum directly to reduce problems with matrix effects. Obviously it is easier to analyze a single compound than several at the same time. In most of these methods ultraviolet (UV) detection has been utilized, although in a few procedures, fluorescence or laser-induced fluorescence (LIF) detection has been used. The majority these methods have been validated for their linearity, detection limits, accuracy, and precision. A few of these methods used sample extraction although most injected serum with or without acetonitrile treatment. Use of on-line sample clean up and concentration for drugs is a very attractive procedure due to its simplicity and speed. It has been described by Strausbauch et al. *(47)* and Morita *(48)* and reviewed by Guzman et al. *(49)*.

Growing interest in the analysis of drugs by CE is indicated by the publication of several review articles *(50–54)* in addition to a whole journal issue dedicated to CE and drug analysis *(55)*. The practical aspects of TDM analysis by CE has been described *(50)*. Studies, that have dealt primarily with TDM are discussed more in detail later, whereas other studies of general interest are listed in Table 1.

8.1. Anti-Epileptic

The two antiepileptic drugs, phenobarbital and phenytoin, were among the first drugs to be analyzed by CE for TDM. They have been analyzed using both CZE and MEKC. Several of the antiepileptic drugs (ethosuximide, phenytoin, primidone, valproic acid, phenobarbital, and carbamazepine) were analyzed by MEKC after extraction with ethyl acetate in phosphate buffer, 25 m*M*, pH 8.0, containing SDS *(56)*. The separation was completed in 14 min. Barbiturates, i.e., phenobarbital, pentobarbital, amobarbital, and butalbital, in serum and urine were measured by Thormann et al. *(13)* by

Table 1
List of Miscellaneous Drugs Analyzed by CE

Compound	Buffer/conditions	Refs.
Amikacin	MEKC Phosphate/borate, pH 7.0, derivatized, fluorescence	*(106)*
Antibiotics	Several MEKC phosphate/borate with SDS	*(107)*
Antiarrythmic	Several MEKC extraction	*(57)*
β-Blockers	MEKC SDS 50 mM in 100 mM borate buffer, pH 8.1	*(108)*
β-Blockers	CZE phosphate buffer, pH 3.1	*(108)*
β-Blockers	MEKC phosphate, pH 7.0, with N-acetyltrimethylammonium br.	*(109)*
Cefixime	CZE phospahte 50 mM, pH 6.8	*(110)*
Cyclosporine	MEKC phosphate/borate, SDS, acetonitrile, 200 nm	
111OH-coumarin	CZE Phosphate pH 7.5, extraction,	*(112)*
Cytosine-β-D-arabinoside	CZE citrate 40 mM, pH 2.5, extraction	*(113)*
Fosfomycin	CZE borate buffer, 254 nm	*(114)*
Fluorocytosine	MEKC phosphate/borate, pH 9.2, 210 nm	*(115)*
Glipizide	MEKC concentration on the capillary	*(47)*
Glyburide	MEKC concentration on the capillary	*(47)*
Heparinoid mimetics	MEKC phosphate buffer with SDS	*(116)*
Methotrexate	CZE Tris-MES buffer, pH 6.7, extraction LIF detection	*(117)*
Methoxytacrine	CZE serum/urine phosphate 240 nm with	*(118)*
	Nicotinic acid CZE borate 10 mM, pH 9.3,	
	phosphate, 10 mM, pH 2.3, 254 nm	*(119)*
Suramin	CZE Capso buffer 63 mM, pH 9.7, 254 nm	*(120)*
Suramin	CZE Tris borate, pH 8.6	*(121)*
Tomoxifin	CZE acetate, acetonitrile, methanol, extraction	*(122)*
Tacrine	CZE serum/urine phosphate 240 nm	*(118)*
Taxol	MEKC Tris-borate, pH 8.5, 100 mM SDS, extraction, 230 nm	*(123)*
Theophylline	MEKC phosphate, 20 mM , pH 11.0, 40 mM SDS	*(74)*

MEKC using borate, phosphate, and SDS at pH 7.8. Serum could be injected directly on the capillary, whereas urine required extraction. Evanson and Wikotorwicz *(57)* also separated several anti-epileptic drugs by MEKC using a borate buffer, pH 9.3, containing SDS and 30% acetonitrile. Serum samples were injected after solid-phase extraction with separation completed in about 15 min. Pentobarbital was analyzed by CZE in about 5 min after acetonitrile deproteinization using an electrophoresis buffer of 300 mM

borate at pH 8.5 *(58)*. The epoxy and the diol metabolites of carbamazepine, difficult to detect by HPLC or immunoassays, in addition to the parent compound, were quantitated by MEKC in about 3 min using borate buffer and SDS *(59)*.

Most of the recent antiepileptic drugs, such as gabapentin, felbamate, zonisamide, and lamotrigine, have not had commercial immunoassays developed. Gabapentin (neurotin), which is similar to the neurotransmitter gamma amino butyric acid, can be derivatized by incorporating fluorescamine into the deproteinization reagent. Separation was achieved within 12 min using UV detection at 200 nm with a sensitivity of 1 mg/L *(60)*.

Felbamate, a neutral compound, was analyzed by MEKC after addition of an internal standard and then directly injecting serum into the capillary *(1)*. The assay was rapid (about 5 min), with sensitivity of 5 mg/L (Fig. 1), with no interferences noted. Phenobarbital was also analyzed using the same method. In both cases CE was much faster than the HPLC method.

Zonisamide, a new antiepileptic drug, was determined in serum using (MEKC) with detection by diode array. A high correlation ($r = 0.981$) was found between the zonisamide levels in human serum and those obtained by HPLC. The serum levels of phenobarbital, phenytoin, and carbamazepine have also been measured using the same method *(61)*.

Lamotrigine, another antiepileptic drug, is a basic compound. In general, basic compounds are difficult to analyze by either GC or HPLC, usually requiring derivatization. CE can analyze most basic drugs quite easily in pure aqueous solutions. Their analysis in serum, however, is more difficult than that of acidic compounds. Deproteinization by acetonitrile followed by the addition of acetic acid to lower the pH below the pK_a of the compound being analyzed and also below the pH of the separation buffer was necessary in order to obtain a good separation.

8.2. Anti-Arrhythmic

The majority of anti-arrhythmic drugs are basic compounds and many also act as antihypertensive agents. These compounds migrate rapidly and are seen in the first part of the electropherogram. However, they can be difficult to separate since they tend to bind to the capillary walls, making analysis and especially stacking difficult. Recently *(24)*, we have shown that buffers containing amines and zwitterions are useful not only in analysis but also stacking of these compounds. The analysis of procainamide and *N*-acetylprocainamide is a good example of stacking of basic drugs on the capillary. In this method, which correlated well with immunoassay, about 10% of the capillary volume was injected with sample *(63)*. Using the same method, urinary procainamide also has been analyzed by CE *(64)*.

Lukkari et al. *(65)* separated after urine extraction 10 β-adrenergic blockers, i.e., propranolol, oxyprenalol, and nadolol. CE also determined Amiodarone, a highly hydrophobic compound, in buffers with a high content of organic solvents *(22,66)*. Using "Field Amplified Injection," the sensitivity for amiodarone analysis was increased by several orders of magnitude *(22)*. The method compared well to HPLC. MEKC was also used by Evanson and Wikotorwicz *(57)* to separate procainamide, *N*-acetylprocainamide, disopyramide, and chlorodisopyramide.

8.3. Analgesics

Many analgesics such as ibuprofen, salicylates, and acetaminophen are available without a prescription. Because of their wide therapeutic windows, routine monitoring of these drugs is not necessary. However, acetaminophen overdoses are occasionally encountered and in cases, careful monitoring of acetaminophen levels and half-life is very important. High doses near the toxic level of ibuprofen have also been advocated recently for the treatment of cystic fibrosis *(67)*. Hence, monitoring the serum level is important. Many methods have been described for the analysis of these drugs in either tablet or pure form. We measured ibuprofen *(68)* and ketoprofen *(2)* in serum by CZE after acetonitrile deproteinization using borate buffers. Watzug and Lloyd *(11)* and Kunkel *(69)* described the direct serum analysis of acetaminophen and salicylic acid by MEKC using borate buffer containing SDS. Goto et al. *(70)* measured salicylic acid in serum by CZE and found that the results compared quite well to fluorescence polarization immunoassay.

8.4. Antidepressants

Antidepressants, such as the tricyclics, trazdone, and Prozac, are commonly used to treat anxiety and depression. Since these basic, hydrophobic drugs are present in serum at low levels they are very difficult to measure regardless of methodology. In order to separate by HPLC the use of a well-deactivated column with a high plate number is important. Lomon et al. *(71)* used CE to separate seven antidepressant drugs in aqueous media using a CAPSO buffer at pH 9.5. The zwitterionic buffer, CAPSO, along with methanol decreases the adsorption of these compounds to the capillary wall. We have also shown that amine-containing buffers are important for the stacking of these compounds in order to improve their detection *(24)*. Additionally, Harrell et al. *(72)* separated seven antidepressant drugs using a synthetic nonionic forming micelle polymer in about 15 min.

8.5. Anti-Asthmatic

Theophylline, a drug used in the treatment of asthma, has a narrow therapeutic window. Because of this narrow window, it is important to know the serum concentration in order to determine whether it is in the therapeutic or toxic range. Additionally, theophylline and the closely related compound, caffeine, are frequently used to treat apnea in newborns. Like the antiepileptic drugs, these compounds have been analyzed by either MEKC or CZE. MEKC allows direct injection of serum, urine, or saliva in a borate buffer, pH 9.0, in the presence of SDS with separation in about 15 min *(73)*. We obtained a good correlation ($r = 0.98$) to immunoassay when theophylline was measured by CZE in borate buffer, pH 8.5 *(15)*. Zhao et al. *(74)* determined caffeine and its metabolites by MEKC, and Johansson et al. *(75)* used CZE to measure theophylline in phosphate-borate buffers. Caffeine, dyphylline, theobromine, and theophylline have also been separated by MEKC in borate buffer, pH 9.3 containing SDS and 30% acetonitrile *(57)*.

8.6. Renal Function and Contrast Agents

In clinical labs, renal function is routinely estimated by measuring the creatinine clearance. This test is convenient but it is known to be inaccurate especially when a significant loss (>50%) in renal function occurs. In research several iodinated compounds such as iothalamic acid and iohexol are used to provide a better measurement of renal clearance using either serum or urine. Iohexol was rapidly assayed (<5 min) by CZE after deproteinization of serum by acetonitrile *(76)*. Values as low as 5 mg/L can be measured by this technique. Isovue, another candidate compound for the measurement of renal function, was also measured by CZE after acetonitrile deproteinization *(77)*. Landers et al. *(78)* used CE to quantitate iothalamic acid in serum and in a timed urine collection to measure the glomerular filtration rate. The test correlated well with an isotopic reference method.

9. CE AND IMMUNOASSAY

Many drugs, such as tacrolimus and digoxin, remain far below the detection limits of CE or HPLC without extraction and subsequent concentration. In response to this limitation, Chen and Evangelista *(79,80)* described a method that has potential for better sensitivity along with simultaneous detection of several drugs. This method is based on a combination of immunoassay, laser-induced fluorescence (LIF), and CE. In this system, fluorescent-labeled drug conjugates antibodies of known specificity and the unknown samples were mixed. After the reaction is completed, CE separates the free drug (including the fluorescent-labeled drug) from the bound. The quantity of drug in the unknown sample that can be estimated from a standard curve established using the same methodology. Cortisol, an endogenous substance and a drug, has also been quantitated using a similar approach *(81,82)*.

Recently, Steinmann and Thormann *(83)* described an assay using MEKC, LIF, and commercial Fluorescence Polarization Assay reagents to separate a variety of drugs. The free and bound tracers for the different drugs were separated in phosphate-borate buffer containing SDS. The feasibility of simultaneous determination of several drugs was also demonstrated. A similar method was also described for the analysis of digoxin using the commercial reagent from an enzyme immunoassay kit *(84)*. Additionally, Chiem and Harrison *(85)* described a microchip CE method to separate the reaction products of a reaction of an antibody and theophylline within approx 40 s. The buffer system consisted of tricine, pH 8.0, with 0.01% (w/v) Tween 20, and 40 m*M* NaCl, allowing adequate separation for theophylline and for the theophylline-antibody complex. Reproducibility of migration times was 1–1.5%.

10. SPECIAL FEATURES OF ANALYSIS

In addition to measurement of the serum drug levels, other pharmacological parameters are important in TDM such as protein binding, half-life, ionization, and metabolism. The following represent some interesting studies related to TDM, which were performed by using CE.

10.1. Chiral Separation

Although isomers have very close chemical structures, they can exhibit different biological effects or can be metabolized differently *(86)*. These isomers can also show differential binding to serum proteins. Giacomini et al. *(88)* have shown that the coadministration of racemic disoprymide affected the clearance of the d-isomer due to the more avid binding of its isomer to serum proteins. Also the S form of verapamil has less binding to serum proteins increasing its plasma clearance to twice that of the R form *(89)*. Thus, several proteins, including those found in human serum, such as transferrin, have been utilized in CE for chiral separation of a variety of drugs *(87)*.

Chiral separations have generated great interest in CE because of low cost, ease of analysis, speed, and the high resolution relative to HPLC. Unfortunately, most of the chiral separations described are performed on drugs to check for purity in pharmaceutical preparations. A few studies, however, have been performed on separations from biological samples. For example, Srinivassan and Bartlett *(90)* described a stereoselective method for serum phenobarbital using cyclodextrin and solid phase extraction. Ohara et al. *(91)* also described a method using CE to determine the enantioselective determination of the basic drug verapamil that was not bound to serum proteins. Nishi *(92)* reviewed the separation of enantiomers

Table 2
List of Some Drugs Analyzed in Serum/Plasma by Chiral Separation

Drug	Comments	Refs.
Bupivacaine	βCD, Extraction	*(124)*
Cicletanine	γCD, borate with SDS (plasma contained S+;urine R-)	*(125)*
Hexobarbital	βCD phosphate, pH 7.0 with SDS	*(126)*
Ibuprofen	Maltrin M040 (TAPS-Tris pH 7.8)	*(127)*
Phenobarbital	Hydroxy propyl CD with solid phase extraction	*(90)*
Warfarin	Glucidex Tris phosphate, pH 7.0	*(128)*
Warfarin	Modified βCD Phosphate, pH 8.3	*(37)*
Verpamil	Trimethyl-βCD at pH 2.5, frontal analysis	*(91)*
Verapamil	Trimethyl-βCD	*(129)*

of drugs by electrokinetic chromatography using chiral micelles and proteins. In addition, Fanali *(93)* and Bojarski and Aboul-Enein *(94)* reviewed the identification of chiral drugs by CE including those present in biological fluids. Table 2 lists some of the drugs analyzed in serum for chirality.

D'Hulst and Verbeke *(95)* and Altria et al. *(96)* showed that a limit of detection of <1% and 0.1% of the total drug level, respectively, can be obtained for the minor enantiomer levels. Thus, CE offers a very rapid, low cost, and excellent separation for chiral separations, but the reproducibility falls short of that of HPLC *(94,96,97)*.

10.2. Physico-Chemical Properties of Drugs

The pK_a of a compound or drug can also be measured using CE by measuring its mobility as a function of pH *(98)*. Schmutz and Thormann *(99)* determined how the physical and chemical properties of 25 drugs would effect their analysis by MEKC. They found that compounds, which did not bind tightly to proteins in addition to those with a low pK_a, dissociated easily from the bound proteins and migrated as sharp peaks.

10.3. Free Drugs

Most drugs bind to serum proteins while the unbound fraction (free) of the drug is thought to be the active form. Thus, it is important to measure and understand the drug-protein interaction. This is especially important in such disorders as renal failure where the amount of the free drug changes as a result of uremia and binding protein concentrations.

The free, bound, percentage of binding, and the binding constant can be determined based on several well-established techniques such as dialysis, filtration, and size exclusion. CE can extend these techniques to measure free drugs. For example, several free drugs were measured after filtration through special membranes *(17)*. The problem with this method of measurement is that free drugs are present at a much lower concentration than the total drug. Thus, in order to measure these low levels, concentration or stacking steps may be necessary. For example, in the analysis of phenytoin, acetonitrile is added to the filtrate to concentrate the drug on the capillary (*see* Fig. 2).

In addition to the previous techniques, CE based on changes in the electrophoretic mobility *(100,101)* can measure drug binding. Kraak et al. *(100)* described three different methods for measuring protein-drug binding by CE. The first is based on the Hummel-Dryer method in which the capillary is filled with a buffer containing the drug giving a large background signal. The sample, which contains the drug, protein, and buffer, is injected. The bound drug migrates differently from the free drug, producing a negative peak. The area of the negative peak is a measure of the bound drug. The second method is based on the vacancy method where as the capillary is filled with mixture of the buffer, the drug, and the protein. This also causes a large background signal. The sample that contains only the buffer is injected. Both the free and the bound drug migrate separately and each gives a negative peak. The third method depends on the frontal analysis. In this method the capillary is filled with the buffer. Different concentrations of the drug in the presence and absence of a fixed binding protein concentration are incubated at 25°C followed by injection of a large amount of sample (~5–7% of the capillary volume). The free drug, the complex and the protein gives each a frontal, plateau-shaped peak. The free-drug concentration can be calculated *(102)* from the height of the frontal peak as follows:

$$E = (D/S) \times P \tag{1}$$

where D = Height free drug concentration, E = free drug concentration, S = concentration of the pure standard, and P = drug peak height in presence of the protein.

The concentration of the bound drug can be calculated by subtracting the free drug from the total. The percentage and the binding association constant can be also calculated from a Scatchard plot of this data *(91,101–103)*. Kraak et al. *(100)* concluded that the frontal analysis appeared to be the preferred method for drug binding. It is more reproducible and gives a smooth Scatchard curve compared to the other two techniques.

Binding of drugs to a specific carrier is also a promising approach to target drugs to specific organs. Protein binding can alter the metabolism or delivery of the drug to the target organ. Naproxen conjugated to albumin is an example of such drug targeting. Albrecht et al. *(104)* have shown that naproxen, a nonsteriodal anti-inflammatory drug, can be determined in serum using MEKC as free, albumin conjugated, and lysine conjugated. Samples were injected and separated in a borate/phosphate buffer containing SDS with LIF detection. This method has also been extended to measurement of this drug in liver and kidney tissue *(105)*.

11. CONCLUSION

In general, CE is a versatile analytical technique capable of analyzing a wide variety of drugs both charged and uncharged. CE is most useful in TDM to analyze new drugs rather than for those with established immunoassays. The cost of operation is much less than that of HPLC. In addition to analyzing a drug and its metabolites, CE can be used for analysis of the bound, free drugs, isomers, and measure the physicochemical properties.

As stated in this and previous chapters one of the main limitations of the CE is poor sensitivity. For the most part this can be overcome by preconcentration (either on or before the capillary) or by the use of special flow cells. Using these methods, sensitivities close to that of the HPLC can be obtained. In addition, several relatively simple methods for sample stacking on the capillary for CZE and MEKC have been described in the last few years. However, because of the need to measure drugs at lower and lower serum levels, there is still a need for further studies addressing new stacking methods, flow cells, and detectors (i.e., LIF).

Precision is the other area of CE that is still in need of improvement. By addition of multiple internal standards, using mobility data and a better understanding the sources of the variation, the precision of CE has become much better. Again the goal is to match or surpass the precision of HPLC. Although CE is faster than HPLC, shorter and narrower capillaries, (i.e., microchips) together with high voltage would further speed analysis.

Overall, analysis of drugs (especially newly developed drugs) by CE will keep on growing because of the continued need to monitor the serum levels of these new drugs.

REFERENCES

1. Shihabi, Z. K. and Oles, K. S. (1994) Felbamate measured in serum by two methods: HPLC and capillary electrophoresis method. Clin. Chem. 40, 1904–1908.
2. Friedberg, M. A. and Shihabi, Z. K. (1997) Ketoprofen analysis in serum by capillary electrophoresis. J. Chromatogr. B 695, 193–198.
3. Scholl, J. B. and DeZwaan, J. (1997) Micellar electrokinetic chromatography as a generalized alternative to high-performance liquid chromatography for purity determination of a class of investigational antibacterial drugs. J. Chromatogr. B 695, 147–156.

4. Hsu, L. C., Constable, D. J., Orvos, D. R., and Hannah, R. E. (1995) Comparison of high-performance liquid chromatography and capillary zone electrophoresis in penciclovir biodegradation kinetic studies. J. Chromatogr. B 669, 85–92.

5. Tomlinson, A. J., Benson, L. M., Landers, J. P., Scanlan, G. F., Fang, J., Gorrod, J. W., and Naylor, S. (1993) Investigation of metabolism of the neuroleptic drug haloperidol by capillary electrophoresis. J. Chromatogr. A 652, 417–426.

6. Wynia, G. S., Windhorst, P. C., Post, P. C., and Maris, F. A. (1997) Development and validation of a capillary electrophoresis method within pharmaceutical quality control environment and comparison with high –performance liquid chromatography. J. Chromatogr. A 773, 339–350.

7. Heeren, F., Tanner, R., Theurillat, R., and Thormann, W. (1996) Determination of Fluconazole in human plasma by micellar electrokinetic capillary chromatography with detection at 190. J. Chromatogr. A 745, 165–172.

8. Altria, K. D. and Bestford, J. (1996) Main component assay of pharmaceuticals by capillary electrophoresis: considerations regarding precision, accuracy, and linearity data. J. Cap. Electro. 3, 13–23.

9. Shihabi, Z. K. (1997) Effect of sample matrix on capillary electrophoresis, in Handbook of Electrophoresis, 2nd ed. (Landers, J. P., ed.), CRC, Boca Raton, FL, pp. 457–477.

10. Mazzeo, J. R. (1977) Micellarr electrokinetic chromatography, in Handbook of Electrophoresis, 2nd ed. (Landers, J. P., ed.), CRC, Boca Raton, FL, pp. 49–73.

11. Watzig, H. and Lloyd, D. K. (1995) Effect of pH and sodium dodecyl sulfate concentration on the analytical window in the direct-injection analysis of plasma samples by capillary electrophoresis. Electrophoresis 16, 57–63.

12. Thormann, W., Minger, A., Molteni, S., Caslavska, J., and Gebauer, P. (1992) Determination of substituted purines in body fluids by micellar electrokinetic capillary chromatography with direct sample injection. J. Chromatogr. 593, 275–288.

13. Thormann, W., Meier, P., Marcolli, C., and Binder, F. (1991) Analysis of barbiturates in human serum and urine by high-performance capillary electrophoresis-micellar elektrokinetic capillary chromatography with on-column multi-wavelength detection. J. Chromatogr. 545, 445–460.

14. Garcia, L. L. and Shihabi, Z. K. (1993) Sample matrix effects in capillary electrophoresis. I-Basic considerations. J. Chromatogr. A 652, 465–469.

15. Shihabi, Z. K. (1993) Sample matrix effects in capillary electrophoresis. II-Acetonitrile deproteinization. J. Chromatogr. A 652, 471–475.

16. Ueda, T., Maekawa, T., Sadamitsu, D., Oshita, S., Ogino, K., and Nakamura, K. (1995) The determination of nitrite and nitrate in human blood plasma by capillary zone electrophoresis. Electrophoresis 16, 1002–1004.

17. Thormann, W. (1996) Drug monitoring by capillary electrophoresis, in Handbook of Analytical Therapeutic Drug Monitoring and Toxicology (Wong, S. H. and Sunshine, I., eds.), CRC Press, Boca Raton, FL, pp. 1–19.

18. Shihabi, Z. K. (1995) Sample stacking by acetonitrile-salt mixtures. J. Cap. Elec. 2, 267–271.

19. Lloyd, D. K. (1996) Capillary electrophoretic analyses of drugs in body fluids: sample pretreatment and methods for direct injection of biofluids. J. Chromatogr. A, 735, 29–42.

20. Friedberg, M. A., Hinsdale, M., and Shihabi, Z. K. (1997) Effect of pH and ions in the sample on stacking in capillary electrophoresis. J. Chromatogr. A 781, 35–42.

21. Burgi, D. S. and Chien, R.-L. (1991) Optimization in sample stacking for high-performance capillary electrophoresis, Anal. Chem. 63, 2042–2047.

22. Zhang, C. X., Aebi, Y., and Thormann, W. (1996) Microassay of amiodarone and desethylamiodarone in serum by capillary electrophoresis with head-column field-amplified sample stacking. Clin. Chem. 42, 1805–1811.

23. Shihabi, Z. K. (1996) Peptide stacking by acetonitrile-salt mixtures for capillary zone electrophoresis. J. Chromatogr. A 744, 231–240.

24. Shihabi, Z. K. (1998) Stacking of weakly cationic compounds by acetonitrile for capillary electrophoresis. J. Chromatogr. A 817, 25–30.

25. Bachmann, J. B. K. (1996) Investigation of matrix effects in capillary zone electrophoresis. J. Chromatogr. A 734, 319–330.

26. Gebauer, P., Thormann, W., and Bocek, P. (1992) Sample slf-stacking in zone electrophoresis. J. Chromatogr. 608, 47–57.

27. Gebauer, P., Thormann, W., and Bocek, P. (1995) Sample self-stacking and sample stacking in zone electrophoresis with major sample components of like charge: general model and scheme of possible modes. Electrophoresis 16, 2039–2050.

28. Quirino, J. P. and Terabe, S. (1997) On-line concentration of neutral analytes for micellar electrokinetic chromatography. I. Normal stacking mode. J. Chromatogr. A 781, 119–128.

29. Liu, Z, Sam, P., McClure, J., Grainger, J., and Patterson, D. G. (1994) Field-amplified sample stacking in micellar electrokinetic chromatography for on-column sample concentration of sample neutral molecules. J. Chromatogr. A 673, 125–132.

30. Quirino, J. P. and Terabe, S. (1997) On-line concentration of neutral analytes for micellar electrokinetic chromatography. II. reversed electrode polarity stacking mode. J. Chromatogr. A 791, 255–267.

31. Quirino, J. P. and Terabe, S., (1998) On-line concentration of neutral analytes for micellar electrokinetic chromatography. 3. Stacking with reverse migration micelles. Anal. Chem. 70, 149–157.

32. Shihabi, Z. K. and Hinsdale, M. E. (1995) Some variables affecting reproducibility in capillary electrophoresis. Electrophoresis 16, 2159–2163.

33. Dose, E. V. and Guichon, G. A. (1991) Internal standardization technique for capillary zone electrophoresis. Anal. Chem. 63, 1154–1158.

34. Siren, H., Jumppanen, J. H., Manninen, K., and Reikkola, M.-L. (1994) Introduction of migration indices for identification: chiral separation of some β-blockers by using cyclodextrins in micellar elektrokinetic capillary chromatography. Electrophoresis 15, 779–784.

35. Kurosu, Y., Sato, Y., Shisa Y., and Iwata, M. (1998) Comparison of the reproducibility in migration times between a constant current and a constant–

voltage mode of operation in capillary zone electrophoresis. J. Chromatogr. A 802, 391–394.

36. Jumppanen, J. H. and Reikkola, M.-L. (1995) Marker techniques for high-accuracy identification in CZE. Anal. Chem. 67, 1060–1066.

37. Gareil, P., Gramond, J. P., and Guyon, F. (1993) Separation and determination of warfarin enantiomers in human plasma samples by capillary zone electrophoresis using a methylated beta-cyclodextrin-containing electrolyte. J. Chromatogr. 615, 317–325.

38. Watzig, H. (1995) Appropriate calibration functions for capillary electrophoresis. I. Precision and sensitivity using peak areas and heights J. Chromatogr. A 700, 1–7.

39. Watzig, H. and Dette, C. (1993) Precise quantitative capillary electrophoresis. Methodological and instrumental aspects. J. Chromatogr. 636, 31–38.

40. Baumann, K. and Watzig, H. (1995) Appropriate calibration functions for capillary electrophoresis II. Heteroscedasticity and its consequences. J. Chromatogr. A 700, 9–20.

41. Kunkel, A., Degenhardt, M., Schrim, B., and Watzig, H. (1997) Performance of instruments and aspects of methodology and validation in quantitative capillary electrophoresis: an update. J. Chromatogr. A 768, 17–27.

42. Smith, S. C., Strasters, J. K., and Khaledi, M. G. (1991) Influence of operating parameters on reproducibility in capillary electrophoresis. J. Chromatogr. 559, 57–68.

43. Llyod, D. K. and Watzig, H. (1995) Sodium dodecyl sulfate solution is an effective between-run rinse for capillary electrophoresis of samples in biological matrices. J. Chromatogr. B 663, 400–405.

44. Kelley, M. A., Altria, K. D., and Clark, B. J. (1996) Approaches used in the reduction of buffer electrolysis effects for routine capillary electrophoresis procedures in pharmaceutical analysis. J. Chromatogr. A 768, 73–80

45. Altria, K. D., Hadgett, T. A., and Bryant, S. M. (1997) Validated capillary electrophoresis method for the analysis of a range of acidic drugs and excipients. J. Pharm. Biomed. Anal. 15, 1091–1101

46. Altria, K.D., Rudd, D.R., Kelly, M.A., Hadgett, T., Gill, I., and Frake, P. (1995) Validated capillary electrophoresis method for the assay of a range of basic drugs. J. Pharm. Biomed. Anal. Chem 13, 951–957.

47. Strausbauch, M., Xu, S., Ferguson, J., Nunez, M., Machacek, D., Lawson, G., et al. (1995) Concentration separation of hypoglycemic drugs using solid–phase extraction–capillary electrophoresis J. Chromatogr. A 717, 279–291.

48. Morita, I. and Sawada, J. (1993) Capillary electrophoresis with on-line sample pretreatment for the analysis of biological samples with direct injection. J. Chromatogr. 641, 375–381.

49. Guzman, N. A, Park, S. S., Schaufelberger, D., Hernandez, L., Paez, X., Rada, P., et al. (1997) New approaches in clinical chemistry: on-line analyte concentration and microreaction capillary electrophoresis for the determination of drugs, metabolic intermediates, and biopolymers in biological fluids. J. Chromatogr. B 697, 37–66.

50. Shihabi, Z. K. (1997) Therapeutic drug monitoring by capillary electrophoresis, in Handbook of Capillary Electrophoresis Applications (Shintani, H. and Polonsky, J. eds.), Chapman and Hall, London, pp. 386–408.
51. Oda, R. P., Roche, M. E., Landers, J. P., and Shihabi, Z. K. (1997) Capillary electrophoresis for the analysis of drugs in biological fluids, in Handbook of Electrophoresis, 2nd ed. (Landers, J. P., ed.), CRC Press, Boca Raton, FL, pp. 639–674.
52. Thormann, W., Zhang, C.-X., and Schultz, A. (1996) Capillary electrophoresis for drug analysis in body fluids. Therp. Drug Monit. 18, 506–520.
53. Thormann, W., Molteni, S., Caslavska, J., and Schmutz, A. (1994) Clinical and forensic applications of capillary electrophoresis. Electrophoresis, 15, 3–12.
54. Shihabi, Z. K. (1998) Review: therapeutic drug monitoring by capillary electrophoresis. J. Chromatogr. A 807, 27–36.
55. Cohen, A. S., Terabe, S., and Deyl, Z. (1996) Capillary electrophoretic separation of drugs. J. Chromatogr. 735, 1–447.
56. Lee, K.-J., Heo, G. S., Kim, N. J., and Moon, D. C. (1992) Analysis of antiepileptic drugs in human plasma using micellar electrokinetic capillary chromatography. J. Chromatogr. 608, 243–250.
57. Evenson, M. A. and Wiktorowicz, J. E. (1992) Automated capillary electrophoresis applied to therapeutic monitoring. Clin. Chem. 38, 1847–1852.
58. Shihabi, Z. K. (1993) Serum pentobarbital assay by capillary electrophoresis. J. Liq. Chromatogr. 16, 2059–2068.
59. Hartter, S., Jensen, B., Heimke, C., Leal, M., Weigmann, H., and Unger, K. (1998) Micellar electrokinetic capillary chromatography for therapeutic drug monitoring of carbamzepine and its main metabolite. J. Chromatogr. B 712, 253–258.
60. Garcia, L. L., Shihabi, Z. K., and Oles, K. S. (1995) Determination of gabapentin in serum by capillary electrophoresis. J. Chromatogr. B 669, 157–162.
61. Makino, K., Oishi R., Kataoka, Y., Futagami, K., Sueyasu, M., and Goto, Y. (1997) Micellar electrokinetic capillary chromatography of therapeutic drug monitoring of zonisamide. J. Chromatogr. B 695, 417–425.
62. Shihabi, Z. K. and Oles, K. S. (1996) Serum lamotragine analysis by capillary electrophoresis. J. Chromatogr. B 683, 119–123.
63. Shihabi, Z. K. Serum procainamide analysis based on acetonitrile stacking by capillary electrophoresis. Electrophoresis (In Press).
64. Vragas, G., Havel, J., and Hadasova, E. (1997) Direct determination of procainamide and N-acetylprocainamide by capillary zone electrophoresis in pharmaceutical formulations and urine. J. Chromatogr. A 772, 271–276.
65. Lukkari, P., Siren, H., Pantsar, M., and Riekkola, M.-L. (1993) Determination of ten β-blockers in urine by micellar electrokinetic capillary chromatography. J. Chromatogr. 632, 143–148.
66. Zhang, C.-X., Heeren, F. V., and Thormann, W. (1995) Separation of hydrophobic, positively chargeable substances by capillary electrophoresis. Anal. Chem. 67, 2070–2077.

67. Konstan, M. W., Byard, P. J., Hoppel, C. L., and Davis, P. B. (1995) Effect of high-dose of ibuprofen in patients with cystic fibrosis. N. Engl. J. Med. 332, 848–854.

68. Shihabi, Z. K. and Hinsdale, M. E. (1996) Analysis of ibuprofen in serum by capillary electrophoresis. J. Chromatogr. B, 683, 115–118.

69. Kunkel, A., Gunter, S., and Watzig, H. (1997) Quantitation of acetaminophen and salicylic acid in plasma using capillary electrophoresis without sample pretreatment. Improvement of precision. J. Chromatogr. A 768, 125–133.

70. Goto, Y., Oishi, R., Shuto, H., Kataoka, Y., and Makino, K. (1998) Determination of salicylic acid in human serum with capillary zone electrophoresis. J. Chromatogr. B 706, 329–35.

71. Salomon, K., Burgi, D. S., and Helmer, J. C. (1991) Separation of seven tricyclic antidepressants using capillary electrophoresis. J. Chromatogr. 549, 375–385.

72. Harrell, C. W., Dey, J., Foley, J. P., and Warner, I. M., (1998) Enhanced separation of antidepressant drugs using a polymerized nonionic surfactant as a transient capillary coating. Electrophoresis 19, 712–718.

73. Thormann, W., Minger, A., Molteni, S., Caslavska, J., and Gebauer, P. (1992) Determination of substituted purines in body fluids by micellar electrokinetic capillary chromatography with direct sample injection. J. Chromatogr. 593, 275–288.

74. Zhao, Y. and Lunte, C. E. (1997) Determination of caffeine and its metabolites by micellar electrokinetic capillary electrophoresis. J. Chromatogr. B 688, 265–274.

75. Johnsson, M., Rydberg, M., and Schmekel, B. (1993) Determination of theophylline in plasma using different capillary electrophoretic systems. J. Chromatogr. A 652, 487–493.

76. Shihabi, Z. K. and Constantinescu, M. S. (1992) Iohexol in serum determined by capillary electrophoresis. Clin. Chem. 38, 2117–2120.

77. Shihabi, Z. K., Rocco, M. V., and Hinsdale, M. E. (1995) Analysis of the contrast agent iopamidol by capillary electrophoresis. J. Liq. Cromatogr. 18, 3825–3832.

78. Bergert, J. H., Liedtke, R. R., Oda, R. P., Landers, J. P., and Wilson, D. M. (1997) Development of a nonisotopic capillary electrophoresis-based method for measuring glomerular filtration rate. Electrophoresis 18, 1827–1835.

79. Chen, F.-T. A. and Evangelista, R. A. (1994) Feasibility studies for simultaneous immunochemical multianalyte drug assay by capillary electrophoresis with laser-induced fluorescence. Clin. Chem. 40, 1819–1822.

80. Evangelista, R. A. and Chen, F.-T. A. (1994) Analysis of structural specificity in antibody-antigen reactions by capillary electrophoresis with laser-induced fluorescence detection. J. Chromatogr. A 680, 587–591.

81. Schmalzing, D., Nashabeh, W., Yao X., and Mhatre, R. (1995) Capillary electrophoresis-based immunoassay for cortisol in serum. Anal. Chem. 67, 606–612.

82. Schmalzing, D., Nashabeh, W., and Fuchs, M. (1995) Solution-phase immunoassay for determination of cortisol in serum by capillary electrophoresis. Clin. Chem. 41, 1403–1406.

83. Steinmann, L. and Thormann, W. (1996) Characterization of competitive binding, fluorescent drug immunoassays based on micellar electrokinetic capillary chromatography. Electrophoresis 17, 1348–1356.

84. Liu, X., Xu, Y., and Ip, M. P. (1995) Capillary electrophoretic enzyme immunoassay for digoxin in human serum. Anal. Chem. 67, 3211–3218.

85. Chiem, N. and Harrison, D. J. (1997) Microchip-based capillary electrophoresis for immunoassays: analysis of monoclonal antibodies and theophylline. Anal. Chem. 69, 373–378.

86. Wainer, I. W. (1996) Toxicology through a looking glass, in Handbook of Analytical Therapeutic Drug Monitoring and Toxicology (Wong, S. H. and Sunshine, I., eds.), CRC Press, Boca Raton, FL, pp. 21–34.

87. Schmid, M. G., Gubitz, G., and Kilar, F. (1998) Stereoselective interaction of drug enantiomers with human serum transferrin in capillary zone electrophoresis. Electrophoresis 19, 282–287.

88. Giacomini, K. M., Nelson, W. L., Pershe, R. A., Valdivieso, L., Turner-Tamiyasu, K., and Blaschke, T. F. (1986) In vivo interaction of enantiomers of disopuramide in human subjects. J. Pharmacokin. Biopharm. 14, 335–356.

89. Gross, A. S., Heuer, B., and Eichelbaum, M. (1988) Stereoselective protein binding of verapamil enantiomers. Biochem. Pharmacol. 37, 4623–4627.

90. Srinivasan, K. and Bartlett, M. G. (1997) Capillary electrophoresis stereoselective determination of R-(+)-and S-(-)-phenobarbital from serum using hydroxy propyl-ψ-cyclodextrin, solid phase extraction and ultraviolet detection. J. Chromatogr B. 703, 289–294.

91. Ohara, T., Nakagawa, T., and Shibukawa, A. (1995) Capillary electrophoresis/frontal analysis for microanalysis of enantioselective protein binding of a basic drug. Anal. Chem. 67, 3520–3525.

92. Nishi, H. (1996) Enantiomer separation of drugs by electrokinetic chromatography. J. Chromatogr. A 735, 57–76.

93. Fanali, S. (1996) Identification of chiral drug isomers by capillary electrophoresis. J. Chromatogr. A 735, 77–121.

94. Bojarski, J. and Aboul-Enein, H. Y. (1997) Application of capillary electrophoresis for the analysis of chiral drugs in biological fluids. Electrophoresis 18, 965–969.

95. D'Hulst, A. and Verbeke, N. (1994) Quantitation in chiral capillary electrophoresis: theoretical and practical considerations. Electrophoresis 15, 854–863.

96. Altria, K. D., Goodall, D. M., and Rogan, M. M. (1994) Quantitative applications and validation of the resolution of enantiomers by capillary electrophoresis. Electrophoresis 15, 824–827.

97. Penn, S. G., Liu, G. Begrton, F. T., Goodall, D. M., and Loran J. S. (1994) Systemic approach to treatment of enantiomeric separations in capillary electrophoresis and liquid chromatography. I. Initial evaluations using propranolol and dansylated aminoacids. J. Chromatogr. A 680, 147–155.

98. Cleveland, J. A., Benko, M. H., Gluck, S. J., and Walbroehl, Y. M. (1993) Automated pKa determination at low solute concentrations by capillary electrophoresis. J. Chromatogr. A 652, 301–308.

99. Schmutz, A. and Thormann, W. (1994) Assessment of impact of physico-chemical drug properties on monitoring levels by micellar electrokinetic capillary chromatography with direct serum injection. Electrophoresis 15, 1295–1303.

100. Kraak, J. C., Bush, S., and Poppe, H. (1992) Study of protein-drug binding using capillary electrophorsis. J. Chromatogr. A 608, 257–264.

101. Gomez, F. A., Mirkovich, J. N., Dominguez, V. M., Liu, K. W., and Macias, D. M. (1996) Multiple-plug binding assays using affinity capillary electrophoresis. J. Chromatogr. A 727, 291–299.

102. McDonnell, P. A, Caldwell, G. W., and Masucci, J. A. (1998) Using capillary electrophoresis/frontal analysis to screen drugs interacting with human serum proteins. Electrophoresis 19, 448–454.

103. Shibukawa, A. and Nakagawa, T. (1996) Theoretical study of high-performance frontal analysis: a chromatographic method for determination of drug-protein binding interaction. Anal. Chem. 68, 447–454.

104. Albrecht, C., Reichen, J., Visser, J., Meijer, D. K. F., and Thormann, W. (1997) Differentiation between naproxen, naproxen-protein conjugates, and naproxen-lysine in plasma via micellar electrokinetic capillary chromatography: a new approach in the bioanalysis of drug targeting preparations. Clin. Chem. 43, 2083–2090.

105. Albrecht, C. and Thormann, W. (1998) Determination of naproxen in liver and kidney tissues by electrokinetic capillary chromatography with laser-induced fluorescence detection. J. Chromatogr. A 802, 115–120.

106. Oguri, S. and Miki, Y. (1996) Determination of amikacin in human plasma by high-performance capillary electrophoresis with fluorescence detection. J. Chromatogr. B 686, 205–210.

107. Nishi, H., Fukuyama, T., and Matsuo, M. (1990) Separation and determination of apoxicillin in human plasma by micellar electrokinetic chromatography with direct sample injection. J. Chromatogr. 515, 245–255.

108. Bretnall, A. E. and Clarke, G. S. (1996) Selectivity of capillary electrophoreis for the analysis of cardiovascular drugs. J. Chromatogr. A 745, 145–154.

109. Lukkari, P., Siren, H., Pantsar, M., and Riekkola, M.-L. (1993) Determination of ten β-blockers in urine by micellar elektrokinetic capillary chromatography. J. Chromatogr. 632, 143–148.

110. Honda, S., Taga, A., Kakehi, K., and Koda, S., Okamoto, Y. (1992) Determination of cefixime and its metabolites by high-performance capillary electrophoresis. J. Chromatogr. 590, 364–368.

111. Huie, R., Wang, H. P., Van Dreal, P., and Wong, S. S. (1995) Quantitation of cyclosporine using capillary electrophoresis. Clin. Chem. 41, S116.

112. Bogan, D. P., Deasy, B., O'Kennedy, R., Smyth, M. R., and Fuhr, U. (1995) Determination of free and total 7-hydroxycoumarin in urine and serum by capillary electrophoresis. J. Chromatogr. B 663, 371–378.

113. Lloyd, D. K., Cypess, A. M., and Wainer, I. W. (1991) Determination of cytosine-β-D-arabinoside in plasma using capillary electrophoresis. J. Chromatogr. 568, 117–124.

114. Baillet, A., Pianetti, G. A., Taverna, M., Mahuzier, G., and Baylocq-Ferrier, D. (1993) Fosfomycin determination in serum by capillary zone electrophoresis with indirect ultraviolet detection. J. Chromatogr. 616, 311–318.

115. Schultz, A. and Thormann, W. (1994) Rapid determination of the antimycotic drug flucytosine in human serum by micellar electrokinetic capillary chromatography with direct sample injection. Ther. Drug Monit. 16, 483–490.

116. Mayer, S. and Schleimer, M. (1996) Quantitative determination of heparinoid mimetics in human and rat plasma by micellar electrokinetic chromatography. J. Chromatogr. A 730, 297–303.

117. Roach, M., Gozel, P., and Zare, R. N. (1988) Determination of methotrexate and its major metabolite, 7-hydroxymethotrexate using capillary zone electrophoresis and laser induced fluorescence detection. J. Chromatogr. 426, 129–140.

118. Vargas, M. G., Havel, J., and Patocka, J. (1998) Capillary zone electrophoresis determination of some drugs against Alzheimer's disease. J. Chromatogr. A 802, 121–128.

119. Zarzycki, P. K., Kowalski, P., Nowakowska, J., and Lamparczyk, H. (1995) High-performance liquid chromatographic and capillary electrophoretic determination of free nicotinic acid in human plasma and separation of its metabolites by capillary electrophoresis. J. Chromatogr. A 709, 203–208.

120. Garcia, L. L. and Shihabi, Z. K. (1993) Suramin determination by capillary electrophoresis. J. Liq. Chromatogr. 16, 2049–2057.

121. Hettiarachchi, K. and Cheung, A. P. (1995) Precision in capillary electrophoresis with respect to quantitative analysis of suramin. J. Chromatogr. A 717, 191–202.

122. Sanders, J. M., Burka, L. T., Shelby, M. D., Newbold, R. R., and Cummingham, M. L. (1997) Determination of tamoxifen and metabolites in serum by capillary electrophoresis using a nonaqueous buffer system. J. Chromatogr. B 695, 181–185.

123. Hempel, G., Lehmkuhl, D., Krumpelmann, S., Blaschke, G., and Boos, J. (1996) Determination of paclitaxel in biological fluids by micellar electrokinetic chromatography. J. Chromatogr. A 745, 173–179.

124. Soini, H., Riekkola, M.-L., and Novotny, M. V. (1992) Chiral separations of basic drug and quantitation of bupivcaine enantiomers in serum by capillary electrophoresis with modified cyclodextrin buffers. J. Chromatog. 608, 265–274.

125. Prunonsa, J., Obach, R., Diez-Cascon, A., and Gouesclou, L. (1992) Determination of cicletinine enantiomers in plasma by high-performance capillary electrophoresis. J. Chromatogr. 574, 127–133.

126. Francotte, E., Cherkaoul, S., and Faupel, M. (1993) Separation of the enantiomers of some racemic nonsteroidal aromatase inhibitors and barbiturates by capillary electrophoresis. Chirality, 5, 516–526.

127. Soni, H., Stefansson, M., Reikola, M. L., and Novotny, M. V. (1994) Maltooligosaccharides as chiral selectors for the separation of pharmaceuticals by capillary electrophoresis. Anal. Chem. 66, 3477–3484.

128. D'Hulst, A. and Verbeke, N. (1994) Separation of the enantiomers of coumarinic anticoagulant drugs by capillary electrophoresis using maltodextrins as chiral modifiers. Chirality 6, 225–229.

129. Dethyl, J.-M., De Broux, S., Lesne, M., Longstreth, J., and Gilbert, P. (1994) Stereoselective determination of verapamil and norverapamil by capillary electrophoresis. J. Chromatogr. B 654, 121–127.

18

Applications of Capillary Zone Electrophoresis in the Analysis of Metal Ions of Clinical Significance

Lokinendi V. Rao, John R. Petersen, Amin A. Mohammad, and Anthony O. Okorodudu

1. INTRODUCTION

For centuries, many metals, specifically metals such as aluminum, cadmium, arsenic, lead, selenium, and chromium, have been recognized as toxic. Although toxic exposures to large numbers of people are not common, chronic low-level exposure does occur. This happens more frequently to individuals than to large population groups. In a study conducted in 1994 *(1)* on a large general medical population, 0.6% of the patients were identified has having some physical finding or exposure concern, suggesting a need to check for an underlying heavy-metal toxicity. Interestingly, the incidence of heavy-metal poisoning appears to be approximately the same as the more common in-born errors of metabolism. Similar to many of the in-born errors of metabolism, when identified early the problems caused by heavy-metal exposure is readily treatable. Conversely, if exposure is not identified, reduced, and treated, serious, sometimes irreparable, damage occurs to nervous, renal, and cardiovascular systems. Because metal toxicity is readily treatable if identified early enough, the determination of metal concentrations in the body fluids or body tissues is of considerable importance in health care.

Atomic absorption spectrometry with flame or electrothermal atomization furnace, inductively coupled plasma emission spectroscopy *(2)*, and high-performance liquid chromatography-mass spectrometry (HPLC-MS) *(3)* are state-of-the-art techniques currently used to measure metals in biological fluids *(4)*. Ion chromatographic methods, although capable of separating all of the important metal ions in one run, has not found widespread

From: *Clinical and Forensic Applications of Capillary Electrophoresis*
Edited by: J. R. Petersen and A. A. Mohammad © Humana Press Inc., Totowa, NJ

acceptance because of the difficulty in running the assay. Capillary zone electrophoresis (CZE), which is fast, uses small sample size, and is relatively easy to perform, should overcome most of the drawbacks of classical chromatography. It is a highly efficient separation method for ionized species based on the combined effects of electrophoresis and electroosmosis. It is also capable of handling proteinacious samples easier than classical chromatography because of the absence of a stationary phase (5).

2. CADMIUM

Cadmium is a metal that is used routinely in industry. It is used in electroplating, the production of nickel-based rechargeable batteries, as a common pigment in organic-based paints, and strangely enough, tobacco products. Breathing cadmium vapors can lead to nasal epithelial deterioration and pulmonary congestion resembling chronic emphysema (6). Also accumulation of cadmium in tissues, i.e., chronic exposure, causes renal damage, which gets progressively worse over time. The chemical forms of cadmium in tissues can be divided into two groups: metallothionein (MT) bound and non-MT-bound. Cadmium accumulates in the body mainly as the bound form. The nonbound form, which is the toxic form of cadmium, can be detected in tissues before sufficient amounts of MT can be produced to sequester cadmium or after cadmium exposure greater than the organ's ability to synthesize adequate MT. To limit the exposure to cadmium, in 1992 the National Institute of Occupational Safety and Health (NIOSH), mandated that employees exposed to cadmium in the workplace be monitored (7). The concentration of cadmium can be measured in blood (standardized to liters of whole blood) or urine (standardized to µg of cadmium per gram urine creatinine). Normally the blood cadmium concentration is <5 µg/L of whole blood and for urine the cadmium concentration is <3 µg/g creatinine.

Graphite-furnace, atomic-absorption spectrometry is the most widely used technique for cadmium determination. Although the detection limit of this method is <0.2 µg/L, analytical difficulties in the analysis of blood cadmium are reflected by the lack of consistent results of external-quality assessment programs (8). Because of the aging that occurs with the graphite tubes used, significant alterations of tube properties can sometimes lead to drifting of the signal. Electroanalytical methods based on anodic-stripping voltametry (9) are also available to quantitate the cadmium level. For this technique, the detection limit is <0.1 µg/L, although a rather large volume of whole blood (>0.5 mL) is needed. Isotope-dilution inductively coupled mass spectrometry (ICPMS) (8) improved both accuracy and precision with detection limits of 0.11 µg/L. However, after sample pretreatment, which is

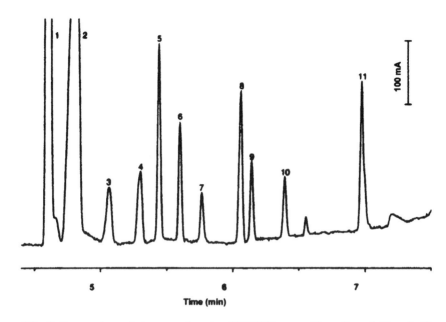

Fig. 1. Separation of nine metals using HEDTC as auxiliary ligand. Fused silica capillary 75 um × 60 cm, 52 cm to detector. BGE 60 mM MOPS, 30 mM TRIS, 10 mM SDS, 0.1 mM HEDTC, pH 7.2; applied voltage 20 kV; temperature 2°C; detection 254 nm; injection hydrostatic 10 s at 10 cm height, 10 µM each metal. 1 = EOF; 2 = ligand oxidation product; 3 = Cd^{2+}; 4 = Pb^{2+}; 5 = Pt^{2+}; 6 + Co^{2+}; 7 = Ni^{2+}; 8 = Bi^{2+}; 9 = Cr^{2+}; 10 = Cu^{2+}; 11 = Hg^{2+}. Reproduced with permission from ref. *(11)*.

needed to eliminate background absorbance and interferences, the detection limit is reduced to 0.3 µg/L.

The use of capillary electrophoresis (CE) to separate and detect metals is currently being investigated. Using micellar electrokinetic capillary chromatography (MEKC) Saitoh et al. in 1989 separated a variety of metals using sodium dodecyl sulfate (SDS) and a complexing agent (4-(2-Pyridylazo) resorcinol) *(10)*. Cadmium, however, gave poor peak shape, low efficiency, and poor selectivity. However, after optimizing the conditions *(11)*, cadmium, along with eight other metals were well separated with good peak shapes (Fig. 1). Cheng et al. in 1995 (12) reported a successful separation of cadmium with a new buffer that contained no complexing agent. By using an UV active substance, 2-aminopyridine, and a 75 µm i.d. fused silica capillary, the authors reported good separation efficiency with a detection limit for cadmium of 0.6 mg/L. Tnierbaev et al. *(13)* were also able to use MEKC to separate and quantitate nine metal chelates, including cadmium, within 15 min *(see* Fig. 2)

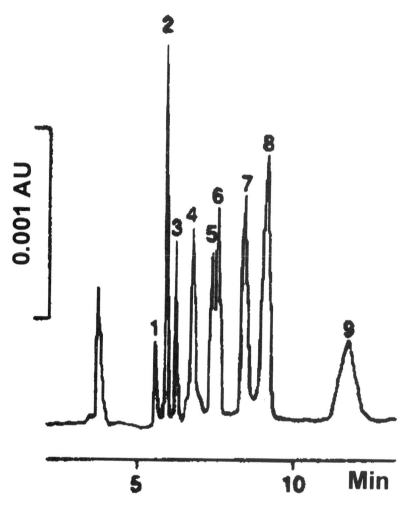

Fig. 2. Micellar CE separation of metal chelates of PAR. Capillary 50 cm; 42 cm to detector) × 75 µm; 10 mM ammonium phosphate, 75 mM SDS, 0.0001 M PAR, pH 8.0; voltage 15 kV; injection 30 s (hydrostatic); detection 254 nm. 1 = Cr^{3+} (0.24 mM); Co^{2+} (0.06 mM); 3 = Cu^{2+} (0.08 mM); 4 = Pb^{2+} (0.08 mM); 5 = Ni^{2+} (0.08 mM); 6 = Fe^{2+} (0.08 mM); 7 = Zn^{2+} (0.16 mM); 8 = Fe^{3+} (0.08 mM); 9 = Cd^{2+} (0.24 mM). The first peak is acetone. Reproduced with permission from ref. *(13)*.

3. ALUMINUM

Aluminum accumulates in blood and, if not filtered by the kidney, binds avidly to proteins, such as albumin. It is rapidly distributed throughout the leads to the accumulation of aluminum at two sites; bone *(14)* and brain *(15)*. In patients with normal renal function, serum aluminum is normally lower than 6 µg/L. However, kidney dialysis patients who are exposed to high levels of aluminum in the form of oral phosphate binders, albumin administration, and dialysis water. Since the kidney filters aluminum, it is very important to monitor aluminum levels in this group of patients to prevent toxicity. Patients with serum aluminum levels >60 µg/L, but >100 µg/L, have been identified as candidates for late onset of aluminum overload disease and thus treatment. Since treatment is not without its side affects, it is important to obtain an accurate measurement. Normally analysis of aluminum is routinely performed by atomic-absorption spectrophotometry with electrothermal atomization after the specimen is mixed with matrix modifier *(16)*. In addition to increases in aluminum concentrations in dialysis patients, Perl *(17)* also reported that aluminum is accumulated in the neurofibrillary tangle of the patients with Alzheimer's disease.

Very little has been done to separate and detect aluminum using CE. In 1993, Shi and Fritz *(18)*, used CZE to separate 27 metal ions in 6 min using lactic acid as an the complexing agent. However, no peak could be detected for either Al (III) or Fe (III). Later, the same authors *(19)* used an acidic pH of 3.2 and nicotinamide formate buffer, to obtain a good peak for Al (III) (*see* Fig. 3).

4. ARSENIC

Arsenic is one of the best-known, and perhaps infamous, of the metal toxins. It can exist in a number of different forms *(20)*. Some these forms are toxic, whereas others are not. The toxic forms are the inorganic species, As (III) and As (V). Monomethyl arsine (MMA) and dimethyl arsenine (DMA) are partially detoxified metabolites. Serum arsenic is only elevated for a short time (<4 h) after administration. It then disappears into the phosphate pool *(21)*. The toxic forms of arsenic, As (III) and As (V), are be found in urine shortly after ingestion, peaking at 10 h, and returning to normal in 20–30 h. The primary mechanism for arsenic toxicity is related to sulfhydryl binding. Arsenic also interferes with the activity of several enzymes of the heme biosynthetic pathways.

Since urine is concentrated by the kidney it is the sample of choice for arsenic analysis. Arsenic is routinely analyzed by using ICP-MS *(22)* or anodic-stripping voltametry. Although CE has not been used in the routine analysis of arsenic there have been a few articles that have dealt with the separation and detection of arsenic. One dealt with separation of arsenic, arsenate, and organoarsenic anions by CZE *(23)*. From this report, it can be concluded that separation in the co-electroosmotic mode is preferred with detection often being direct UV photometric detection (190 nm). The use of

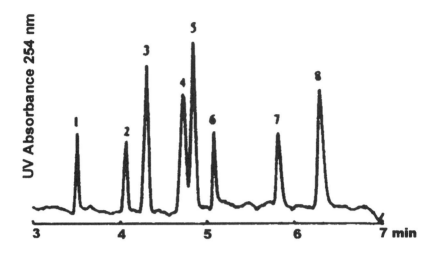

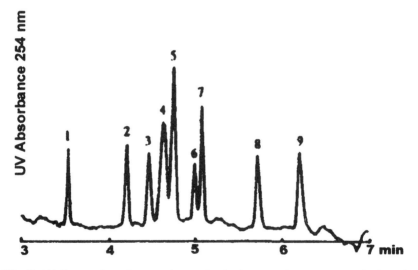

Fig. 3. (A) Separation of a sample standard mixture using an uncomplexing electrolyte. Electrolyte, 8 mM nicotinamide, pH 3.2, adjusted with formic acid; applied voltage, 25 kN; injection time 40 s. 1 = K$^+$ (1.5 ppm); 2 = Ba^{2+} (1.5 ppm); 3 = Sr^{2+} and Ca^{2+} (0.8 ppm); 4 = Mg^{2+} (0.5 ppm) and Na$^+$ (0.8ppm); 5 = Al^{3+} (0.8 ppm); 6 = Cu^{2+} (0.8 ppm); 7 = Li$^+$ (0.2 ppm); 8 = VO^{2+} (2 ppm). **(B)** Separation of the same sample standard mixture using an uncomplexing electrolyte with 18-crown-6. Electrolyte, 8 mM nicotinamide, 0.6 mM 18-crown-6, pH 3.2, adjusted with formic acid; applied voltage, 25 kN; injection time 40 s. 1 = K$^+$ (1.5 ppm); 2 = Ca^{2+} (0.8 ppm); 3 = Sr^{2+} (1.5 ppm); 4 = Mg^{2+} (0.5 ppm) and Na$^+$ (0.8 ppm); 5 = Al^{3+} (0.8 ppm); 6 = Cu^{2+} (0.8 ppm); 7 = Ba^{2+} (1.5 ppm); 8 = Li$^+$ (0.2 ppm); 9 = VO^{2+} (2 ppm). Reproduced with permission from ref. *(19)*.

ICP-MS, employed as a post–column detection technique in CZE, enhanced sensitivity, and selectivity of the system. With this system, Michalke and Schramel *(24)* were able to separate and detect in a single run six arsenic species. Detection limits were calculated according to IUPAC recommendations to be 15 µg As/L for As (III) and As (V) or 0.015 µg/mL. This is more than adequate to quantitate levels (0.1–0.5 µg/mL) associated with chronic poisoning. Separately, Huang and Whang *(25)* were able to separate and detect five arsenic species using indirect fluorescence detection with an assay time of 8 min. The detection limits for their method was between 0.04 and 0.16 µg/mL, and although not as good as ICP-MS, was still adequate to detect arsenic concentrations (0.1 µg/mL) associated with chronic poisoning.

5. LEAD

Lead is a heavy metal commonly found in the environment with no known physiological significance in humans *(26)*. It is found in high concentrations in many paints, leaded gasoline, drinking water, food, soil, and dust. Lead is absorbed primarily through the GI tract, lungs, after ingestion, or inhalation of lead-contaminated substances. High doses are known to adversely affect many systems of the body *(27)*. A typical diet in United States constitutes approx 300 µg of lead per day, of which 1–10% is absorbed. As per CDC guidelines *(28)*, a blood level of 10 µg/dL is considered toxic in children. The WHO has also defined whole blood levels >30 µg/dL in adults as an indication of significant exposure. Levels of >55 µg/dL can cause death, brain damage, kidney failure, seizures, and anemia.

Analysis of lead is routinely performed by atomic-absorption spectrometry after the specimen has been mixed with matrix modifier *(29)*. The use of palladium over magnesium/phosphate modifier has also tremendously improved the detection limit to 0.1 µg/L for a 10 µL-injection volume. This can be done with a precision of 2.2%. Stable isotope dilution gas chromatography-mass spectrometry (GC-MS) has also been exploited with a detection limit of 0.1 µg/L *(27)*. An alternate method currently in use is anodic stripping voltametry, with an analysis time of 90 s. Although fast, this method has a lower limit of detection of 1 µg/dL with precision of only 10% *(27)*.

Although CE has not been used to detect the presence of lead in biological fluids by using an ultramicroelectrode as an electrochemical detector, it is possible detect and quantitate lead. Polesello and Valsecchi *(30)* reviewed recent advances in electrochemical detection in CE for the analysis of inorganic compounds. By using an end-column ultramicroelectrode with a 10–25 µm capillaries a lead-detection limit of $2 \times 10^{-5} M$ was achieved. Although the sensitivity needs to be increased by two orders of magnitude to be clinically useful, it does show the feasibility of using CE in the detection of lead. Perhaps by using ICP-MS or indirect florescence detection in addition to a preconcentration step, it would be possible to achieve the sensitivity needed clinically.

6. SELENIUM

Selenium is both an essential and toxic element, and plays an important role in environmental analysis as well as in health studies. Sufficient selenium supplementation can protect against heart disease and has a possible role for cancer prevention *(31)*. The absence of selenium correlates with a loss of glutathione peroxidase activity and is associated with damage to cell membranes resulting from accumulation of free radicals. The normal daily dietary intake of selenium is 0.01 and 0.04 ppm. Selenium is accumulated such that the normal concentration in human blood is 95–160 µg/L (0.015 ppm). In the selenium deficiency, the serum concentration is <40 µg/L. Selenium toxicity in humans is not known to be a significant problem except in acute overdose cases and selenium is not classified as a human teratogen. Biological and toxicological effects of selenium are strongly dependent on its chemical form *(32)*, thus there is an increasing interest in the differentiation of selenium species, both organic and inorganic.

Analysis of selenium is routinely performed by atomic-absorption spectrometry after the specimen is mixed with matrix modifier *(33)*. The high resolving power of CE makes it potentially valuable for separation and detection of the various selenium species. CZE separation of selenium anions has been the subject of several reports and reviews *(23)*. The preferred way to separate the various species of selenium is the co-electroosmotic mode with direct photometric detection. The absorption properties of selenite (+2 oxidation state) are significantly higher than the selenate (+8 oxidation state) at 200 nm, giving detection limits of 2 and 0.4 ppm, respectively. Indirect photometric detection for the separation of selenate, selinite, selenocystine, and selenomethionine in combination with electrokinetic injection, which selectively injects and concentrates ions, provided highly sensitive detection for inorganic selenium ions. Further, coupling ICP-MS with CE affords specific multi-element detection, in addition to providing extremely sensitive detection of the various metals. Thus, use of CE, specifically CZE, with ICP-MS *(32)* was applied to selenium speciation providing the possibility to analyze six selenium species in a single run. With this method, detection limits were found to be as 10–20 µg/L of inorganic species and 35–50 µg/L for organic selenium species, which is within the limits needed to be clinical useful.

7. CHROMIUM

Chromium is used extensively in the manufacture of stainless steel, chrome plating, leather tanning, as a dye for printing, and textile manufacture, and as such can possess a significant occupational health hazard *(34)*. The toxic form is Cr 6+. Inhalation of dust particles containing this metal causes erosion of the epithelium of the nasal passages and has also been associated with squamous-cell carcinoma of lung *(35)*. Cr 6+ is rapidly reduced to Cr 3+, which has no known toxicity *(36)*. Because of the rapid disaparence of the toxic form of chromium monitoring biological specimens for Cr 6+ is neither practical nor clinically useful in attempting to detect chromium toxicity. Thus, measurement of chromium (Cr 3+) in urine can be used to assess exposure to chromium, although the concentration of Cr 3+ may not indicate specific exposure to Cr 6+. However, monitoring the air at the manufacturing site for the presence of Cr 6+ is useful way to test for Cr 6+ exposure.

Chromium is also known as "glucose-tolerance factor" since it is required for insulin activity *(37)*. Existing technology can not measure chromium deficiency, because the lower limit of normal range of chromium in blood challenges the detection limit (0.2 ng/mL) of atomic absorption techniques.

Chromium has been measured by CZE. In this method separation of Cr (IV) or Cr (III) requires complexation with either cyclohexanediaminetetraacetic acid (CDTA) or ethyldiaminetetraacetic acid (EDTA) to to cause the chromium species to migrate towards the cathode. Using CDTA and direct detection at 240 nm gave 19 and 59 ppb (ng/mL) detection levels for Cr (VI) and Cr (III), respectively. About 10-fold lower detection limits noted when EDTA used *(23)*. Although the limit of sensitivity for the method using EDTA is good, another one to two orders of magnitude is still required for CE to be clinical useful.

8. CONCLUSION

In conclusion, CZE analysis of heavy metals is still under research and development. Although promising, the techniques that have been used still do not have adequate sensitivity for routine applications in the clinical analysis of biological samples. Depending on the CE technique used, an additional one to two orders of magnitude increase in sensitivity is still needed. Perhaps with the newer electrochemical techniques that are being developed or by using indirect fluorescence techniques additional sensitivity can be gained.

REFERENCES

1. Moyer, T. P. (1994) Incidence of heavy metal toxicity in a clinical population (Abstract). 4th International conference on Therapeutic Drug Monitoring and Toxicology, Vienna, Austria.

2. Ash, O. K. and Komaromy-Hitler, G. L. (1997) Analysis of clinical specimens using inductively coupled plasma mass spectrometry, in Handbook of Analytical Therapeutic Drug Monitoring and Toxicology. (Wong, S. H. Y. and Sunshine, I., eds.), CRC Press, Boca Raton, FL pp. 109–125.

3. Nuttall, K. L. and Gordon W. H. (1995) Inductively coupled plasma mass spectrometry for trace elemental analysis with clinical laboratory. Ann. Clin. Lab. Sci. 25, 264–271.

4. Taylor, A. (1997) Detection and monitoring of disorders of essential trace elements. Ann. Clin. Biochem. 33, 486–510.

5. Buchberger, W., Winna, K., and Turner, M. (1994) Application of capillary zone electrophoresis in clinical chemistry. Determination of low molecular-mass ions in body fluids. J. Chromatogr. A 671, 375–382.

6. Hertz-Picciotto, I. and Hu, S. W. (1994) Contribution of cadmium in cigarettes to lung cancer: an evaluation of risk assessment methodologies. Arch. Environ. Health 49, 297–302.

7. Occupational exposure to cadmium. (1992). Fed. Regist. 57 42, 102–142.

8. Daher, R. T. (1995). Trace metals (lead and cadmium exposure screening). Anal. Chem. 67, 405R–410R.

9. Ostapczuk, P. (1992) Direct determination of cadmium and lead in whole blood by potentiometric stripping analysis. Clin. Chem. 38, 1995–2001.

10. Saitoh, T., Hoshino, H., and Yotsuyanagi, T. (1989) J. Chromatogr. 469, 175–181.

11. Macka, M. and Haddad, P. R. (1997) Determination of metal ions by capillary electrophoresis. Electrophoresis 18, 2482–2501.

12. Cheng, K., Nordmeyer, F. R., and Lamb, J. D. (1995) A novel buffer system for separation of metal cations by capillary electrophoresis with indirect UV detection. J. Cap. Electrophor. 2, 279–285.

13. Timerbaeu, A. R., Semenova, O. P., Jandik, P., and Bonn, G. K. (1994) Metal ion capillary electrophoresis with direct UV detection. Effect of a charged surfactant on the migration behavior of metal chelates. J. Chromatogr. 671, 419–427.

14. Buchinsky, D. A., Sprague, S. M., and Hallegot, P. (1995) Effects of aluminum on bone surface ion composition. J. Bone Mineral res. 10, 1988–1997.

15. Erasmus, R. T., Savory, J., Wiilis, M. R., and Herman, M. M. (1993) Aluminum neurotoxicity in experimental animals. Ther. Drug Monit. 15, 582–592.

16. Brown, S., Bertholf, R. L., Willsis, M. R., and Savory, J. (1984) Electrothermal atomic absorption spectrometric determination of aluminum in serum with a new technique for protein precipitation. Clin, Chem. 30, 1216–1218.

17. Perl, D. P. (1980) Alzheimer's disease: X-ray spectrometric evidence of aluminum accumulation in neurofibrilliary tangle bearing neurons. Science 208, 297–299.

18. Shi, Y. and Fritz, J. S. (1993) J. Chromatogr. 640, 473–478.

19. Shi, Y. and Fritz, J. S. (1994) New electrolyte systems for the determination of metal cations by capillary zone electrophoresis. J. Chromatogr. A 671, 429–435.

20. Tabocova, S., Hunter, E. S., and Gladen, B. C. (1996) Developmental toxicity of inorganic arsenic in whole embryo; culture oxidation state, dose, time and gestational age dependence. Toxicol. Appl. Pharmacol. 138, 298–307.

21. Hindmarsh, J. T. and McCurdy, R. F. (1986) Clinical and environmental aspects of arsenic toxicity. Crit. Rev. Clin. Lab. 23, 315–347.

22. Nixon, D. E. and Moyer, T. P. (1996) Routine clinical determination of lead, arsenic, cadmium and thallium in urine and whole blood by inductively coupled plasma mass spectrometry. Spectrochim. Acta 51B, 13–25.

23. Kaniansky, D., Masar, M., Marak, J., and Bodor, R. (1999) Capillary electro-phoresis of inorganic anions. J. Chromatgr. A 834, 133–178.

24. Michalke, B. and Schramel, P. (1998) Capillary electrophoresis interfaced to inductively coupled mass spectrometry for element selective detection in arsenic speciation. Electrophoresis 19, 2220–2225.

25. Huang, Y. M. and Whang, C. W. (1998) Capillary electrophoresis of arsenic compounds with indirect fluorescence detection. Electrophoresis 19, 2140–2144.

26. Lockitch, G. (1993) Perspectives on lead toxicity. Clin. Biochem. 26, 371–381.

27. Daher, R. T. (1995) Trace metals (lead and cadmium exposure training). Anal. Chem. 67, 405R–410R.

28. Roper, W. L., Houk, V. N., Falk, H., and Binder, S. (1991) Preventing lead poisoning in young children. A statement by the CDC, Atlanta, GA. USDHHS, Publ PB92–155076/HDM.

29. Parson, P. J. and Slavin, W. (1993) A rapid Zeeman graphite furnace atomic absorption spectrometric method for determination of lead in blood. Spectrochim. Acta 48B, 925–939.

30. Polesello, S. and Valsecchi, S. H (1999) Electrochemical detection in the capillary electrophoresis analysis of inorganic compounds. J. Chromatogr. A 834, 103–116.

31. Fleming, C. R., Mc Call, J. T., and O' Brien, J. F. (1984) Selenium status in patients receiving home parenteral nutrition. J.P.E.N. 8, 258–262.

32. Michlake, B. and Schramel, P. (1998) Application of CZE-inductively coupled plasma mass spectrometry and capillary isoelectric focussing and capillary iso-electric focussing-inductively coupled to MS for Selenium speciation. J. Chromatogr. A 807, 71–80.

33. Jacobson, B. E. and Lockitch, G. (1988) Direct determination of Selenium in serum by graphite-furnace atomic absorption spectrometry with deuterium background correction and a reduced palladium modifier. Age specific refer-ence ranges. Clin. Chem. 34, 709–714.

34. Alpoim, M. C., Geraldes, C. F., Oliveira, C. R., and Lima, M. C. (1995) Molecu-lar mechanisms of chromium toxicity. Oxidation of hemoglobin. Biochem. Soc. Trans. 23, 255–281.

35. Cohen, M. D., Kargain, B., Klein, C. B., and Costa, M. (1993) Mechanism of chromium carcinigenecity and toxicity. Crit. Rev. Toxicol. 23, 255–281.

36. Tsalev, D. L., and Zaprianov, Z. K. (eds.) (1984). Atomic Absorption Spectrometry in Occupational and Environmental Health Practice. CRC Press, Boca Raton, FL.

37. Morris, B. W., Griffiths, H., and Kemp, G. J. (1988) Effect of glucose loading on concentrations of chromium in plasma and urine of healthy adults. Clin. Chem. 34, 1114–1116.

19
Clinical and Forensic Drug Toxicology
Analysis of Illicit and Abused Drugs in Urine by Capillary Electrophoresis

Wolfgang Thormann and Jitka Caslavska

1. INTRODUCTION: ANALYSIS OF URINARY DRUGS IN CLINICAL AND FORENSIC TOXICOLOGY

Clinical and forensic toxicology is concerned with the detection, identification, and measurement of toxic compounds and their metabolites in human body fluids and tissues. Most often the toxic compounds are drugs taken either accidentally or intentionally in quantities sufficient to cause an adverse reaction or death. Analysis and identification of a possible drug or drug combinations, toxicological drug screening and confirmation should encompass as many different classes of drugs as possible. The most important classes being salicylate, paracetamol, antiepileptics, antidepressants, neuroleptics, hypnotics (benzodiazepines, barbiturates, diphenhydramine), digoxin, and theophylline, as well as many illicit drugs, such as opiates, methadone, D-lysergic acid diethylamide (LSD), cocaine, and/or its major metabolite benzoylecgonine, cannabinoids and amphetamines. Currently, urinary drug monitoring has established itself as the basis of clinical and forensic toxicology. It is also the method of choice for drug testing of employees at the workplace, athletes at sports events (such as the Olympics), and patients in drug-substitution programs. Since positive urine tests for an illegal drug can result in severe penalties and drastically change the life of the presumed abuser, urine drug testing must be as free from error as possible. Positive results from an initial screening process should always be confirmed by another method that is more selective and possibly also more sensitive than that used for rapid screening. Furthermore, monitoring of drugs and metabolites in urine is a useful approach for the assessment of drug metabolism and to investigate the patient's compliance.

From: *Clinical and Forensic Applications of Capillary Electrophoresis*
Edited by: J. R. Petersen and A. A. Mohammad © Humana Press Inc., Totowa, NJ

Comprehensive approaches, such as immuno- and chromatographic assays, for the analysis of illicit and licit drugs in urine, have been developed and are routinely used in clinical and forensic laboratories all over the world *(1–4)*. Typically, immunological techniques, including those based on fluorescence-polarization immunoassay (FPIA), enzyme-multiplied immunoassay technique (EMIT), cloned enzyme donor immunoassay (CEDIA), and kinetic interaction of microparticles in solution (KIMS), are employed because of their ease of use (reagents for a number of drugs of abuse are available in kit form) and speed of analysis. Immunoassays, however, often lack specificity and sometimes sensitivity. Thus, they are inappropriate for confirmation of the presence of a specific drug or metabolite. Moreover, most commercial immunoassays are by nature unsuitable for the simultaneous monitoring of multiple drugs and metabolites. Chromatographic approaches, such as thin-layer chromatography (TLC), high-performance liquid chromatography (HPLC), and gas chromatography (GC), can provide results for multiple components. These methods typically require extensive sample pretreatment, are characterized by a modest sample throughput, and are difficult to automate. Despite the widespread use of TLC as a screening method in forensic science, due to difficulties inherent with the technique, it is not routinely used in clinical laboratories. HPLC, on the other hand, is widely applied for drug screening *(5)*. Automated HPLC with multiwavelength detection is commercially available *(6)* and has been successfully employed as a drug profiling system for emergency toxicology *(7)*. Although these methods are useful for screening, gas chromatography with mass spectrometry (GC-MS, *(8)*), and to a minor extent, liquid chromatography with mass spectrometry (LC-MS) *(9,10)*, are employed for confirmatory testing in clinical and forensic laboratories.

Capillary electrophoresis (CE) has been used to separate and identify many drugs, including drugs of abuse, in a variety of body fluids, including urine. Thus many CE-based assays for drugs of toxicological interest have emerged *(11–15)*. A comprehensive concept for toxicological drug screening and confirmation has also been developed and applied to the monitoring of drugs of abuse in patient urine *(16–18)*. In this chapter, CE-based assays for analysis of illicit and abused drugs and their major metabolites in urine are described (Table 1). Usually two CE methods are employed: capillary zone electrophoresis (CZE) and micellar electrokinetic capillary chromatography (MECC). A detailed explanation of these CE methods can be found in Chapter 2. Examples discussed in this chapter come from data gathered in our laboratory and were selected to provide insight into the strategies employed for sample preparation and drug detection. The monitoring of drugs in blood by CE is discussed in Chapters 17 and 20.

Table 1
Selected Screening and Confirmation Assays for Illicit and Abused Drugs in Urine

Drugs, metabolites	CE method(s)	Urine preparation	Solute detection	Reference assay(s)	Ref(s)
Barbiturates	MECC	EXI	UV-MWD	EMIT	(19)
Barbiturates (butalbital)	MECC	EXI	UV	various methods	(20)
Salicylate	MECC, CZE	DSI, dilution	UV-MWD	Trinder	(21)
Salicylic acid, gentisic acid, salicyluric acid	MECC	DSI, dilution	UV, F, UV, F, LIF	Trinder	13,22
Salicylic acid, gentisic acid, salicyluric acid	Non-aq. CZE	EXI, H-EXI	UV	–	(23)
Nonopioid analgesics (paracetamol, salicylate, antipyrine, ibuprofen, naproxen, propyphenazone, and metabolites)	CZE, MECC	DSI, H	DAD, MS	–	(24)
Paracetamol and metabolites	CZE	DSI	UV, DAD, MS	–	(25)
11-nor-Δ⁹-tetrahydrocannabinol 9-carboxylic acid	MECC	H-EXI	UV-MWD	FPIA	(26)
Methadone, EDDP	CZE	DSI, EXI	UV-MWD	EMIT, GC-MS	(27)
Methadone, EDDP	Chiral CZE	EXI	UV	–	(28,29)
Methadone, EDDP	CZE	DSI, EXI	UV-MWD, MS	GC-MS	(30)
Benzodiazepines	MECC	H-EXI	UV-MWD	EMIT, GC-MS	(31)
Benzoylecgonine, opiates, methaqualone, amphetamine, methamphetamine	MECC	EXI	UV-MWD	EMIT	(16,17)
Cocaine and major classes of illicit and abused drugs	MECC, CZE	EXI	UV-MWD	EMIT, FPIA, GC-MS	(18)
Opiates (morphine, codeine, dihydrocodeine, pholcodine)	CZE	EXI	UV	HPLC	(32)

Compound	Mode	Sample injection	Detection	Confirmation	Ref.
Ephedrine, norephedrine	CZE	DSI (dilution)	UV	–	(33)
Amphetamine, methamphetamine, designer drugs, methadone, ephedrines, and metabolites	CZE	EXI	UV-MWD	EMIT	(34)
Amphetamine, methamphetamine, designer drugs, methadone and metabolites	Chiral CZE	EXI	UV-MWD	FPIA, EMIT	(35)
Amphetamine and analogs, methadone, EDDP	CZE	EXI,DSI	UV-MWD, MS		(36)
MDMA (Ecstasy) and metabolites	Chiral CZE	DSI, EXI, H-EXI	UV	–	(13,37)
MDMA (Ecstasy) and metabolites	CZE	DSI, EXI, H-EXI	UV	–	(13)
Methaqualone	MECC	EXI	UV	GC-MS	(38)
LSD	CZE	EXI	LIF	RIA	(39)
β-blockers (oxprenolol)	MECC	DSI (dilution), EXI	UV	(GC-MS)	(40)
Tricyclic antidepressants and antipsychotics, amiodarone	MECC	EXI	UV	–	(41)
Furosemide, piretanide	MECC	EXI	UV, UV-DAD	–	(42)
Diuretics	CZE	EXI	UV	GC-MS	(43)
Dihydrocodeine and metabolites	MECC	DSI, EXI, H-EXI	UV-MWD		(44)
Dextromethorphan, levomethorphan, dextrorphan, levorphanol	Chiral MECC	EXI	UV		(45)
Dextromethorphan and metabolites	MECC, CZE	H	UV-MWD, UV	HPLC	(46,47)
Haloperidol (various metabolites)	CZE	EXI	MS, DAD	–	(48)

Abbreviations: CZE, capillary zone electrophoresis; DAD, diode array detection; DSI, direct sample injection; EMIT, enzyme multiplied immunoassay technique; EXI, extract injection; F, fluorescence detection; FPIA, fluorescence polarization immunoassay; GC-MS, gas chromatography-mass spectrometry; H, hydrolysis; HPLC, high-performance liquid chromatography; LIF, laser induced fluorescence detection; MECC, micellar electrokinetic capillary chromatography; MS, mass spectrometry; MWD, multiwavelength detection using a fast scanning detector, RIA, radioimmunoassay.

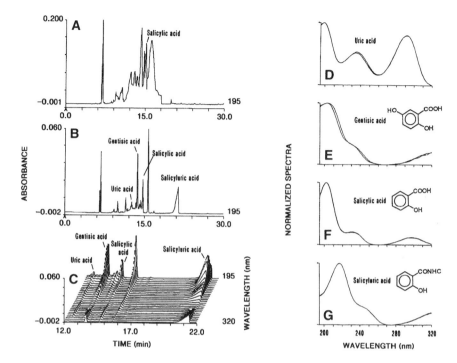

Fig. 1. Analysis of salicylate, salicyluric acid, and gentisic acid by direct urine injection and multiwavelength absorbance detection. MECC data for directly injected (**A**) and 10-fold diluted patient urine (**B,C**) obtained in a buffer composed of 75 m*M* SDS, 6 m*M* sodium tetraborate and 10 m*M* disodium hydrogenphosphate (pH about 9.1). A homemade instrument featuring a 75-μm ID untreated fused silica capillary of 70 cm effective (90 cm total) length and a fast-scanning multiwavelength detector was employed. Sample was applied via gravity, the voltage was 20 kV, and the current was about 80 μA. Absorbance data were gathered between 195 and 320 nm with a 5-nm interval. (**D–G**) depict spectral identity proofs for uric acid (endogenous marker), gentisic acid, salicylic acid, and salicyluric acid, respectively.

2. ANALYSIS OF URINARY DRUGS AND METABOLITES BY CE WITH OPTICAL DETECTION

2.1. Assays with No or Minimal Sample Detection

When using CE, urine specimens can often be injected directly into the separation column or may require only minimal pretreatment, such as dilution, centrifugation, or filtration. The data depicted in Fig. 1 represents MECC data of a urine from a patient with suspected salicylate intoxication. The patients sample tested markedly positive (>1 m*M*) for salicylate employing the modified spectrophotometric method of Trinder *(21)*. Using a fluorescence polarization immunoassay (FPIA), the serum of the same patient was found to contain 3.0 mM salicylate, a value that is above the recommended therapeutic range of 1.1–2.2 mM. After direct urine injection (Fig. 1A), MECC revealed an overloaded, completely unresolved electropherogram in which the presence of salicylate was difficult to identify. However, after 10-fold dilution (Fig. 1B,C), clear separation of salicylate and two of its metabolites, gentisic acid and salicyluric acid, were obtained. In addition, an endogenous marker substance, uric acid, could also be identified. For all four compounds, there was excellent agreement of the absorbance spectra with those of pure compounds (Fig. 1D–G) allowing identification as well as purity assessment of these zones. Comparison of panels A and B also reveals the impact of the sample matrix, showing that detection time by itself is not adequate for analyte identification. However, in conjunction with multiwavelength detection it is possible to identify analytes unambiguously. Analysis of the same sample by CZE at pH 8. 3 also gave comparable data *(21)*.

Currently, the most popular optical detection method is on-column UV absorbance. However, due to the short optical pathlength within the detection cell, the lowest detectable concentration (without preconcentration or stacking of solutes) is in the 1–10 μM (low μg/mL) range. This sensitivity is 1–2 orders of magnitude less than found using HPLC. Other optical detection techniques include fluorescence (F) and laser-induced fluorescence (LIF). When compared to UV absorption detection, sensitivity enhancement using F and LIF can be between 10- and 1000-fold, respectively *(49)*. These two detection modes can also provide increased selectivity that is useful for identification of selective analytes. This is nicely shown with the data presented in Fig. 2A, MECC data obtained with 10-fold diluted urine of the patient with suspected salicylate intoxication. Both UV absorption data (wavelength of 220 nm) and the fluorescence data (emission wavelength of 450 nm) reveal the presence of salicylate. By using fluorescence detection molecules of similar structure, including the metabolites salicyluric acid and gentisic acid, can be detected recognized. Thus the simultaneous monitoring of UV absorption and fluorescence provides valuable information for drug monitoring as well as for the determination of metabolites. Comparison of Fig. 2A and B shows that LIF detection provides a significantly higher sensitivity compared to that obtained by UV and F detection. The same urine used in Fig. 2A was analyzed after 30-fold dilution with water and detected with a HeCd laser (excitation 325 nm line). Using various narrow bandfilters (emission), it can be shown that salicylic acid, salicyluric acid, and gentisic acid have differences in their emission spectrum. Recording multiple electropherograms with different filters can provide multiwavelength fluores-

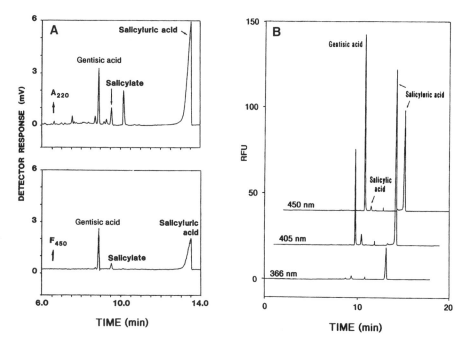

Fig. 2. Monitoring of urinary salicylate and metabolites by CE with fluorescence detection. Sample and buffer were the same as for Fig. 1. **(A)** Simultaneously collected MECC absorbance (at 220 nm, upper graph) and fluorescence (at 450 nm, lower graph) data obtained for 10-fold diluted urine. A homemade instrument featuring a 75 μm ID capillary of 50 cm effective (70 cm total) length and a tunable UV-VIS detector that was adapted for simultaneous fluorescence and absorbance detection was employed *(22)*. Sample was applied via gravity, the voltage was 20 kV and the current was about 90 μA. **(B)** MECC data of 30-fold diluted patient urine obtained with LIF detection having an air-cooled HeCd laser (Liconix, Santa Clara, CA) which emits at 325 nm (power level: about 5 mW) and bandpass filters of 366, 405, and 450 nm (from bottom to top, presented with an *x*-axis offset of 1 min and a *y*-axis shift of 20 RFU). The data were collected on a P/ACE 5510 capillary electrophoresis system (Beckman Instruments, Fullerton, CA, USA) that was equipped with an untreated fused silica capillary of 75 μm ID and 40 cm effective (47 cm total) length. The sample was pressure injected, a constant voltage of 15 kV was applied (current about 70 μA) and the capillary temperature was maintained at 20°C.

cence data, permitting analyte identification. Thus, instrumentation with wavelength-resolved fluorescence detection *(50,51)* (which is not currently commercially available) would provide straightforward data that could be employed for spectral identification in a way comparable to UV absorption, as seen in Fig. 1.

Although LIF provides the highest sensitivity, it is of limited use as there are only a few laser lines available for elute excitation and there are only a limited number of the compounds of interest that fluoresce without derivatization. Using laser-induced resonance energy transfer as described by Petersen et al. *(52)*, the LIF application range can be expanded to nonfluorescing solutes. In this approach, the energy absorbed by a donor molecule is transferred to an acceptor compound (e.g., terbium or europium) which subsequently fluoresces. The feasibility of this method was demonstrated in a CZE setup by detecting salicylic acid, gentisic acid, salicyluric acid and 4-aminosalicylic acid after direct injection of fortified urine. A HeCd laser (325 nm) was used and the terbium ion luminescence at 547 nm was monitored *(52)*. In the absence of terbium, no fluorescence at 547 nm was detected. The analysis of drugs of abuse in real world samples, however, has not yet been studied. The same is true for CE configurations with indirect fluorescence or absorbance detection, which have been employed extensively in other applications *(53,54)*.

2.2. Assays Based on Extraction, Hydrolysis, and Stacking

For elutes that cannot be monitored by direct sample injection or after minimal sample pretreatment have to be extracted and often concentrated. Depending on application, analytes may also have to be hydrolyzed (Table 1). Conventional liquid-liquid or solid-phase extraction procedures are typically employed when extraction is found to be necessary. Another method that is being investigated and thus not yet used routinely for analyte concentration is on-line extraction and preconcentration of analytes *(55,56)*. On-column preconcentration can also be attained by various electrokinetic injection and stacking procedures *(see below)*.

To show the impact of sample preparation, CZE data for urinary Ecstasy (3,4-methylenedioxymethamphetamine or MDMA) is shown in Fig. 3. The urine was from a patient who received 1.5 mg racemic MDMA/kg body weight and was collected 12 h after drug administration. After direct injection of untreated urine, MDMA (22.5 µg/mL) could be determined easily (Fig. 3A). By using solid-phase extraction (2 mL urine with reconstitution in 200 µL of 10-fold diluted running buffer) MDMA and its metabolite 3,4-methylenedioxyamphetamine (MDA) could be detected (Fig. 3B). However, the major metabolite, 4-hydroxy-3-methoxymethamphetamine (HMMA, a compound that is mainly excreted as conjugates *[37]*), could only be monitored after enzymatic hydrolysis prior to solid-phase extraction (Fig. 3C). These data illustrate the impact of the various extraction procedures. With extraction, interfering endogenous substances are removed and elutes of interest concentrated by reconstitution of the dried extract in a volume that

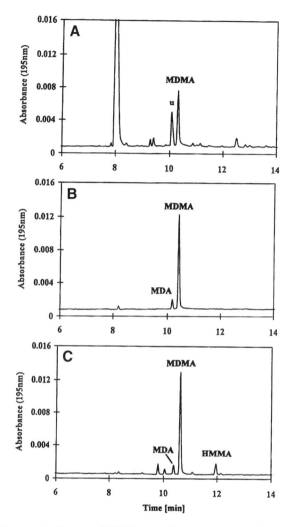

Fig. 3. CZE assay for Ecstasy (MDMA) and its major metabolites in human urine. Data shown were obtained after direct urine injection (**A**), solid-phase extraction (**B**), and enzymatic hydrolysis and solid-phase extraction (**C**) of a urine that was collected 12 h after ingestion of 1.5 mg racemic MDMA per kg body weight. The data were collected on a BioFocus 3000 capillary electrophoresis system (Bio-Rad Laboratories, Hercules, CA) that was equipped with an untreated 50-μm ID fused silica capillary of 55.4 cm effective (60 cm total) length. The sample was pressure-injected, a constant voltage of 22 kV (current about 60 μA) was applied, the temperatures of cartridge and carousel were maintained at 20°C and detection was effected at 195 nm. A 75 m*M* phosphate buffer at pH 2.5 was employed. Solid-phase extraction was executed as described in *(37)* and hydrolysis of HMMA conjugates was effected with 60 μL of β-glucuronidase/arylsulfatase from Helix pomatia per mL of urine and incubation at 37 °C for 16 h. MDMA, 3,4-methylenedioxymethamphetamine (Ecstasy); MDA, 3,4-methylenedioxyamphetamine; HMMA, 4-hydroxy-3-methoxymethamphetamine; u, unidentified endogenous compound. Reprinted with permission from ref. *(13)*.

is smaller than the initial urine volume. After hydrolysis, metabolites can be analyzed that—because of lack of a specific extraction process or lack of appropriate reference substances—could otherwise not be monitored.

Many assays have been developed that are based on pretreatments (Table 1). Of particular interest is an assay for multiple classes of drugs that include opiates, methadone, cocaine, and benzoylecgonine, amphetamine and analogs, methaqualone, 11-nor-Δ^9-tetrahydrocannabinol-9-carboxylic acid (THC), benzodiazepines, barbiturates, diphenhydramine, and so on. This assay was developed in our laboratory and has been used to analyze urine samples received for drug screening from the local University Hospital. It is based on a two-step, solid-phase extraction with a copolymeric sorbent *(17)* followed by analysis of the two concentrated extracts by MECC or CZE with on-column fast scanning spectral detection. The spectral information obtained in this approach is used to help identify the substances. From the same aliquot of urine the two-step extraction procedure allows analysis, of barbiturates, some benzodiazepines, THC and methaqualone (in the first eluate), as well as opiates, cocaine and benzoylecgonine, selected benzodiazepines or their metabolites, methadone and its primary metabolite 2-ethylidene-1,5-dimethyl-3,3-diphenylpyrrolidine (EDDP), diphenhydramine and amphetamines (in the second eluate) *(18)*. MECC data of a urine specimen from a hospitalized patient that was found to be 1) markedly positive for cocaine, opiates, methaqualone, and methadone using EMIT; 2) EMIT negative for amphetamines, barbiturates, and benzodiazepines; and 3) positive for cannabinoids employing an FPIA immunoassay, are depicted in Fig. 4. Using 5 mL urine and the two-step extraction procedure with methylene chloride as first elutant (Fig. 4A) and methylene chloride/isopropyl alcohol (80:20) containing 10% NH_3 as second elutant (Fig. 4B,C), the presence of methaqualone, benzoylecgonine, and opiates was confirmed. Peak assignment was achieved through comparison of retention times and absorption spectra of eluting peaks with those of computer-stored control runs (Fig. 4D). The presence of 6-acetyl morphine (peak 13 in Fig. 4B,C) indicates the possible consumption of heroin. The peak denoted with M (Fig. 4A) was found to have the same normalized spectrum as methaqualone. Furthermore, peaks M_1 and M_2 (Fig. 4A,B, respectively) were determined to have spectra that are very similar to that of methaqualone. Thus, the assay is assumed to confirm not only the presence of methaqualone, but also some of its many metabolites. For detection of THC, the urine would have to be hydrolyzed prior to extraction *(18,26)*. Methadone and EDDP (which were found in the second fraction) elute in the micelle peak (Fig. 4B,C) and, therefore, would have to be analyzed by CZE *(18,27)*.

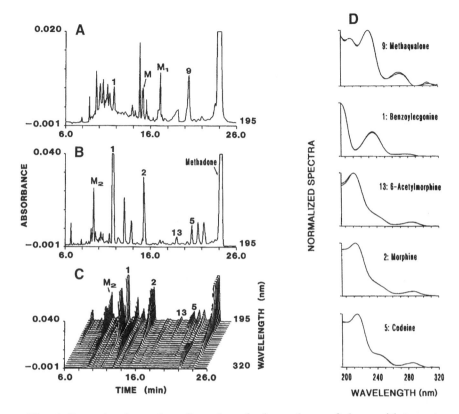

Fig. 4. Screening for and confirmation of urinary drugs of abuse with two-step extraction and polychrome absorbance detection. MECC electropherograms obtained after two-step, solid-phase extraction of a patient urine that has been found positive for methaqualone, opiates, benzoylecgonine, and methadone by screening with EMIT-dau. MECC data of the first fraction (**A**), the second fraction (**B,C**) and spectral identity proofs (**D**) for methaqualone *(9)*, benzoylecgonine *(1)*, 6-acetyl-morphine *(13)*, morphine *(2)* and codeine *(5)* are shown. Instrument and buffer were the same as for Fig. 1. M, M_1, and M_2 are metabolites of methaqualone. Reprinted with permission from ref. *(13)*.

Compared to GC-MS, CE instrumentation is less expensive and some-what simpler to operate. However, in addition to the structural information provided by MS, the GC-MS detection sensitivity is higher than that of MECC and CZE with on-column UV absorption detection. Nevertheless, for most compounds, the sensitivity of our MECC and CZE assays (about 50 ng/mL with application of 5 mL urine) is equal to or better than those of commercial immunoassays, which are typically employed for rapid urine screening. LSD is an exception as the required cutoff value for that compound is 0. 5 ng/mL. In the two-step extraction procedure, LSD appears in the second fraction with a comparable detection limit as that for other illicit substances (data not shown). Thus, this generalized procedure is not adequate for analysis of LSD in the required concentration range. However, electroinjection in conjunction with LIF has recently been shown to permit the determination of urinary LSD in the low ppb concentration level *(39)*. Also the two-step extraction procedure in combination with CE was found to be capable of recognizing false-negative results from immunological screening processes *(13,31)*.

Electrophoretic mass transport is highly regulated, allowing charged solutes to be concentrated (stacked) across an electrolyte discontinuity. This also includes the boundary initially produced between sample and running buffer. In CE, this inherent feature of electrophoresis may take place when the sample compounds encounter isotachophoretic conditions (isotachophoretic sample stacking is based on differences in electrophoretic mobilities) or when the conductivity of the sample is less than that of the buffer (field-amplified sample stacking). After hydrodynamic sample introduction, stacking techniques are not only dependent on sample composition, but also on the sample volume injected and are thus limited by the capillary volume. Experimentally determined enhancement factors associated with these on-column stacking techniques typically do not exceed 100. Head-column, field-amplified sample stacking (also referred to as field-amplified sample injection) associated with electrokinetic sample introduction takes place at the tip of the column removing the limitation of injection volume. It is typically performed with a sample of low conductivity and a short plug of water at the capillary inlet. During electroinjection, analytes are stacked at the interface between the low-conductivity zone and the running buffer. With this type of injection, very little sample solvent is co-injected because the net electroosmotic velocity is typically much smaller than the local electrophoretic transport. Using this approach, a 1000-fold sensitivity enhancement can easily be obtained and ng/mL drug levels can be determined using UV absorption detection *(57)*. Based on this principle, a microassay for urinary dihydrocodeine and nordihydrocodeine *(58)* employing microliter urine volumes has recently been developed. In addition, Taylor et al. *(32)* and Wey and Thormann *(59)* demonstrated that a lower detection limit is obtained when extracted opiates are injected electrokinetically instead of hydrodynamically. The same was found to be true for analysis of urinary amphetamines *(60)*. It is important to realize that detection limits in CE are not only dependent on the type of optical detector used *(see* Fig. 2), but also on the matrix of the sample and the injection procedure employed.

2.3. CE-Based Immunoassays for Urinary Drugs of Abuse

The combination of immunochemistry and CE has lead to the emergence of a number of competitive binding drug assays using labeled drugs as fluorescent tracers. These procedures incubate small amounts of urine (20–50 μL), antibody solution, and tracer prior to application of an aliquot of the mixture onto the capillary. After separation of the unbound fluorescent tracer and antibody-tracer-complex by CZE or MECC, detection is by LIF detection. Chen and co-workers reported the feasibilities for immunological determination of urinary morphine and PCP *(61)*, in addition to morphine, PCP, THC, and benzoylecgonine *(62)* by CZE using drug-cyanine conjugates as tracers and LIF detection with a He-Ne laser (excitation: 543 or 633 nm; emission: 590 or 690 nm). Other approaches employed fluorescein-labeled tracers and LIF detection with an Ar ion laser (excitation: 488 nm; emission: 520 nm). Using this approach, monitoring of urinary benzoylecgonine by CZE *(13)*, urinary methadone *(30)*, and amphetamines *(34)* by MECC- and CZE-based immunoassays, and a CZE four-analyte immunoassay for urine screening *(63)* using reagents from Abbott's TDxFLx FPIA kits (*see* Chapter 12), is possible. Furthermore, Choi et al. described the use of various antibodies for CZE-based immunological analysis of methamphetamine in urine *(64,65)*.

Typically the automated solution-based immunoassays for drugs of abuse that are in widespread use are based on FPIA, EMIT, CEDIA, and KIMS. All of these methods represent one analyte immunoassays (e.g., for methadone or benzoylecgonine) or assays for one group of analytes, such as opiates and amphetamines. Other approaches, such as those with discrete placement of antibodies in spatially separated zones on a solid support onto which binding of different antigens can take place (e.g., the Triage 7 and 8 systems comprising immunoassays for seven and eight analytes or group of analytes, respectively *(66)* permit simultaneous screening for multiple components or multiple groups of analytes. Alternately, the Testcup-5 system of Roche Diagnostic Systems combines a cup for urine collection and a panel with five assays *(67)*. These noninstrumental multianalyte immunoassays were developed for on-site testing of drugs of abuse. CE has also been found suitable for the performance of simultaneous immunoassays of more than one analyte (or more than one group of analytes) in a single sample *(61–63)*. Our four-analyte CE-based immunoassay uses four different sets of reagents, namely those for methadone (M), opiates (O), the cocaine metabolite benzoylecgonine (C) and amphetamine/methamphetamine (A) and was thus referred to as the MOCA assay. It was applied to the screening of drugs of abuse in fortified blank urines, commercial-quality

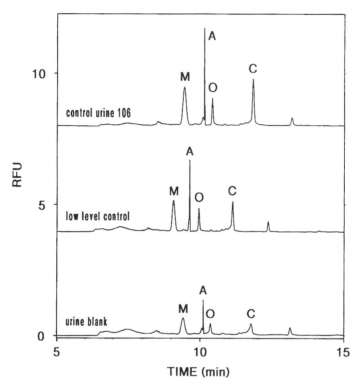

Fig. 5. CZE four-analyte immunoassay. MOCA four-analyte immunoassay data obtained with blank urine (bottom graph), a positive, low-level control sample (center graph), and the external quality control urine 106 of the UKNEQAS for drugs of abuse in urine scheme (top graph) using Abbott's TDxFLx FPIA reagents for methadone, amphetamine/methamphetamine, opiates, and cocaine metabolite. Samples were composed of 25 μL aliquots of urine, antibody solutions, and tracer solutions. The data were collected on a P/ACE 5510 capillary electrophoresis system (Beckman Instruments, Fullerton, CA) equipped with an untreated fused-silica capillary of 75 μm ID and 40 cm effective (47 cm total) length. The applied voltage was 13 kV (currents about 87 μA) and the capillary temperature was maintained at 20°C. The sample carousel was at ambient temperature. Solute detection was effected by LIF using an air-cooled argon ion laser (Ion Laser Technology, Salt Lake City, UT) at 488 nm (operated at 5 mW) and a 520 nm bandpass filter. The buffer was composed of 50 mM sodium tetraborate, pH 9.3, M, free tracer of methadone; A, free tracer of amphetamine; O, free tracer of the opiate morphine; C, free tracer of the cocaine metabolite benzoylecgonine.

control urines and patient samples and was validated *(63)*. Data obtained with the MOCA assay were found to be quantitative and to be in agreement with data resulting from routine urinary screening using EMIT and FPIA.

The electropherograms depicted in Fig. 5 were obtained with a blank urine (bottom graph), with a low-level control urine containing 300 ng/mL methadone, 250 ng/mL morphine, 500 ng/mL D-amphetamine, and 500 ng/mL benzoylecgonine (center graph) and with the external quality control urine No. 106 (upper graph). For all four analytes, small peaks for the free tracers were noted when the urine blank was analyzed. Significantly increased responses for the free tracers were obtained with both the low-level control urine and the external-quality control urine that is known to contain all four classes of drugs (chromatographic data for methadone, free morphine, benzoylecgonine and amphetamine being 2.29, 5.64, 2.46, and 2.38 µg/mL, respectively) *(63)*. Thus, the multianalyte CE immunoassay provides meaningful data and can be used to screen patient urines for the various classes of drugs of abuse. In this case, threshold values of the peak heights relative to the peak height of an internal standard should be defined and applied for urine classification *(63)*.

CE-based multianalyte immunoassays are limited by the ability of CE to separate labeled antigens from each other and from the antibody-antigen complexes. CE-based immunoassays are simple, rapid, sensitive, and reliable approaches for multianalyte screening of drugs in body fluids. The principle employed lends itself to configure custom-made screening reagents that include the specific antibodies and the labeled tracers. To increase versatility, but at the expense of instrumental complexity, strategies with different tagging of tracers together with LIF detection with multiple laser lines and/or wave-length resolved fluorescence detection could represent interesting approaches for simultaneous selective detection of many different types of solutes.

3. CHIRAL CE OF URINARY DRUGS AND METABOLITES: ASSAYS FOR ENANTIOMER SCREENING OF MISUSED, ABUSED, AND BANNED SUBSTANCES

CE has proven to provide a simple, inexpensive, and effective approach for the separation of enantiomers after the addition of a chiral selector to the buffer. The separation by CE of the enantiomers of several drugs of interest in toxicology and doping control has been investigated. By using various cyclodextrins it was possible to effect the chiral differentiation of the optical isomers of racemethorphan and racemorphan *(45)*, amphetamines, cathine, cathinone, cocaine, and others *(68)*, as well as of urinary mephenytoin and phenytoin *(69)*, urinary methadone *(28,29)*, urinary MDMA (Ecstasy) *(37)*, and various amphetamines in urine *(35)*.

Chiral discrimination has a number of possible applications in clinical and forensic toxicology. For example the antitussive dextromethorphan (an allowed drug) and the narcotic analgesic levomethorphan (a banned drug), are the d-(+) and l-(-) isomers of 3-methoxy-*N*-methylmorphinan, respectively. Aumatell and Wells *(45)* demonstrated that these enantiomers could easily be distinguished using a chiral CZE assay that was developed for urinary analysis of the optical isomers of racemethorphan and racemorphan. Distinction of these compounds is not only of interest in forensic science (such as the elucidation of the cause of death after intake of levomethorphan), but also for the treatment of intoxicated patients. In addition, dextrorphan (allowed drug) and levorphanol (banned drug) can easily be separated by MECC using β-cyclodextrin as chiral selector *(45)*. Other compounds, such as (+)-propoxyphene (a narco-analgetic and a controlled substance) and (-)-propoxyphene (an antitussive and an allowed compound), have been separated by chiral CE *(68)*. Finally, the ability to separate the enantiomers of amphetamine and methamphetamine has forensic applications as well *(35)*. The S-(+) enantiomers (d-enantiomers) of amphetamine and methamphetamine have about five times more psychostimulant activity than the R-(-) enantiomers (l-enantiomers) and are thus banned or controlled substances, whereas R-(-)-methamphetamine is found in the Vicks Inhaler® sold in the United States. Furthermore, selegiline (a prescribed drug administrated to treat Parkinson patients) is known to metabolize to the R-(-) enantiomers of methamphetamine and amphetamine.

Recently *(35)* we developed a assay comprising a pH 2.5 buffer containing 8.3 m*M* (2-hydroxypropyl)-β-cyclodextrin (OHP-β-CD) as chiral selector. This assay was able to separate enantiomers from urinary extracts containing methamphetamine, amphetamine, methadone together with its major metabolite EDDP, in addition to 3,4-methylenedioxymethamphetamine (Ecstasy) and other designer drugs (Fig. 6). Enantiomer identification was based on comparison of UV absorption data (as for Figs. 1 and 4) along with comparison of the electropherograms with those obtained by re-running spiked extracts. The suitability of the chiral electrokinetic capillary method for drug screening and confirmation is demonstrated with the data presented in Fig. 6B. Analysis of the unhydrolyzed quality control urine 106 in the achiral buffer revealed the presence of amphetamine, methadone, and EDDP (top graph of Fig. 6B, *[34]*). By using the chiral assay it was possible to show that both enantiomers were present for all three compounds (bottom graph of Fig. 6B). These data indicate that a much-increased resolution is obtained with the chiral buffer (Fig. 6A). Furthermore, morphine (Fig. 6B) and other substances found in alkaline urinary extracts can only be monitored in the chiral buffer *(35)*. Using the chiral assay to analyze a urine from a patient on selegiline pharmacotherapy, the presence of the R-(-)-enantiomers of methamphetamine and amphetamine could be unambiguously identified *(35)*. Thus, ingestion of an R-enantiomer or other drugs that

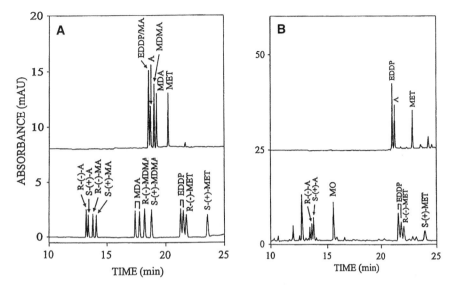

Fig. 6. Chiral separations of amphetamines, methadone, and EDDP. Achiral (top graphs, 195 nm) and chiral (bottom graphs, 195 nm) CE data of **(A)** a mixture of standard compounds and **(B)** the extract of quality control urine 106. For the data of (A), standard compounds were dissolved in water at a concentration of about 5 μg/mL (achiral data) and 10 μg/mL (chiral data) of each enantiomer. For the data of panel (B), alkaline urinary extracts were prepared as described in ref. *(35)*. The achiral buffer employed was composed of 75 m*M* KH$_2$PO$_4$ and 1% ethanolamine (adjusted to pH 9.2 with 1 *M* HCl, whereas the chiral buffer comprised 75 m*M* KH$_2$PO$_4$, pH 2.5, and 8.3 m*M* OHP-β-CD. The BioFocus 3000 with 50 μm ID capillaries of 95.4 cm (achiral assay) and 55.4 cm (chiral assay) effective lengths was used. A, amphetamine; MA, methamphetamine; MET, methadone; MO, morphine. For further details, refer to ref. *(35)*.

metabolize to the R-enantiomers can be distinguished from the ingestion of S-(+)-enantiomers (due to drug abuse) or prescribed drugs that metabolize to the S-enantiomers of methamphetamine and amphetamine. The approach is simple, reproducible, inexpensive, and reliable (being free of interferences of other major basic drugs that are frequently found in toxicological urines) and can be used to screen for and confirm urinary enantiomers in a routine laboratory.

4. ANALYSIS AND CONFIRMATION OF URINARY DRUGS AND METABOLITES BY CE-MS

Interfacing a CE with a mass spectrometer (MS) has been shown to be an attractive approach, analogous to the use of LC-MS *(9,10)*, to gather structural information of compounds, and to use the MS as a CE detector *(70,71)*. Currently there are few published articles discussing CE-MS monitoring of drugs in urine. The best examples are CE-MS determination of urinary *N*-1-hydroxyethylflurazepam (the major metabolite of flurazepam) *(72)*, halo-peridol *(48)*, anti-inflammatory drugs (ibuprofen, flurbiprofen) and their metabolites *(73)*, paracetamol and metabolites *(24,25,74)*, nonopioid anal-gesics *(24)*, methadone *(30,36)*, and methylphenidate *(75)*. In addition, the feasibility of using MS as the detector for the enantiomers of terbutaline spiked into a urine blank has been demonstrated *(76)*. In this instance the use of the chiral selector (heptakis (2,6-di-*O*-methyl)-β-cyclodextrin) in addition to the use of MS gave the selectively needed to verify the chiral composition in complex matrices.

CE-MS instrumentation employed thus far for urinary confirmation test-ing of drugs of abuse and/or their metabolites uses CE interfaced to a MS with atmospheric pressure electrospray ionization. This is followed by iden-tification of protonated molecular ions and/or their fragments using a triple quadrupole *(30)* or an ion trap *(36)* MS. In the first approach, fragmentation of methadone and EDDP was determined by MS-MS. Confirmation was achieved with in-source fragmentation employed. The first quadrupole was operated in the selected ion monitoring mode by switching between the respective parent/daughter ion masses for methadone (m/z = 310, 265) and EDDP (m/z = 278, 249, 234). The CE-MS-MS approach has been success-fully applied to the confirmation of methadone and EDDP in urines that were positive for methadone using CE-based immunoassays, FPIA, EMIT, and CE with UV absorption detection *(30)*. Using an ion trap MS, the pres-ence of amphetamine, MDMA, MDA, methadone, EDDP and morphine in urine could easily be confirmed by the full ion scan mode followed by MS-MS of the protonated molecular ions *(36)*. An example is the alkaline extract of the quality control urine 106 in Fig. 7 where the presence of amphetamine, methadone, EDDP and morphine could unambiguously be confirmed by CE-MS. In addition, CE-MS was shown to be capable of detecting amphetamine and nicotine, compounds that co-migrated under the conditions employed. This was not the case using CZE with UV detection (Fig. 7A) *(36)*. After sample extraction, urinary drug concentrations of 50–100 ng/mL can be detected by CE-MS, comparable to that observed by CE with UV detection. This sensitivity is sufficient for confirmatory testing of most urinary drugs of abuse. The use of a volatile buffer (Figure 7A) was not found to be a limitation in the separation. CE-MS instrumentation with a single quadrupole MS does not permit unambiguous confirmation since no structural proof via fragmentation is possible. A single quadrupole MS can, however, be used as detector.

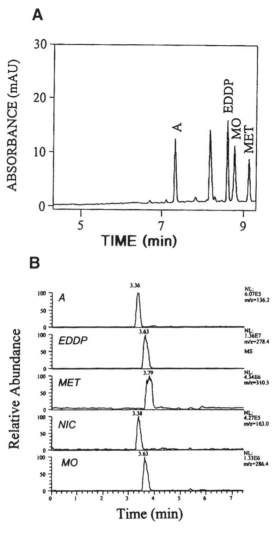

Fig. 7. CZE and CE-MS data of urinary amphetamine, methadone, and EDDP. The buffer employed was composed of ammonium acetate/acetic acid (20 mM each, pH 4.6). The alkaline urinary extract of quality control urine 106 was analyzed (**A**) by CZE with UV absorbance detection using the BioFocus 3000 and (**B**) by CE-MS with the Cristal CE system model 310 coupled to the Finnigan MAT LCQ via a CE atmospheric pressure, electrospray-ionization interface. The BioFocus was equipped with an untreated 50-μm ID fused silica capillary of 60 cm total length (55.4 cm to the detector), sample was injected by applying positive pressure of 4 psi × s, a constant voltage of 20 kV (current about 15 μA) was applied, the temperatures of cartridge and carousel were maintained at 20°C. CE-MS measurements were made with stabilization of the electrospray using a sheath liquid flow of 3 μL/min methanol/water/acetic acid (60/39/1 [v/v]), a 75-μm ID capillary of 70 cm length, sample injection of 200 mbar for 6 s and a separation voltage of 30 kV. A, amphetamine; MET, methadone; NIC, nicotine; MO, morphine.

5. CONCLUSION

As is shown by the examples presented in this chapter, CE provides high-quality data that would be of interest to clinical and forensic drug toxicologists. The obvious tests to be replaced by CE involve methodologies that are too expensive, inaccurate, and/or prone to interferences. Prime examples include applications that require enantiomeric resolution, methods that consume high amounts of organic solvents, and assays that lack specificity. Before widespread adoption of CE assays in clinical and forensic drug toxicology can occur, however, validation and the quality assurance aspects of CE based assays have to be addressed. This is especially important for assays that are used for screening and/or confirmation of the presence or absence of illicit, abused, and banned drugs in urine. Initially, data with quality control urines was collected and published *(34–36,63)*. In this work, data produced by electrokinetic capillary assays were found to be in agreement with the results of other techniques. Despite these encouraging results, additional efforts in exploring the use of CE in the clinical and forensic areas needs to be continued. Of critical importance is that analysis of a large number of external quality control urines, e.g., those offered by Cardiff Bioanalytical Services (UKNEQAS for drugs of abuse, Cardiff, UK) or College of American Pathologists (CAP), should be undertaken.

Currently the use of optical detection is the most popular detection mode employed. UV absorbance in the single and multiwavelength formats as well as fluorescence and laser-induced fluorescence has been successfully used in a number of publications (Table 1). Also, based upon the commercial availability of benchtop instrumentation, the use of MS is currently increasing and soon will establish itself as the detection method of choice for confirmation testing. Thus far, electrochemical detection *(77)*, which is highly sensitive and selective, has received only cursory evaluation for detection of drugs in urine. This is mostly due to the lack of commercial detectors. The use of amperometric detection, however, has recently been demonstrated for the analysis of urinary promethazine and thioridazine *(78)*.

Analysis of illicit and abused urinary drugs and their metabolites by CE offers many attractive features. CE offers separation methods that are amenable to the analysis of ionic (CZE, MECC) and neutral (MECC) solutes, including compounds that are difficult to analyze by GC. Furthermore, CE provides extremely high efficiency, resolving power, and separation speed when compared to HPLC. CE is also complementary to existing analytical methods, such as HPLC, GC, and high-throughput, automated immuno- and photometric assays. CE methods performed in capillaries of 25–75 µm ID are considered nanoscale separation techniques, the capillary and sample plug volumes being 0.1–5 µL and 1–10 nL, respectively. Versatility, high efficiency, and the possibility of direct urine injection or minimal sample preparation are appealing features for clinical and forensic analysis. Although CE is appealing for routine clinical and forensic use, the limit of detection is somewhat not as good as that of other separation techniques (including HPLC). This often calls for either on-line or off-line preconcentration of analytes prior to analysis. Fortunately, electrophoretic techniques feature a unique concentration effect (inherent to electrophoretic mass transport and very rarely seen in other separation techniques), which can provide compensation for the lack of sensitivity. Having instrumentation with a single fused silica capillary (as was the case for all the data presented in this chapter), sample throughput is limited since analyses can only be performed in a sequential mode. Having multiple capillaries in parallel would allow increased sample throughput and/or to permit the simultaneous analysis of a urinary extract in different buffers *(18)*. Alternatively, the use of microchips in the single or multilane formats would provide even faster analyses and thus the highest throughput.

ACKNOWLEDGMENTS

The authors acknowledge valuable discussions with Rudolf Brenneisen, Steven R. Binder, Ira S. Lurie, and France Tagharo the technical assistance provided by Regula Theurillat and the support provided by the lab technicians of the departmental drug-assay laboratory. This work was sponsored by the Swiss National Science Foundation.

REFERENCES

1. Taylor, W. J. and Diers Caviness, M. H. (1986) A textbook for the clinical application of TDM, Abbott Laboratories, Irving, TX.
2. Moffat, A. C. (ed.) (1986) Clarke's Isolation and Identification of Drugs in Pharmaceuticals, Body Fluids and Post-Mortem Material, 2nd ed. Pharmaceutical Press, London.
3. DeCresce, R., Mazura, A., Lifshitz, M., and Tilson, J. (1989) Drug testing in the workplace, ASCP Press, Chicago, IL.
4. Wong, S. H. Y. and Sunshine, I. (eds.) (1997) Handbook of Analytical Therapeutic Drug Monitoring and Toxicology, CRC, Boca Raton, FL.
5. Binder, S. R. (1996) Analysis of drugs of abuse in biological fluids by liquid chromatography. Adv. Chromatogr. 36, 201–271.
6. Adams, A. K., Essien, H., and Binder, S. R. (1991) Identification of drugs in physiological fluids following on-line liquid chromatographic purification and analysis. Ann. Biol. Clin. 49, 291–297.
7. Sadec, N., Francois, G., Petit, B., Dutertre-Catella, H., and Dumontet, M. (1997) Automated liquid-chromatographic analyzer used for toxicology screening in a general hospital: 12 months' experience. Clin. Chem. 43, 498–504.

8. Gerhards, P., Bons, U., Sawazki, J., Szigan, J., and Wertmann, A. (1997) GC/MS in der klinischen Chemie. VCH Verlagsgemeinschaft, Weinheim, Germany.
9. Hoja, H., Marquet, P., Verneuil, B., Lotfi, H., Pénicaut, B., and Lachâtre, G. (1997) Application of liquid chromatography-mass spectrometry in analytical toxicology: a review. J. Anal. Tox. 21, 116–126.
10. Maurer, H. H. (1998) Liquid chromatography-mass spectrometry in forensic and clinical toxicology. J. Chromatogr. B 713, 3–25.
11. Thormann, W., Zhang, C.-X., and Schmutz, A. (1996) Capillary electrophoresis for drug analysis in body fluids. Ther. Drug Monit. 18, 506–520.
12. Thormann, W. (1997) Capillary electrophoresis for drug analysis in body fluids, in Handbook of Analytical Therapeutic Drug Monitoring and Toxicology, (Wong, S. H. Y. and Sunshine, I., eds.), CRC, Boca Raton, FL, pp. 1–19.
13. Thormann, W., Aebi, Y., Lanz, M., and Caslavska, J. (1998) Capillary electrophoresis in clinical toxicology. Forensic Sci. Int. 92, 157–183.
14. Lurie, I. S. (1995) Analysis of seized drugs by capillary electrophoresis, in Analysis of Addictive and Misused Drugs (Adamovics, J. A., ed.), Marcel Dekker, New York, pp. 151–219.
15. Tagliaro, F. and Smith, F. P. (1996) Forensic capillary electrophoresis. Trends Anal. Chem. 15, 513–525.
16. Wernly, P. and Thormann, W. (1991) Analysis of illicit drugs in human urine by micellar electrokinetic capillary chromatography with on-column fast scanning polychrome absorption detection. Anal. Chem. 63, 2878–2882.
17. Wernly, P. and Thormann, W. (1992) Drug of abuse confirmation in human urine using stepwise solid-phase extraction and micellar electrokinetic capillary chromatography. Anal. Chem. 64, 2155–2159.
18. Steinmann, L. and Thormann, W. (1995) Toxicological drug screening and confirmation by electrokinetic capillary techniques: concept of an automated system. J. Cap. Electrophor. 2, 81–88.
19. Thormann, W., Meier, P., Marcolli, C., and Binder, F. (1991) Analysis of barbiturates in human serum and urine by high-performance capillary electrophoresis-micellar electrokinetic capillary chromatography with on-column multi-wavelength detection. J. Chromatogr. 545, 445–460.
20. Ferslew, K. E., Hagardorn, A. N., and McCormick, W. F. A. (1995) Application of micellar electrokinetic capillary chromatography to forensic analysis of barbiturates in biological fluids. J. Forensic Sci. 40, 245–249.
21. Caslavska, J., Lienhard, S., and Thormann, W. (1993) Comparative use of three electrokinetic capillary methods for the determination of drugs in body fluids. Prospects for rapid determination of intoxications. J. Chromatogr. 638, 335–342.
22. Caslavska, J., Gassmann, E., and Thormann, W. (1995) Modification of a tunable UV-visible capillary electrophoresis detector for simultaneous absorbance and fluorescence detection: profiling of body fluids for drugs and endogenous compounds. J. Chromatogr. A, 709, 147–156.
23. Hansen, S. H., Jensen, M. E., and Bjørnsdottir, I. (1998) Assay of acetylsalicylic acid and three of its metabolites in human plasma and urine using non-

aqueous capillary electrophoresis with reversed electroosmostic flow. J. Pharm. Biomed. Anal. 17, 1155–1160.

24. Heitmeier, S. and Blaschke, G. (1999) Direct assay of nonopioid analgesics and their metabolites in human urine by capillary electrophoresis and capillary electrophoresis-mass spectrometry. J. Chromatogr. B 721, 109–125.

25. Heitmeier, S. and Blaschke, G. (1999) Direct determination of paracetamol and its metabolites in urine and serum by capillary electrophoresis with ultraviolet and mass spectrometry detection. J. Chromatogr. B 721, 93–108.

26. Wernly, P. and Thormann, W. (1992) Confirmation testing of 11-nor-delta^9-tetrahydrocannabinol-9-carboxylic acid in urine with micellar electrokinetic capillary chromatography. J. Chromatogr. 608, 251–256.

27. Molteni, S., Caslavska, J., Allemann, D., and Thormann, W. (1994) Determination of methadone and its primary metabolite in human urine by capillary electrophoretic techniques. J. Chromatogr. B 658, 355–367.

28. Lanz, M. and Thormann, W. (1996) Characterization of the stereoselective metabolism of methadone and its primary metabolite via cyclodextrin capillary electrophoretic determination of their urinary enantiomers. Electrophoresis 17, 1945–1949.

29. Frost, M., Köhler, H., and Blaschke, G. (1997) Enantioselective determination of methadone and its main metabolite 2-ethylidene-1,5-dimethyl-3,3-diphenylpyrrolidine (EDDP) in serum, urine and hair by capillary electrophoresis. Electrophoresis 18, 1026–1034.

30. Thormann, W., Lanz, M., Caslavska, J., Siegenthaler, P., and Portmann, R. (1998) Screening for urinary methadone by capillary electrophoretic immunoassays and confirmation by capillary electrophoresis-mass spectrometry. Electrophoresis 19, 57–65.

31. Schafroth, M., Thormann, W., and Allemann, D. (1994) Micellar electrokinetic capillary chromatography of benzodiazepines in human urine. Electrophoresis 15, 72–78.

32. Taylor, R. B., Low, A. S., and Reid, R. G. (1996) Determination of opiates in urine by capillary electrophoresis. J. Chromatogr. B 675, 213–223.

33. Chicharro, M., Zapardiel, A., Bermejo, E., Perez, J. A., and Hernández, L. (1993) Direct determination of ephedrine and norephedrine in human urine by capillary zone electrophoresis. J. Chromatogr. 622, 103–108.

34. Ramseier, A., Caslavska, J., and Thormann, W. (1998) Screening for urinary amphetamine and analogs by capillary electrophoresis immunoassays and confirmation by capillary electrophoresis with on-column multiwavelength absorbance detection. Electrophoresis 19, 2956–2966.

35. Ramseier, A., Caslavska, J., and Thormann, W. (1999) Stereoselective screening for and confirmation of urinary enantiomers of amphetamine, methamphetamine, designer drugs, methadone and selected metabolites by capillary electrophoresis. Electrophoresis 20, 2726–2738.

36. Ramseier, A., Siethoff, C., Caslavska, J., and Thormann, W. (1999) Confirmation testing for urinary amphetamines and designer drugs by capillary electrophoresis-ion trap mass spectrometry. Electrophoresis 21, 380–387.

37. Lanz, M., Brenneisen, R., and Thormann, W. (1997) Enantioselective determination of 3,4-methylene-dioxymethamphetamine and two of its metabolites in human urine by cyclodextrin-modified capillary zone electrophoresis. Electrophoresis 18, 1035–1043.

38. Plaut, O., Girod, C., and Staub, C. (1998) Analysis of methaqualone in biological matrices by micellar electrokinetic capillary chromatography. Comparison with gas chromatography-mass spectrometry. Forensic Sci. Intl. 92, 219–227.

39. Frost, M., Köhler, H., and Blaschke, G. (1997) Determination of LSD in blood by capillary electrophoresis with laser induced fluorescence detection. J. Chromatogr. B 693, 313–319.

40. Lukkari, P., Sirén, H., Pantsar, M., and Riekkola, M.-L. (1993) Determination of 10 β-blockers in urine by micellar electrokinetic capillary chromatography. J. Chromatogr. 632, 143–148.

41. Aumatell, A. and Wells, R. J. (1995) Determination of cardiac antiarrhytmic, tricyclic antipsychotics and antidepressants in human and animal urine by micellar electrokinetic capillary chromatography using a bile salt. J. Chromatogr. B 669, 331–344.

42. Lalljie, S. P. D., Barosso, M. B., Steenackers, D., Alonso, R. M., Jiménez, R. M., and Sandra, P. (1997) Micellar electrokinetic chromatography as a fast screening method for the determination of the doping agents furosemide and piretanide in urine. J. Chromatogr. B 688, 71–78.

43. Jumppanen, J., Sirén, H., and Riekkola, M.-L. (1993) Screening for diuretics in urine and blood serum by capillary zone electrophoresis. J. Chromatogr. A 652, 441–450.

44. Hufschmid, E., Theurillat, R., Martin, U., and Thormann, W. (1995) Exploration of the metabolism of dihydrocodeine via determination of its metabolites in human urine using micellar electrokinetic capillary chromatography. J. Chromatogr. B 668, 159–170.

45. Aumatell, A. and Wells, R. J. (1993) Chiral differentiation of the optical isomers of racemethorphan and racemorphan in urine by capillary zone electrophoresis. J. Chromatogr. Sci. 31, 502–508.

46. Caslavska, J., Hufschmid, E., Theurillat, R., Desiderio, C., Wolfisberg, H., and Thormann, W. (1994) Screening for hydroxylation and acetylation polymorphisms in man via simultaneous analysis of urinary metabolites of mephenytoin, dextromethorphan and caffeine by capillary electrophoretic procedures. J. Chromatogr. B 656, 219–231.

47. Li, S., Fried, K., Wainer, I. W., and Lloyd, D. K. (1993) Determination of dextromethorphan and dextrorphan in urine by capillary zone electrophoresis: application to the determination of debrisoquin-oxidation metabolic phenotype. Chromatographia 35, 216–222.

48. Tomlinson, A. J., Benson, L. M., Johnson K. L., and Naylor, S. (1994) Investigation of drug metabolism using capillary electrophoresis with photodiode array detection and on-line mass spectrometry equipped with an array detector. Electrophoresis 15, 62–71.

49. Albin, M., Grossmann, P. D., and Moring, S. E. (1993) Sensitivity enhancement for capillary electrophoresis. Anal. Chem. 65, 489A–497A.

50. Timperman, A. T., Khatib, K., and Sweedler, J. V. (1995) Wavelength-resolved fluorescence detection in capillary electrophoresis. Anal. Chem. 67, 139–144.
51. Timperman, A. T. and Sweedler, J. V. (1996) Capillary electrophoresis with wavelength-resolved fluorescence detection. Analyst 121, 45R–52R.
52. Petersen, J. R., Bissell M. G., and Mohammad, A. A. (1996) Laser induced resonance energy transfer—a novel approach towards achieving high sensitivity in capillary electrophoresis. I. Clinical diagnostic application. J. Chromatogr. A 744, 37–44.
53. Foret, F., Křivánkovč L., and Bocek, P. (1993) Capillary zone electrophoresis. VCH Publishers, Weinheim, Germany.
54. Engelhard, H., Beck, W., and Schmitt, T. (1996) Capillary Electrophoresis: Methods and Potentials. Vieweg, Braunschweig, Germany.
55. Strausbauch, M. A., Xu, S. J., Ferguson, J. E., Nunez, M. E., Machacek, D., Lawson, G. M., et al. (1995) Concentration and separation of hypoglycemic drugs using solid-phase extraction-capillary electrophoresis. J. Chromatogr. A 717, 279–291.
56. Guzman, N. A., Park, S. S., Schaufelberger, D., Hernandez, L., Paez, X., Rada, P., Tomlinson, A. J., and Naylor, S. (1997) New approaches in clinical chemistry: on-line analyte concentration and microreaction capillary electrophoresis for the determination of drugs, metabolic intermediates and biopolymers in biological fluids. J. Chromatogr. B 697, 37–66.
57. Zhang, C.-X. and Thormann, W. (1996) Head-column field-amplified sample stacking in binary system capillary electrophoresis: a robust approach providing over 1000-fold sensitivity enhancement. Anal. Chem. 68, 2523–2532.
58. Wey, A. B. and Thormann, W. (1999) Head-column field-amplified sample stacking in binary system capillary electrophoresis: preparation of extracts for determination of opioids in microliter amounts of body fluids. J. Chromatogr. A 853, 95–106.
59. Wey, A. B. and Thormann, W. (1999) Head-column field-amplified sample stacking in binary system capillary electrophoresis: the need for the water plug. Chromatographia Suppl. I 49, S12–S20.
60. Ramseier, A. (1999) Kapillarelektrophorese zur Bestimmung von Amphetamin, Methamphetamin und Designerdrogen im Urin, Pharm Dissertation, University of Bern, Switzerland.
61. Chen, F.-T. A. and Evangelista, R. A. (1994) Feasibility studies for simultaneous immunochemical multianalyte drug assay by capillary electrophoresis with laser induced fluorescence. Clin. Chem. 40, 1819–1822.
62. Chen, F.-T. A. and Evangelista, R. A. (1997) Capillary electrophoresis-based immunoassays, in Handbook of Capillary Electrophoresis Applications. (Shintani, H. and Polonsky, J. eds.), Blackie Academic & Professional, London, pp. 219–239.
63. Caslavska, J., Allemann, D., and Thormann, W. (1999) Analysis of urinary drugs of abuse by a multianalyte capillary electrophoretic immunoassay. J. Chromatogr. A 838, 197–211.
64. Choi, J., Kim, C., and Choi, M. J. (1998) Immunological analysis of methamphetamine antibody and its use for the detection of methamphetamine by capillary electrophoresis with laser-induced fluorescence. J. Chromatogr. B 705, 277–282.

65. Choi, J., Kim, C., and Choi, M. J. (1998) Comparison of capillary electro-phoresis-based immunoassay with fluorescence polarization immunoassay for the immunodetermination of methamphetamine using various methamphet-amine antibodies. Electrophoresis 19, 2950–2955.

66. Buechler, K. F., Moi, S., Noar, B., McGrath, D., Villela, J., Clancy, M., et al. (1992) Simultaneous detection of seven drugs of abuse by the Triage panel for drugs of abuse. Clin. Chem. 38, 1678–1684.

67. Towt, J., Tsai, S. C., Hernandez, M. R., Klimov, A. D., Cravec, C. V., Rouse, S. L., et al. (1995) Ontrak testcup: a novel, on-site, multianalyte screen for the detection of abused drugs. J. Anal Toxicol. 19, 504–510.

68. Lurie, I. S., Klein, R. F. X., Dal Cason, T. A., LeBelle, M. J., Brenneisen, R., and Weinberger, R. E. (1994) Chiral resolution of cationic drugs of forensic interest by capillary electrophoresis with mixtures of neutral and anionic cyclodextrins. Anal. Chem. 66, 4019–4026.

69. Desiderio, C., Fanali, S., Küpfer, A., and Thormann, W. (1994) Analysis of mephenytoin, 4-hydroxymephenytoin and 4-hydroxyphenytoin enantiomers in human urine by cyclodextrin micellar electrokinetic capillary chromatography: simple determination of a hydroxylation polymorphism in man. Electrophore-sis 15, 87–93.

70. Smith, R. D., Wahl, J. H., Goodlett, D. R., and Hofstadler, S. A. (1993) Capil-lary electrophoresis/mass spectrometry. Anal. Chem. 65, 574A–584A.

71. Cai, J. and Henion, J. (1995) Capillary electrophoresis-mass spectrometry. J. Chromatogr. A 703, 667–692.

72. Johansson, I. M., Pavelka, R., and Henion, J. D. (1991) Determination of small drug molecules by capillary electrophoresis-atmospheric pressure ionization mass spectrometry. J. Chromatogr. 559, 515–528.

73. Ashcroft, A. E., Major, H. J., Lowes, S., and Wilson, I. D. (1995) Identification of non-steroidal anti-inflammatory drugs and their metabolites in solid phase extracts of human urine using capillary electrophoresis-mass spectrometry. Anal. Proc. Anal. Commun. 32, 459–462.

74. Ashcroft, A. E., Major, H. J., Wilson, I. D., Nicholls, A., and Nicholson, J. K. (1997) Application of capillary electrophoresis-mass spectrometry to the analy-sis of urine samples from animals and man containing paracetamol and phen-acetin and their metabolites. Anal. Commun. 34, 41–43.

75. Bach, G. and Henion, J. (1998) Quantitative capillary electrophoresis-ion trap mass spectrometry determination of methylphenidate in human urine. J. Chromatogr. B 707, 275–285.

76. Sheppard, R. L., Tong, X., Cai, J., and Henion, J. D. (1995) Chiral separation and detection of terbutaline and ephedrine by capillary electrophoresis coupled with ion spray mass spectrometry. Anal. Chem. 67, 2054–2058.

77. Haber, C. (1997) Electrochemical detection in capillary electrophoresis, in Handbook of Capillary Electrophoresis, 2nd Ed. (Landers, J. P., ed.), CRC, Boca Raton, FL, pp. 425–447.

78. Wang, R., Lu, X., Wu, M., and Wang, E. (1999) Separation of promethazine and thioridazine using capillary electrophoresis with end-column amperometric detection. J. Chromatogr. B 721, 327–332.

20

Screening Biological Specimens for Drugs of Forensic Significance

John C. Hudson, Murray J. Malcolm, and Mauro Golin

1. INTRODUCTION

Since the introduction of capillary electrophoresis (CE) in 1981 *(1)*, there has been a marked increase in the number of applications of CE to the analysis of drugs in various situations. For example, the pharmaceutical industry has made extensive use of CE in analysis of main drug components *(2,3)*, of drug-related impurities *(4)*, of trace impurities in the process stream *(5)*, and of the isomeric composition of numerous drugs *(6)*. At the same time, Lurie *(7)*, and others *(8,9)* have reported on the analysis of drugs of abuse in street preparations. Several workers, notably Thormann *(10)*, Eap et al. *(11)*, and Penalvo et al. *(12)*, have applied CE in one or another of its configurations to the problems of analysis of drugs in urine or plasma. These efforts have mainly been directed toward the goals of therapeutic drug monitoring (TDM), but Caslavska et al. *(13)* have also addressed the application to emergency toxicology. This chapter will focus on CE as a tool for screening biological specimens for drugs of forensic significance. Naturally, information derived from pharmaceuticals, street drugs, and from TDM analysis can be exploited in the development of a comprehensive screening procedure. In forensic analysis a screening procedure, as discussed in detail later, must be comprehensive, fast, inexpensive, and easy to use.

Initially, the screen must be comprehensive. It must detect as many forensically significant drugs as possible in a single analytical pass. In this case, "forensically significant" means, in a broad sense, all drugs that might reasonably be involved in fatal poisonings or in the impairment of human functions such as driving a motor vehicle. With the notable exception of the barbiturates, the vast majority of drugs fitting this description are basic

From: *Clinical and Forensic Applications of Capillary Electrophoresis*
Edited by: J. R. Petersen and A. A. Mohammad © Humana Press Inc., Totowa, NJ

(nitrogenous) compounds. Examples are, amphetamines, antihistamines, narcotic analgesics and tricyclic antidepressants. Until recently, comprehensive screens have utilized gas chromatography with nitrogen-phosphorus detectors (GC-NPD) to screen extracts from biological specimens. Often extracts must be derivatized to make the compounds more volatile. Our focus and the focus of this chapter has been to consider the question: "Can CE replace GC/NPD in a comprehensive drug screen?"

Forensic analysis poses a number of potential problems for any such screening procedure but possibly the most pressing is the type of sample analyzed. For a forensic toxicologist the specimen that must most often be accommodated is whole blood in variable stages of hemolysis and in varying degrees of putrefaction. Simpler specimens such as urine may be available in any given case but any screening procedure must first and foremost be able to handle hemolysed whole blood.

Oda and coworkers *(14)*, note that "in forensic toxicology, the analysis is required to be only qualitative, but without false positive or false negative results." While generally agreeing with this observation most operations confirm all positive screen results by another analysis, usually mass spectrometry. Toxicologists can, therefore, tolerate a few false-positive results at the screening stage. However, a negative screening result may well end analysis in the case. Thus, it is more important that false negative results be minimized. For example, in a GC screen the more precise the retention behavior, the greater the confidence with which potentially positive results can be ruled out. In essence this means that the screening procedure must be reliable and consistent day after day. If CE were to be seriously considered as replacement for GC-NPD, then migration behavior must be comparably precise.

Sensitivity of the screen must be high enough to detect drugs found in forensic specimens at low concentrations. Many of the drugs of forensic interest are used in relatively low dosages which, naturally, give rise to correspondingly low blood concentrations. Therapeutic levels of basic drugs typically range from a few nanograms per milliliter of blood up to a few hundred nanograms per milliliter. Since such levels are well within the sensitivity limits of GC-NPD, it is critical that CE has at least comparable sensitivity.

Ideally, any forensic screening procedure must be robust, fast, inexpensive, and simple to use. The screen should be available with a minimum of fine-tuning, minimal instrument down-time, and low maintenance and operating costs. These conditions also imply that no extensive sample cleanup or preparation should be needed. In addition, no derivatization of the analyte should be required. Such desirable properties are not specific to forensic drug screening. However, since GC-NPD is considered the "gold standard," these are inevitable points of comparison with any potential replacement. The use of CE as a method to screen forensic drugs as outlined earlier will be considered later in more detail. Reference will be made to work done in this laboratory *(15,16)* and to the selected reports of others.

2. THE CE SYSTEM

Most commercially available instruments offer similar capabilities. The main differences appear to be in the degree of automation, sample capacity, flexibility of injection techniques, and detector options. Our early work was done on a Beckman P/ACE 5500 equipped with both a single-wavelength UV and diode array detectors (DAD). More recently, we have used a Beckman System MDQ with a DAD.

For us, the decision to use CE for drug screening was dictated primarily by the need for simplicity. Lurie *(7)* reported separation and detection of drugs of forensic interest in a micellar electrokinetic capillary chromatography (MECC) system. Thormann et al. *(10,17,18)*, Renou-Gonnord and David *(19)*, and Hyotylainen et al. *(20)* have also used MECC successfully for drug detection. Gonzales and Laserna *(21)*, used capillary zone electrophoresis (CZE) to screen for banned drugs in sport. Chee and Wan *(22)* also showed the feasibility of using CZE to screen for 17 basic drugs in urine and plasma. Since our major interest initially was on basic drugs, it seemed reasonable to evaluate CZE, the simplest possible CE configuration. Using the procedure of Chee and Wan, 60 cm (to detector) × 50 μm id at 25 kV or 50 cm (to detector) × 75 μm at 18 kV id uncoated fused silica capillaries were used. The run buffer was 100 mmol/L sodium phosphate at pH 2.38 along with electrokinetic injection, typically 10 kV for 8 s, although the injection time may be varied. Pressure injections have been used but experience suggests that electrokinetic injection is more selective for cations. Considering the rather straightforward extraction methods chosen, such selectivity is beneficial. Typically, separation voltages of 18–25 kV with normal polarity have been used giving a total run times of about 25 min.

This approach to a screen for basic drugs clearly excludes those that are not protonated at pH 2.38. Some of the benzodiazepines (very weak bases) are not detected in this screen. Tomita and Okuyama *(23)* have reported, however, a MECC system (phosphate/borate/SDS/methanol) that can potentially detect and separate benzodiazepines, and presumably other neutral compounds, at concentrations applicable in the forensic toxicology situation.

Detector sensitivity is a matter of great concern in a forensic drug screen because, as noted earlier, the drugs of major forensic interest tend to be present at low concentrations. This places special demands on any analytical system used to analyze samples without any pre-treatment. CZE, with the common UV detectors or DAD, monitoring at wavelengths in the range 200–220 nm, are known to be rather insensitive *(2,10)*. From experience we have found that drug concentrations must be on the order of 0.3 µg/mL of the injected solution to ensure consistent detection while avoiding expensive detector modifications. This is in agreement with reports in which urine *(21,24,25)*, and plasma or serum *(12,17,26)*, were injected directly onto a capillary. Limits of detection in such direct-injection methods have typically been reported to be approx 1 µg/mL. While this is adequate for most acidic drugs, in order to be useful in the analysis of basic drugs of forensic interest, the sensitivity has to be increased 10–100 times. As attractive as direct sample injection is, it cannot work for most basic drugs in our simple instrumental configuration. Thus, sample preparation that provides a pre-concentration step appears to be inevitable.

3. SAMPLE PREPARATION

A useful overview of sample pretreatment has been provided by Lloyd *(28)*. Although pre-concentration of the analyte is an important reason for considering extraction as a preliminary step to CE analysis, it is not the only one. Extraction also eliminates protein, which is important to prevent fouling of the capillary in CZE, and helps to eliminate interferences in MECC *(17)*. Further, it is noted that liquid-liquid extraction practically eliminates the inorganic salts present in the original sample, which can interfere with CE analysis.

The first choice for sample preparation is direct solvent extraction (DSE) of whole blood with a solvent such as 1-chlorobutane/NH_4OH for basic and neutral drugs *(27)*. This is a simple, relatively quick extraction that has long been used to prepare samples for chromatographic screening. For GC-NPD this simple extraction method has been shown to require no additional steps to separate the complex mixture of neutral compounds from basic drugs. Thus, it seemed reasonable that sample preparation for CE analysis also be as simple and easy.

Using 1-chlorobutane/NH_4OH, a direct solvent extraction of 1.0 mL whole blood was performed. The solvent, containing traces of NH_4OH, must be evaporated to about 1 mL before the addition of 10 µL of 1% HCl in MeOH. The resulting HCl salt of the basic drug is less volatile and more water-soluble. The remaining solvent was evaporated to dryness. The residue was redissolved in 30 µL of water, with warming. Our experience indicates that 30 µL is the smallest volume that can be conveniently and consistently handled. The resulting solution is centrifuged at 12,000 rpm for 20 min in 0.2 mL PCR vials to remove any insoluble material, reducing the risk of plugging the CE capillary during injection. The centrifugation step also eliminates filtration that would inevitably results in sample loss. The solution in the PCR vials can be used directly for electrokinetic injection without further processing. This procedure provides a simple but effective cleanup, concentrating the analyte approx 30-fold.

That such a procedure is effective in bringing most basic drugs within the reach of simple CE detection can be illustrated as follows. In practice, we analyze a solution of 20 basic drugs (1 μg/mL) dissolved in water as an instrument performance standard (Fig. 1A). The same drug mixture is also spiked into whole blood at a concentration of 10 ng/mL for each drug. This is the whole blood QC standard analyzed with each batch of cases (Fig. 1B). All drugs are consistently detected in both instances.

Liquid–liquid extraction is not the only way to prepare samples for CE analysis, and it may not be the best. Solid-phase extraction (SPE) has been successfully used to replace DSE *(29–31)* in the preparation of samples. It is also important to note that SPE is more amenable to automation than is DSE. This must be taken into consideration when setting up mass screening methods. In addition to SPE, Palmarsdottir and coworkers *(32,33)*, have demonstrated use of supported liquid membranes to extract basic drugs from plasma, an approach that may offer its own unique advantages.

In keeping with the goal of maximizing sensitivity, a number of special methods of sample injection have been devised. These are techniques by which a larger fraction of the analyte is transferred onto the capillary than is generally possible with simple electrokinetic or pressure injections. Such "preconcentration" methods result in increased sensitivity. Perhaps the simplest of these methods is called stacking, in which sample components are injected from a matrix of lower ionic strength than the run buffer (*see* Chapter 2 for a more detailed description). The example procedure described above in which the sample, dissolved in water, is injected into the run buffer comprising 100 mmol/L sodium phosphate, pH 2.38, is an example of a stacking procedure. A more powerful method has been reported by Palmarsdottir et al. *(32)*, in the analysis of bambuterol where sensitivity was increased about 400 times by a double-stacking procedure after preconcentration using a supported liquid membrane (SLM). The reported limit of detection in this assay was <1 ng/mL of plasma. In addition, Eap et al. *(11)* reported a method for determining mianserin in plasma that uses both liquid–liquid extraction and on-capillary preconcentration to obtain a limit of quantitation of 5 ng/mL. If such methods can be generally applied,

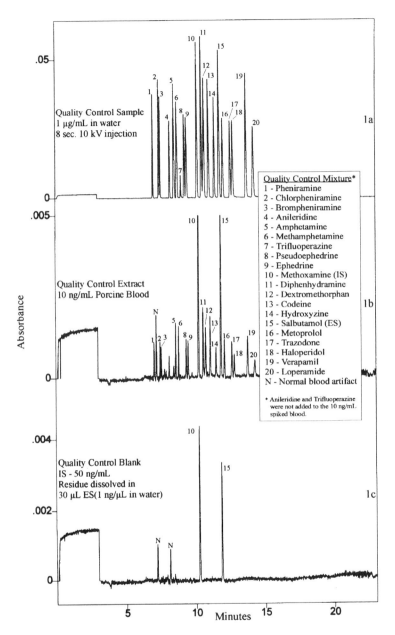

Fig. 1. Quality controls for basic drugs. Whole blood samples (1 mL) were extracted with 5 mL 1-chlorobutane plus 0.2 mL ammonia. The residue is redissolved in methanol (1% HCl), evaporated, and dissolved in 100 mM phosphate, pH 2.38. The sample was injected on a 60 cm (50 cm to detector) × 75 μm fused silica capillary for 8 s at 10 kV. The run buffer was 100 mM phosphate, pH 2.38, a constant voltage (20 or 25 kV) applied, and the temperature held constant at 25°C. **(A)** Quality control sample in water. **(B)** Quality control extract, 10 ng of each drug in procine blood. **(C)** Quality control blank with only 50 ng/mL internal standard added.

they may offer a simple way to further increase sensitivity of a general drug screen for basic drugs.

4. SAMPLE QUALITY

Sample quality (i.e., putrid samples), although of little consequence in most other fields is of considerable concern in forensic toxicology. It is important to know whether the screening method, including sample preparation, functions satisfactorily with fresh specimens and putrid samples. To test the ruggedness of our own sample treatment method, we left spiked whole blood samples at room temperature and compared the results obtained by CZE and GC-NPD. The process of putrefaction can generate artefacts that may mask basic drugs that might be present in the sample (Fig. 2). GC-NPD detects these artefacts which soon renders the chromatogram uninterpretable (Fig. 2). However, corresponding electropherograms are much less affected. This could be due to the fact that most of the artifacts are neutral or weakly basic compounds that are not electrokinetically injected or are practically transparent to UV detectors. Figure 3 illustrates typical case electropherograms including a whole human blood extract from a putrid case containing an overdose level (Fig. 3C).

5. IDENTITY OF PEAKS

In most toxicology laboratories, final identification of a peak will not be made from observed retention or migration behavior. But the decision whether or not to pursue identification will be made solely on the basis of this behavior in either the GC or CE analytical systems. Thus, it is imperative that retention or migration behavior be as reproducible as possible. The more precise the retention behavior, the narrower the window that can be used to decide whether a given peak is a potential positive result. When using a simple UV detector, interpretation of electropherograms and tentative identification of peaks is limited to migration behavior. Use of the DAD adds UV spectral data to migration data and greatly improves the discriminating power of the screen. These two aspects of peak identity are discussed later.

5.1. Migration Behavior

It has been often noted that raw migration time is not highly reproducible. Yang et al. *(34)*, note that this is especially true of micellar systems because the electroosmotic flow (EOF) is a powerful influence on migration in such systems. EOF, in turn, is affected by variables, such as the condition of the interior surface of the capillary, that are difficult to control. Even at pH 2.38 when EOF is reduced almost to zero, raw migration times are less reproducible than is desirable. Migration times have been found to drift with time,

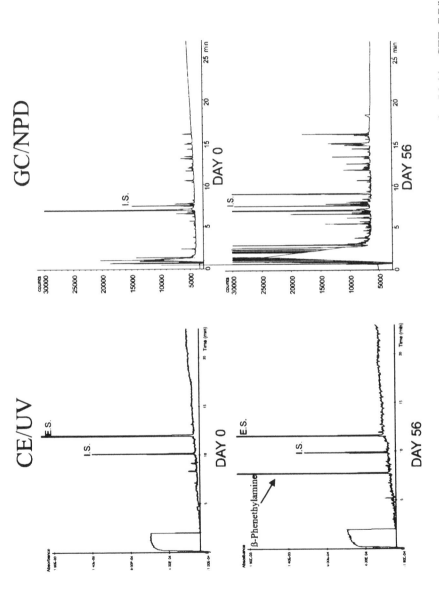

Fig. 2. Comparison results of unpreserved whole human blood stored at room temperature for 56 d by CZE-GC/NPD.

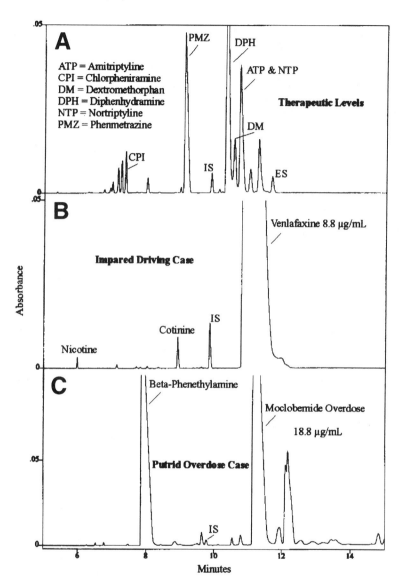

Fig. 3. Whole blood case extracts for (**A**) therapeutic levels of drugs, (**B**) an impaired driving case, and (**C**) an overdose of moclobemide in a putrid sample.

presumably as a result of changes occurring to the inside surface of the capillary. In order to have a good screening procedure, it was clear that it would be necessary to have an expression of migration behavior that was more reproducible than raw migration time. This could be considered analogous to the retention index when using GC.

The analogy with GC (and thin-layer chromatography [TLC]) suggests the expression of relative migration time (RM) as a way to obtain more reproducible results. That is, the migration time of the analyte in question is divided by the migration time of a reference compound analyzed simultaneously. Yang et al. *(34)*, examined the effect of the "migration time ratio", in which they chose a neutral marker as the reference compound. With their test mixture of amino acids, the relative standard deviation (RSD) for simple migration times was 2–5%, whereas the RSD for the migration time ratio in the same system was 1% or less.

Williams and Vigh *(35)*, took the expression of migration behavior a step further, discussing effective mobility (μeff). This quantity may be described as the mobility of the analyte (with dimensions of $cm^2/v.s$) corrected for the mobility of EOF. For us this appeared to offer the most precise expression of migration behavior. For example, we have observed RSD for raw migration time to be about $\pm$ 6%, relative migration about $\pm$ 2%, and for μeff <$\pm$0.3%. We have not observed that the RSD for relative migration and μeff are the same. In all our studies, relative migrations have shown more variation. We have also observed that mobility is independent of capillary diameter and can be reproduced from laboratory to laboratory. Also it should be noted that Ahuja and Foley *(36)* suggested calculation of a migration index for MECC, an index quite analogous to a chromatographic retention index.

In order for a screening procedure based on migration behavior to be useful a list of potential analytes along with their migration data must be available. In this regard we have reported on some 650 drugs and metabolites, giving relative migration and μeff for each *(16)*.

5.2. UV Spectra and Searchable Libraries

It is inevitable that a CE screen for basic drugs will show numerous instances of comigration. Even the best precision noted aforementioned yields, in any statistically sound window, several possibilities of drugs that could be present. With detection by single-wavelength UV detector, such migration information is all that the analyst has to interpret screen results. This does not present an obstacle to confirmation by MS. However more information on individual peaks is always useful and it is easily obtained with the DAD.

Kobayashi et al. *(37)* reported early use of a diode array as a detector for CE, showing the potential of collecting UV spectra on all emerging peaks. Caslavska et al. *(13)* compared three CE methods for rapid determination of drugs in cases of intoxication. They were able to collect UV spectra on peaks and provide rapid results of drug screens by CE. UV spectra were not considered rigorous identification but were sufficient to meet the needs of emergency toxicology. Quick turnaround in such analyses was shown to be possible by CE "provided that instrumentation with a database for peak identification is available" *(13)*. Lilley and Wheat *(24)* have reported use of DAD data and CE, with emphasis on specialized software that allows sophisticated spectral analysis of emerging peaks. This was shown to be particularly effective in eliminating false-positive amphetamine results without the need for MS. In our laboratory, the compounds we have listed by μeff and relative migration *(15,16)* also have their UV spectra stored in a spectral database. A CE system, such as Beckman's MDQ, has software that allows the spectrum from an unknown sample to be searched against stored spectra. This makes drug screening by CE even more powerful and discriminating. However, a detection limit of 10 ng/mL whole blood, referred to earlier, does not apply to searches of UV spectra generated by DAD. Generally, analyte peaks from samples spiked at 40–50 ng/mL are required for meaningful library searches. Also the best matches are obtained, not surprisingly, when the spectra for the unknown and the standard are collected at approximately the same concentration.

6. CONCLUSION

It is now appropriate to return to the question posed at the beginning of this chapter: "Can CE replace GC-NPD in a comprehensive drug screen?" It has been shown *(15,16)* that CZE is capable of analyzing whole blood specimens, whether hemolysed or putrid, by use of a simple liquid–liquid extraction. Detection of basic drugs using a simple UV detector or DAD has been shown to be on the order of 10 ng/mL of whole blood. More powerful sample stacking methods have been shown to increase the detection limit to about 1 ng/mL. Additional improvement in sensitivity is possible but requires a new detector or detector cell and more complicated sample preparation. For a forensic drug screen, however, the ability to detect most basic drugs at 10 ng/mL of blood meets most needs.

The cost of screening basic drug by CE compares favorably to GC-NPD. Initial instrument costs are roughly similar. However, replacement GC columns cost 20–30 times as much as replacement capillaries (i.e., untreated fused silica). Operating costs are roughly similar. For example, both CE and GC-NPD can use the same sample extraction procedure

Total run time of the two methods is, however, significantly different with the CZE screen taking approx 25% less than the run time in a parallel GC-NPD screen. This is primarily because of the shorter time needed by the CZE system to return to initial conditions after an analytical run. Hyotylainen et al. *(20)* describe an approach to CE that may permit even shorter analysis times. Using MEKC, they were able to perform their separations in a short capillary (23 cm). This led to run times of 2 min, an interesting development for those engaged in mass drug screening.

The CZE system can be highly robust, as might be hoped with such a simple system. Aside from physical breakage, which occurs occasionally, capillaries appear to be all but immune to hazards common in GC. In our laboratory, CZE capillaries have been exposed to gross overloading with very complex samples. Adsorption of analyte or contaminant molecules to the capillary appears to be reversible, such that with judicious rinsing between samples with sodium hydroxide, sodium dodecylsulfate, and run buffers or water *(38)*, complete regeneration of the capillary surface is possible. Such rinses that are part of routine screens, take up about 15% of the analysis cycle for each sample. In our hands, one capillary was subjected to over 10,000 injections of pure solutions of drug standards and of whole blood extracts before it needed to be replaced. The capillary performance remained unchanged except for a decrease in the analysis time by about 5 min.

Finally, analyte decomposition, whether due to thermal or other causes, or irreversible absorption of the analyte to the columns, common observations in GC systems, are rarely, if ever, observed in the CZE screen.

From the evidence presented here it would appear that CZE, is capable of providing a comprehensive screen of basic drugs in whole blood and, in some analytical situations, may be the method of choice.

REFERENCES

1. Camilleri, P., ed. (1993) History and development of capillary electrophoresis, in Capillary Electrophoresis: Theory and Practice, CRC, Boca Raton, FL, pp. 1–23.
2. Brunner, L. J., DiPiro, J. T., and Fedman, S. (1995) High performance capillary electrophoresis in the pharmaceutical sciences. Pharmacotherapy 15, 1–22.
3. Holland, L. A., Chetwyn, N. P., Perkins, M. D., and Lunte, S. M. (1997) Capillary electrophoresis in pharmaceutical analysis. Pharma. Res. 14, 372–338.
4. Altria, K. D. (1996) Determination of drug-related impurities by capillary electrophoresis. J. Chromatogr. A 735, 43–56.
5. Johnson, B. D., Grinberg, N., Bicker, G., and Ellison, D. (1997) The quantitation of a residual quaternary amine in bulk drug and process streams using capillary electrophoresis. J. Liq. Chro. Rel. Technol. 20, 257–272.
6. Lin, B., Zhu, X., Koppenhoefer, B., and Epperlein, V. (1997) Investigation of 123 chiral drugs by cyclodextrin-modified capillary electrophoresis. LC/GC 15, 40–46.
7. Lurie, I. S. (1991) Micellar electrokinetic capillary chromatography of illicit drug substances. Anal. Chem. 63, 823–827.
8. Gaus, H. J., Gogus, Z. Z., Schmeer, K., Behnke, B., Kovar, K. A., and Bayer, E. (1996) Separation and identification of designer drugs with capillary electrophoresis and on-line connection with ionspray mass spectrometry. J. Chromatogr. A 735, 221–226.

9. Walker, J. A, Marche, H. L., Newby, N., and Bechtold, E. J. (1996) A free zone capillary electrophoresis method for the quantitation of common illicit drug samples. J.F.S.C.A. 41, 824–829.

10. Thormann, W. (1993) Capillary electrophoresis and electrokinetic capillary chromatography of drugs in body fluids. Chrom. Sci. Ser. 64, 693–704.

11. Eap, C. B., Powell, K., and Baumann, P. (1997) Determination of the enantiomers of mianserin and its metabolites in plasma by capillary electrophoresis after liquid-liquid extraction and on-column sample preconcentration. J. Chromatogr. Sci. 35, 315–320.

12. Penalvo, G. C., Kelly, M., Maillols, H., and Fabre, H. (1997) Evaluation of capillary zone electrophoresis and micellar electrokinetic capillary chromatography with direct injection of plasma for the determination of cefotaxime and its metabolite. Anal. Chem. 69, 1364–1369.

13. Caslavska, J., Lienhard, S., and Thormann, W. (1993) Comparative use of three electrokinetic capillary methods for the determination of drugs in body fluids. J. Chromatogr. 638, 335–342.

14. Oda, R. P., Roche, M. E., Landers, J. P., and Shihabi, Z. K. (1997) Capillary electrophoresis for the analysis of drugs in biological fluids, in Handbook of Capillary Electrophoresis (Landers, J. P., ed.), CRC, Boca Raton, FL, pp. 567–590.

15. Hudson, J. C., Golin, M., and Malcolm, M. J. (1995) Capillary zone electrophoresis in a comprehensive screen for basic drugs in whole blood. Can. Soc. Forens. Sci. J. 28, 137–152.

16. Hudson, J. C., Golin, M., Malcolm, M. J., and Whiting, C. F. (1998) Capillary zone electrophoresis in a comprehensive screen for drugs of forensic interest in whole blood: an update. Can. Soc. Forens. Sci. J. 31, 1–29.

17. Schmutz, A. and Thormann, W. (1993) Determination of phenobarbital, ethosuximide and primidone in human serum by micellar electrokinetic capillary chromatography with direct sample injection. Ther. Drug Mon. 15, 310–316.

18. Zhang, C. X. and Thormann, W. (1994) Determination of drug levels in human serum by micellar electrokinetic capillary chromatography with direct sample injection using different quantitation strategies. J. Cap. Elec. 1, 208–218.

19. Renou-Gonnord, M. F. and David, K. (1996) Optimized micellar electrokinetic chromatographic separation of benzodiazepines. J. Chromatogr. A 735, 249–261.

20. Hyotylainen, T., Siren, H., and Riekkola, M. L. (1996) Determination of morphine analogues, caffeine and amphetamine in biological fluids by capillary electrophoresis with the marker technique. J. Chromatogr. A 735, 439–447.

21. Gonzalez, E. and Laserna, J. J. (1994) Capillary zone electrophoresis for the rapid screening of banned drugs in sport. Electrophoresis 15, 240–243.

22. Chee, G. L. and Wan, T. S. M. (1993) Reproducible and high-speed separation of basic drugs by capillary zone electrophoresis. J. Chromatogr. 612, 172–177.

23. Tomita, M. and Okuyama, T. (1996) Application of capillary electrophoresis to the simultaneous screening and quantitation of benzodiazepines. J. Chromatogr. B 678, 331–337.

24. Lilley, K. A. and Wheat, T. E. (1996) Drug identification in biological matrices using capillary electrophoresis and chemometric software. J. Chromatogr. B 683, 67–76.

25. Zhang, C.-X., Sun, Z.-P., Ling, D.-K., Zheng, J.-S., Guo, J., and Li, X.-Y. (1993) Determination of 3-methylflavone-8-carboxylic acid, the main metabolite of flavoxate, in human urine by capillary electrophoresis with direct injection. J. Chromatogr. 612, 287–294.

26. Perez-Ruiz, T., Martinez-Lozano, C., Sanz, A., and Tomas, V. (1996) Simultaneous determination of diquat and paraquat residues in various matrices by capillary zone electrophoresis with diode array detection. Chromatographia 43, 468–472.

27. Sharp, M. E. (1986) Evaluation of a screening procedure for basic and neutral drugs: n-butyl chloride extraction and megabore gas chromatography. Can. Soc. Forens. Sci. J. 19, 83–101.

28. Lloyd, D. K. (1996) Capillary electrophoretic analysis of drugs in body fluids: sample pretreatment and methods for direct injection of biofluids. J. Chromatogr. A 735, 29–42.

29. Li, C. and Weber, S. G. (1997) Determination of barbiturates by solid-phase microextraction and capillary electrophoresis. Anal. Chem. 69, 1217–1222.

30. Rossi, M. and Rotilio, D. (1997) Analysis of carbamate pesticides by micellar electrokinetic chromatography. J. High. Res. Chromatogr. 20, 265–269.

31. Strausbauch, M. A., Xu, S. J., Ferguson, J. E., Nunez, M. E., Machacek, D., Lawson, G. M., et al. (1996) Concentration and separation of hypoglycemic drugs using solid-phase extraction-capillary electrophoresis. J. Chromatogr. A, 717, 279–291.

32. Palmarsdottir, S., Mathiasson, L., Johnsson, J. A., and Edholm, L. E. (1997) Determination of a basic drug, bambuterol, in human plasma by capillary electrophoresis using double stacking for large volumne injection and supported liquid membranes for sample pretreatment. J. Chromatogr. B, 688, 127–134.

33. Palmarsdottir, S., Lindegard, B., Edholm, L. E., Jonsson, J. A., Mathiasson, L., and Deininger, P. (1995) Supported liquid membrane technique for selective sample workup of basic drugs in plasma prior to capillary zone electrophoresis. J. Cap. Elec. 2, 185–189.

34. Yang, J., Bose, S., and Hage, D. S. (1996) Improved reproducibility in capillary electrophoresis through the use of mobility and migration time ratios. J. Chromatogr. A, 735, 209–220.

35. Williams, B. A. and Vigh, G. (1996) Fast, accurate mobility determination method for capillary electrophoresis. Anal. Chem. 68, 1174–1180.

36. Ahuja, E. S. and Foley, J. P. (1994) A retention index for micellar electrokinetic chromatography. Analyst 119, 353–360.

37. Kobayashi, S., Ueda, T., and Kikumoto, M. (1989) Photodiode array detection in high-performance capillary electrophoresis. J. Chromatogr. 480, 179–184.

38. Lloyd, D. K. and Wätzig, H. (1995) Sodium dodecyl sulphate is an effective between-run rinse for capillary electrophoresis of samples in biological matrices. J. Chromatogr.

Index

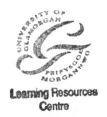